Distinguishing Clinical from Upper Level Management in Social Work

Over the past few decades, as administrative and technological complexity has increased, so has the role and importance of administrative practice in social work. For those making the switch from front-line practice to administration and management there is, therefore, a real need to prepare and enhance the knowledge base and skill set necessary at the executive level. In particular, the importance of budgeting and fiscal management, the need for accountability, negotiation between different and competing organizations, along with an understanding of decision-making, planning, and understanding levels of risk.

Written by two experienced authors within social work education, this practical book presents the interrelated nature of decision-making, and provides a model for understanding what is required in the transition from clinician, to clinical and upper level management. The text covers:

- The difference between clinical and upper level management skills
- The major trends that influence health and human service organizations
- An analysis of the concept of leadership
- The skills needed by clinical managers and upper level managers to administer effectively.

Distinguishing Clinical from Upper Level Management in Social Work is a much needed update to the field of management and administration within human service organizations, and will be important reading for social work students, social service professionals, and other human service providers.

Marvin D. Feit is Professor of Social Work in the Ethelyn R. Strong School of Social Work at Norfolk State University, USA.

Michael J. Holosko is the Pauline M. Berger Professor of Family and Child Welfare at The University of Georgia, School of Social Work, and adjunct instructor at Norfolk State University, USA.

Distinguishing Clinical from Upper Level Management in Social Work

Marvin D. Feit and
Michael J. Holosko

Routledge
Taylor & Francis Group
LONDON AND NEW YORK

First published 2013
by Routledge
4 Park Square, Milton Park, Abingdon, Oxon, OX14 4RN

Simultaneously published in the USA and Canada
by Routledge
605 Third Avenue, New York, NY 10017

Routledge is an imprint of the Taylor & Francis Group, an informa business

British Library Cataloguing in Publication Data
A catalogue record for this book is available from the British Library

Library of Congress Cataloging-in-Publication Data
Feit, Marvin D.
Distinguishing clinical from upper level management in social work / Marvin D. Feit and Michael J. Holosko.
p. cm.
978–0–203–07516–6 (ebook) 1. Social work administration.
2. Social workers—Supervision of. I. Holosko, Michael J. II. Title.
HV40.F366 2013
361.3068'4—dc23
2012031398

ISBN13: 978–0–7890–2538–8 (hbk)
ISBN13: 978–0–7890–2539–5 (pbk)
ISBN13: 978–0–203–07516–6 (ebk)

Typeset in Sabon
by Swales & Willis Ltd, Exeter, Devon

CONTENTS

ACKNOWLEDGEMENTS

In a text of this nature there are many individuals to thank over the three years of its incubation. We want to thank the legions of BSW, MSW, PhD, BA, RN, MA, MSc, and MPH students we have taught collectively over the past 78 years. Yes – you have taught us much more about social work knowledge and understanding than we ever taught you. You were indeed, the inspiration for the perspiration for this text. Another thank you goes to the various waves of reviewers through Sage Publications who offered constructive comments to move this text to the final form.

At the University of Georgia, I [MJH] would like to acknowledge the dedicated work of the graduate student assistants assisting the Berger Chair with this task: Joanna Mitchell, Pauline M. Berger Graduate Assistant, Catherine Patterson, Tisha Abolt Graduate Assistant, Soonok Au, Graduate Assistant. The generosity of Dr. Israel Berger, offering this Chair on behalf of his wife Pauline, made a work of this nature possible, as well as the support given by the Tisha Abolt Graduate Assistant scholarship for this text. To my supportive spouse and partner, thank you so much Deborah Ann Holosko.

At Norfolk State, I [MDF] would like to acknowledge the continued support I have received from my wife, Dr. Nuria M. Cuevas-Feit, who has challenged me to think through my ideas based on practical experience, and to our son, José, who has often provided additional insights to making decisions. My work would not be complete without acknowledging the excellent development of this material if it were not with the insight provided by Dr. Pamela Landon, a valued and cherished colleague for many years, who pushed me to understand the complexity of decisions in the workplace.

PREFACE

This workbook is written to distinguish clinical from upper level management, and centers on what is minimally needed to make the transition from clinician to clinical manager (CM) and/or supervisor, to upper level manager (ULM). It includes the very important dimensions of leadership and decision-making as critical elements which must be addressed, in addition to the knowledge bases of evaluation and financial management. There is presently no significant content in the field of social work which places management, decision-making, and leadership in a specific context, so that one can better understand the key decisions one makes, as they transition through various organizational levels. It is called a workbook because as the text unfolded, many forms, tables, charts, etc., mushroomed, and they are presented herein, as tools that individuals may use to achieve mastery of the respective content areas of program evaluation (PE) and financial management (FM).

The key ingredients which form the basis for decision-making are PE and FM, as they both provide excellent sources of relevant data pertinent to what one wants to accomplish, such as a break-even points, effectiveness, the projected number of clients, or actual clients served, etc. Such data are critical to taking a next step in the decision-making process. For example, this information can provide a CM or ULM with what it would take to be successful, indicate how a unit/ program could be funded, and what might be useful output measures to client access interventions. However, each of these content areas is usually taught as a separate entity, and as part of the overall knowledge base of management or administration course materials.

Our contention is that administration was taught many years ago in schools of social work much better than we do it today, where for example, financial management had been a formative content Master's Degree in

Social Work course. However (and ironically), our current field has not kept abreast with our ever-changing management and administrative reality. This was a main rationale for writing this workbook. The other dimension rarely discussed in this context is that as one moves to higher levels of responsibility, decisions become much more public by default, and may be much more complex, as such decisions involve a level of risk, an understanding of data which may be considered "soft" because it can change at any time, and may include information that one may not have easy access to. While such aspects of making decisions may be mentioned in an MSW curriculum, they are very rarely presented in this interrelated, and/or comprehensive context.

Another important feature of this workbook is that managers at every level can understand clearly that making decisions has to incorporate practical wisdom, as a large component of its base. For certain, one does not learn to be a leader, and/or make decisions in a vacuum or in a classroom, particularly because there are hardly the consequences one might face in the "real" world, such as staff cuts, funding cutbacks, lawsuits, newspaper stories, and/or pressure from constituents. Thus, it is important to distinguish between the different organizational levels as one administers a program and as such, view decision-making as integral to leadership, and as a significant part of administering an organization.

Our contention, based collectively on some 79 years of social work educational experience, is that social workers transition hierarchically in health and human service organizations for reasons that have nothing to do with their supervisory or administrative acumen. The real reasons why they become promoted are typically: a) they are good clinical/front-line workers; b) they are "team players" in the overall organization; c) they have caused "no trouble" in the organization; d) they aspire to do something more than front-line work; and e) no one else was interested in the job and therefore, they were promoted by default. As such, they lack the skill set necessary to do the job effectively at the next administrative level. This was another rationale for writing this workbook.

This text is laid out in seven sequential chapters. Chapter 1 (the introduction) lays the groundwork for both the rationale for the text and its ensuing content. It points out the importance of why clinical and upper level management skills need delineation and also their areas of difference. Chapter 2 presents the scaffolding model that provides the context for the text.

Chapter 3 describes the major trends that influence health and human service organizations at the macro, meso, and micro levels. It reminds one of how such pervasive trends influence all aspects of our client-centered practice. Chapter 4 strips the mask off of the concept of leadership, as it contends that leadership is not a "garbage-can" term that includes any phrase/concept that individuals use to describe it. Through a content analysis of leadership literature, the authors present its five main core attributes. This chapter also provides the rationale for the nesting of PE, FM and decision-making, as the main operational framework of the text.

The two related chapters (5 and 6) provide content that CMs and ULMs minimally need to administer their programs/agencies. They are replete with field-tested charts, forms, and worksheets that both students and agency personnel may use to develop their own knowledge and skills in these areas. They also articulate both "common ground" issues that transcend both of these administrative levels, as well as unique tasks for each level.

Finally, Chapter 7 concludes by presenting how the core leadership attribute of decision-making serves as the umbrella concept under which evaluation and financial management intersect. We refer to this colloquially as "where data meets dollars." Here, we assert that leaders must make informed data-driven decisions, which significantly and positively shape the organizational culture. No other text positions these skill sets in the context of leadership in such a proactive way.

This text is intended to be topical, timely and practical, and its content is deemed essential for both the students and social service professionals to both grasp and understand. But alas, we hope that you, the reader, would be the judge of that!

MJH & MDF

LIST OF FIGURES AND TABLES

FIGURES

TABLES

ABOUT THE AUTHORS

Marvin D. Feit, Ph.D. is Professor of Social Work in the Ethelyn R. Strong School of Social Work at Norfolk State University. He began his academic career at The University of Minnesota School of Social Work, and then joined The University of Tennessee School of Social Work at the Center for the Health Sciences, Memphis, Tennessee. His teaching responsibilities at both institutions included community organization and administration, substance abuse, mental health, financial management, group work, and social work practice. In addition, he also has been a faculty member at Norfolk State University and then became the Director of the Social Work Department at The University of Akron, where he was instrumental in creating the first jointly administered and joint curriculum distance education MSW program with Cleveland State University. He also has been the Director of Social Work at San Francisco State University and the Dean of the Ethelyn R. Strong School of Social Work at Norfolk State University. Dr. Feit received a B.S. in Health and Physical Education from Brooklyn College, City University of New York, a master's degree in Social Work from Columbia University, a Master of Science in Hygiene (M.Sci.Hyg.) from the Graduate School of Public Health at the University of Pittsburgh, and a Ph.D. in Social Work from the School of Social Work at the University of Pittsburgh.

Dr. Feit is the author or co-author of several books and has written many articles and chapters in the areas of group work, substance abuse, health, fiscal management and administration, and practice. Dr. Feit has made numerous presentations at national, state, and local conferences and has served as a consultant to profit and non-profit organizations, federal and state government agencies, and numerous community-based agencies. He is the founding co-editor of the *Journal of Social Work in Public Health*, formerly *Health and Social Policy*, the *Journal of Human Behavior in the Social Environment*, the *Journal of Evidence-Based Social Work*, and the *Journal of Public Child Welfare*. Each journal is published by Taylor and Francis, Inc. which assumed control after purchasing The Haworth Press, Inc. His latest book, *Evidence-Based Interventions in Social Work*, co-authored with John S. Wodarski, Ph.D., was published by Charles C. Thomas, Inc.

Dr. Feit has been a member of the Council on Publications, Council on Social Work Education (CSWE), and has been appointed to the editorial board of the *Journal of Social Work Education*, published by CSWE.

Michael J. Holosko, Ph.D., M.S.W., is the Pauline M. Berger Professor of Family and Child Welfare at The University of Georgia, School of Social Work, and adjunct instructor at Norfolk State University. He has taught across the undergraduate and graduate curriculum in schools of social work (primarily), nursing, public administration, and applied social science in Canada, the United States, Hong Kong, Sweden, Australia, and the US Virgin Islands. He has published extensively in the areas of evaluation, health care, gerontology, social policy, research, music intervention, and spirituality. For the past 32 years, he has been a consultant to a variety of large and small health and human service organizations in the areas of: program evaluation, outcomes, accreditation, organizational development, communication, leadership, visioning, organizational alignment, and stress management. He has published numerous monographs, chapters, articles, and texts in the areas of evaluation, health care, gerontology, social policy, research, music intervention, and spirituality. His recent text, *Pocket Glossary for Commonly Used Research Terms*, written with Bruce Thyer will be developed by Sage publications as a telephone application as well. He serves on the editorial boards of: *Research on Social Work Practice*; *Journal of Health and Social Policy*; *Journal of Human Behavior and Social Environment*; *The Hong Kong Journal of Social Work*; *Journal of Social Service Research* and the *Journal of Evidence-Based Social Work Practice*. For a number of years, he has had both radio and television shows advocating for social justice in North America.

1
INTRODUCTION

In the past several decades, there has been increased attention in social work on administrative practice, as highlighted by Lewis, Lewis, and Soulflee, Jr (1991) and Rapp and Poertner (1992). One of the more significant aspects of this increased attention is the process of becoming an administrator. Perlmutter (1990) best summarized this thrust by calling it "changing hats," which means going from direct practice to administration. The traditional, one-track linear method was precisely the route taken by most social work administrators (Lewis *et al.*, 1991). It remains the same today.

Chess, Norlin, and Jayaratne in 1987 indicated the importance of human service providers preparing themselves for upper level management or administration. At that time they noted that almost half of all graduate-level human service providers were likely to become managers within five years after graduation, and this picture has not changed.

Despite the prominence of the "changing hat" model, very little is known about the new knowledge and skills required in becoming an upper level manager and whether the one-track linear method is the most appropriate educational model. Several early studies provide insight into the process of becoming an administrator. Patti *et al.* (1979) and Scurfield (1981) report a rather surprisingly high degree of continuity in role and in adapting knowledge and skills previously learned in clinical position, with greatest difficulty occurring in the exercise of authority in relationships with subordinates among social work administrators who started from clinical positions. For these and other authors there seems to be continuity in the process of becoming an executive, despite a lack of administrative training.

It has been posited that becoming an executive or chief administrator of a human service organization is problematic and difficult largely because executives moving up an organization are not adequately prepared for the job (Feit, 1979; 1987; and Feit & Landon, 1982). This means that in the process of becoming an administrator there is discontinuity in certain skills and knowledge such as budgeting, evaluating, and working with the board of directors, when one actually becomes an administrator. In other words discontinuity means that these skills are more likely to be needed and subsequently developed when one is in the position, rather than developing a skill over time and sequentially as one moves up the organizational ladder.

The purpose of this text is to provide a model for understanding the transition from clinical to upper level managers. Such a model also identifies new knowledge and skills which may be required of human service administrators as they make the transition from clinical worker, and to present this transition in the context of decision-making and in becoming a leader. It is generally understood that most human service administrators are trained as clinicians and usually have no academic background in upper level management (Gummer, 1990; Perlmutter, 1990). As they move into managerial positions, it is logical to assume that administrators learn their craft either through on-the-job training, continued education courses or a certain combination of these two methods.

It is critical to prepare administrators for the requisite tasks in upper level management and to examine them in the context of becoming a leader. Most of the empirical work upon which the process of becoming an administrator is based was done over three decades ago, and posited by several authors, such as Patti (1979, 1983). Second, in the past two decades there has been a tremendous increase in administrative complexity and technology, such as the application of computers to informational management and the development of different perspectives in managing non-profit organizations.

Third, over thirty years ago Scurfield (1981) suggested that clinical preparation and experience was not relevant to certain technical, theoretical, and organizational aspects of administration, such as budgeting, financial and business administration, administrative theory, and administrative skills. These studies do not discuss the effect of the lack of such training on executives, nor do they suggest when and if the executives eventually learned this material and, if they did, how and where they acquired this experience.

In other words, since political, economic, and social conditions are very different today in regard to non-profit management, particularly when their environments may be characterized by scarcity, ambiguity, and uncertainty (Lewis *et al.*, 1991; and Hasenfeld, 1983), it may be timely to better understand the extent to which upper level human service administrators are adequately prepared for their executive level jobs. The current pressure on executives for accountability, fiscal management requirements when services are more in demand, is increased precisely in the areas identified by researchers that administrators lack training and knowledge. For example, Austin (1985) indicated that the complexity of the nature of human service administration adds to the difficulty in understanding the administrative function. His observations are as accurate today as they were over twenty-five years ago.

Thus, it is generally accepted that aspiring and new upper level executives and administrators do not possess an adequate knowledge base and the requisite skills to function competently in today's world, nor are they prepared to make decisions and to function as leaders. This situation is largely the result of:

1. poor academic background in management
2. the increasing demands for competence in many areas, such as financial management, evaluation, treatment, computer literacy, personnel, planning, and so forth
3. a lack of understanding regarding how human services administrators learn to effectively perform their job as they move up the organizational ladder
4. having to be accountable for making key decisions
5. the increased demand for leadership.

Transition to social work manager and certificates which focus on management are a concept of leadership.

IMPLICATIONS AND DISCUSSION

The first difficulty when becoming an upper level manger is that one often has to learn distinctively new tasks. Moreover, several tasks have to be redefined so as to be useful. Thus, the social work literature which asserts that administration skills tend to be linear and are developed sequentially over time (Austin, 1985; Perlmutter, 1990), are limited in teaching social work students the skills of administration. Indeed, for certain skills, such as budgeting and fiscal management, there is discontinuity, which means that one doesn't learn them in lower organizational positions but they are essential at the executive level.

Austin (1985) noted that two major objectives of the human service administrative function are the provision of effective and efficient services (clinical management) and the maintenance and development of the organization as an essential instrument for service provision (upper level management) (p. 17, parentheses that of authors). The opportunity to pursue an interest in either objective at another time would certainly be available and would be expected in a substantial number of individuals.

It seems clear that becoming an administrator is not simply a matter of "changing hats," or a matter of continuing to build on what has been learned in previous organizational positions, such as supervisor or unit director. In a previous study, administrators responded that budgeting, board relations, supervising, negotiating and planning, in descending order of importance, were the most important new tasks they had to learn, and they wished they had been more adequately prepared. Budgeting and board relations are two areas of task responsibility which administrators do not learn as a function of their position at lower levels in an organization (Feit, 1982; 1987).

Supervising, evaluating, negotiating and planning are tasks of administration which imply continuity in skills learned at lower level organizational positions. However, since these administrators have indicated that these were important new tasks they had to learn, questions may be raised regarding their substance and type of activity as the focus of each task shifts at the different organizational levels. For example, at the supervisory level, one is likely to supervise and evaluate the interventions of direct service workers, provide case consultation, and assist in teaching case management, time management, and so forth to direct service workers. At the executive level, one is likely to hold supervisors accountable for the service(s) provided by workers in their *units*, manage/coordinate the activities of the supervisors in a management team approach, and so forth. Therefore, supervising at the executive level is quite likely to be different from that done at the supervisory level. The same questions may be raised regarding evaluating, negotiating and planning.

Administrators, too, are required to make a shift to upper level management from clinical management if they are to be effective and successful in administering an entire organization. Upper level management centers on the business aspects of administering an organization, and clinical management centers on the effectiveness of the helping process.

New administrators must learn the executive level aspects of supervision, planning, and negotiating which is usually different from the aspects of clinical management. For example, upper level management often requires negotiation between different and/or competing organizational work units (conflict), whereas in clinical management one is usually negotiating between individuals in the same profession or working in the same unit (consensus). Also, in upper level management, administrators would be responsible for designing and implementing then deciding when to begin and end a planning process whereas others complete the tasks. Thus, while the tasks appear to be the same, the aspects of a task are very different. This difference would account for the belief that such tasks as supervising, evaluating, negotiating and planning were familiar; they were actually different tasks one usually has to learn when one first transitions to upper level management.

However, care must be given to attract a diverse population in the clinical and upper level management areas. The clinical background group usually is more diverse, i.e. minorities, and the clarification of role, task, and responsibility in each level of management could make it easier to attract women, minorities, and younger people to upper level management.

SUMMARY

The purpose of the book is to illustrate that becoming an administrator, or going from clinician to administrator, is much more complicated than is suggested in the social work management literature. Becoming an upper level administrator involves the learning of new skills as well as a reorientation to certain skills previously learned at lower level positions. It is very likely that success in becoming an upper level administrator involves making a distinct shift to requisite skills where new and a reorientation to previously learned skills are addressed. In order to respond better to today's functional educational requirements in becoming an effective leader and upper level administrator, it is important to identify the requisite tasks and orientation and key organizational positions, along with an understanding of decision-making and the importance of leadership.

2

A MODEL FOR UNDERSTANDING THE MANAGEMENT AND ADMINISTRATION OF SOCIAL WORK PROBLEMS

A practical model for clarifying the relationship between organizational positions and the task of managing and administering social service programs is needed. Such a model would be valuable in explaining several issues regarding practice and education. In practice, the administrative requirements that are related to the function, task, responsibility, and skills of workers at all organizational levels need to be recognized, understood, and operationalized. In education, this dimension of practice needs to be conceptualized in order to teach upper management and administration effectively.

A major problem hindering the development of such a model has been the way in which management competencies have been conceptualized in the field. Management is usually viewed, discussed, and written about in general terms, as if it were a unitary concept carried out by middle and top level personnel. Efforts to teach social service management effectively have not been particularly helpful because the different managerial levels coupled with the tasks, responsibilities, and skills required have not been related directly to the job requirements of staff and managers at each organizational level. An objective of this chapter is to identify these tasks as they relate to management at each organizational level.

Most organizational literature focusing on management neglects to discuss and to address the difference between the administrative requirements of managing direct service programs and the broader issues of managing human service programs. Many authors in the past several decades base their discussion on the traditional line-staff categorization scheme to delineate clinical and upper level tasks (Holloway, 1980; Perlmutter, 1990; Scurfield, 1981). One key difficulty in the scheme lies in the definition of administrative practice. Scurfield, for example, defined administrative practice as performance in a position that was identified by both the agency and the respondent as one of first-level, middle-level, or top-level administration or management. Such definitions tend to polarize clinical and administrative tasks while blurring attempts to differentiate between the type and complexity of managerial tasks within the various levels of the organizational positions. The purpose of this chapter is to identify the different types of managerial tasks required of each category of worker, so that management as a concept becomes more understandable and practical, and also to make the teaching of administration more relevant.

The literature over the years has tended to be program specific and not easily adaptable to other programs (Patti and Austin, 1987). Other literature deals directly with a specific task or tasks required in upper level administrative practice, such as budgeting (Tuller, 1997; Brent, 2006), and designing management information systems, or with particular aspects of an administrator's job, such as conflict management, leadership skills, monitoring employees, etc. (Feit *et al.*, 1995; Austin, 1985). Such literature remains fragmented and therefore is not adequate for effective upper level administrative responsibility. The complexities of contemporary management of human service organizations are rarely discussed in relation to organizational position and fail to differentiate administrative tasks and other requirements in relation to overall agency management including managing the delivery of service to clients.

In the same literature, upper level management and clinical management have been used interchangeably, thereby implying that they mean the same thing. Greater administrative effectiveness and the development of competent administration in the human service field could be enhanced as the distinction between upper level program management and clinical management is clarified. The purpose of clinical or direct service management is to develop and implement treatment components directly affecting client service. This purpose omits the need for major administrative and business activities to support the clinical components.

On the other hand, upper level management is much broader in scope. Its purpose is to maintain the organization in its larger environment. Consequently, attention must be paid both to operations internally and survival externally. Upper level management must therefore be defined from an organizational perspective, i.e. each administrative problem is viewed based on its effect on all aspects of an organization and fiscal realities and evaluation data are viewed as critical to making decisions. In sum, clinical management becomes a subset of upper level management.

This definitional distinction between managing programs at the upper level and management of clinical treatment or direct services does not result necessarily in assigning administrative responsibilities only to persons holding administrative positions. Indeed, the position taken in this chapter is that management activities are required at all organizational levels, and are a part of every worker's responsibilities. Each level has both clinical and upper level program management decision-making responsibilities. In the context of making appropriate decisions, however, the emphasis, focus, and amount of management responsibilities will differ according to organization level.

The model proposed in Table 2.1 illustrates major components in the clinical and program management of human service programs at key organizational levels. It is intended to clarify the distinctions in management tasks and responsibilities, as well as identify the knowledge needed in relation to making the transition to different organizational positions. Such clarification provides a sound, rational basis for understanding and teaching social service administration more effectively. When illustrating the many requirements of upper level management, attention can be given to developing this key aspect of management in its curriculum and in the social work and human relations field. It also provides a better understanding of instruction for management of the clinical process.

Table 2.1 reflects a fact that in human service programs, treatment and administration are the two major orientations. Imposed on these two orientations are the jobs held by individuals, usually arranged in the hierarchical structure. Thus, one would expect to find clinicians on one side of an orientation continuum and the executive director and top level administrators on the other. Between these two positions lie a host of other key organizational positions, such as clinical supervisors, a director of clinical practice, a program director, or a director of social services. In effect, Table 2.1 indicates that each organizational position can be placed in one of the four specified categories (Feit and Landon, 1982) and illustrates the transition from one position to another.

CLINICAL MANAGEMENT

While the positions obviously differ in each category, each position contains certain managerial activities. For example, in addition to providing direct treatment, a clinician has to perform certain administrative tasks, such as writing client progress notes, preparing client summaries, determining the degree of intervention needed in each case, evaluating their own practice, and seeking ways to improve interpersonal skills, etc. Most of these administrative tasks fall within the parameter of clinical activities while only a few are program management oriented. The separation of these administrative tasks by management responsibility in a clinician's job is shown in the first category of Table 2.1

As one moves to a position of supervision of clinical workers or a unit supervisor, the job as well as the nature of the program management responsibilities and related administrative tasks changes naturally. For example, one must now evaluate the performance of workers, assist workers in managing their cases, supervise workers' activities, conduct individual performances, call attention to gaps in service, help design and implement new services or modify existing services, and communicate administrative and policy

		Principal Managerial or Administrative Task		
Primary Responsibility	Primary Management Orientation	Primary Organizational Position	Clinical	Upper Level
Treatment	Clinical	Direct Service Personnel Social worker Clinical intake Outreach counselor Group worker Community worker	Write client progress notes Write agency reports on service Prepare client summaries Evaluate one's own practice, Seek ways to improve interpersonal skills Attend meetings Present cases at staff meetings or case conferences Gather data for supervisory or management needs	Manage case load Participate in agency evaluation or research studies Participate in external public relations as assigned Complete required program reports
Treatment	Clinical	Supervisor Supervising workers Supervisor of unit Pediatric surgery Psychiatry Surgery Supervisor of group services	Help workers with their cases Identify gaps in service Organize interdisciplinary work Assign cases to workers Help workers manage their case loads Review client summaries Initiate needed clinical changes upward	Evaluate worker performance Supervise clinical workers Communicate administrative and policy changes Organize group data based on single cases Prepare unit reports Assist in the design and implementation of new services or modification of existing services
Clinical Admin. Management	Clinical	Department director Director of Social Services Director of Research & Evaluation	Organizing continuing education experiences for workers Direct and coordinate work units Design and implement a treatment system	Assist in making decisions about services offered Monitor activities of interdepartmental work groups Prepare reports Participate in management team meetings to design and implement the evaluation services Help to design and implement the evaluations of services

			Assess client/worker activity data monitor unit output	Help establish service objectives Supervise unit heads Evaluate unit head management Help prepare internal management and activity forms Develop budget and unit costs data Insure that agency policies are viable Plan new services Present programs to larger public as assigned
Agency Admin./ Upper Level Management	Program	Administrator Executive director deputy director	Monitor the effectiveness of treatment Delegate clinical administration appropriately Respond to external critique program	Provide overall program leadership Manage multidiscipline work units Account for fiscal matters Secure funds Maintain program policies Design an internal management and control system Design and implement a planning process Insure proper evaluation strategies Use or purchase of equipment Work with various community groups Work with Board of Directors Meet external reporting requirements Deal with the public and the media Prepare reports Hold staff meetings Work with other agencies

Table 2.1 Distinguishing between upper level management and clinical management by managerial requirements, organizational position, and primary orientation

changes to staff. These are tasks which clearly need not be addressed when working directly with clients.

It is important to recognize some unique aspects of people in these positions. First, these supervisors tend to reflect more of an interest and concern with treatment. They supervise a group of clinical personnel who are now in a position from which they emerged. Second, they face many new program management-oriented tasks for which they are often ill-prepared. Third, they must now assess and translate individual concerns to group data and vice versa. It is these last two aspects of their job which are often a source of much difficulty.

As a supervisor, the concept of a group task and application of related skills become an additional and prominent factor in effective performance. For example, supervisors need to know how staff groups operate, how labor is divided among workers and how to supervise and motivate different types of workers. Additionally, supervisors must be able to group data based on single cases (is required to present issues from a management perspective), so that decisions involving policy considerations and affecting many workers can be made. In summary, and as Patti and Austin (1987) note, a supervisor of a clinical work unit has to make the transition from a direct service provider to a direct service administrator while retaining a primary and strong treatment orientation.

A major and distinct shift in emphasis in administrative orientation occurs in the third management category, the departmental or program director's level. In this category, the primary orientation and identification is clinical and involves direct service and supervising clinical supervisors. Personnel in this category is one level removed from direct service and one organizational level closer to top management. They are usually members of an executive's immediate management team and view organizational issues from that perspective. The primary focus of their world is internal, and relates directly to the development of clinical effectiveness and the translation of organizational issues to direct service issues or vice versa.

Department directors are expected to assume greater administrative and managerial responsibility, accountability, and authority, and to provide leadership and direction to their subordinates. Hence, their managerial tasks differ but continue, in large measure, to be a natural progression of administrative promotion. While they are expected to continue with their administrative tasks, their assignments take on an added importance and tend to have large scale organizational impact. For example, administrative foci might include making decisions about the kind of services provided by their respective departments, monitoring of activities by the various interdepartmental work groups, developing plans to evaluate clinical services, setting service objectives, designing and implementing treatment systems, and developing unit cost financial accountability systems. These activities are upper level management in orientation. The top management level retains superordinate authority in this area but usually delegate all but final monitoring functions to personnel at this level.

In summary, three key organizational position categories have been described which together constitute the management of clinical programs. In each category three basic areas have been covered: the primary orientation of workers, the typical job held by persons in each category, and a listing and clarification of the major clinical and program management requirements that go along with each position. This sorting of managerial or administrative requirements and the relating of them to organizational positions illustrate the complexity of clinical management and provide the basis for understanding the inherent difficulty in teaching management as a unitary concept. At the same time, it lays the foundation for distinguishing and clarifying what upper management entails.

UPPER LEVEL MANAGEMENT

The fourth category discusses the tasks and qualifications of the administrators of human service programs and provides a picture of administrative responsibility not ordinarily illustrated in texts. This category is typified most by upper level administrators, executives, i.e., those with the authority for the entire organization. Programs, like administrative responsibilities, permeate all organizational levels, however. Top management is accountable to a board of directors or a similar group, and its job consists of relating to a variety of community or constituent groups, as well as providing organizational direction and maintaining internal control. The focus of work relates to the external and internal requirements of the organization.

This category exemplifies the distinction between upper level management and managing clinical programs (Feit & Landon, 1982). It is noted by the break in the administrative task line of progression depicted in Figure 2.1, and by the minimal responsibility in this area for lower level personnel indicated in Table 2.1. A top level or high level or upper level administrator must be concerned with the increasing accountability requirements and complexities of managing human service programs which are demanded by both funding agencies and the public. Moreover, they must understand the application of new technologies which may have only an apparent indirect bearing on clinical practice. Indeed, as requirements and knowledge increase in an extremely wide range of administrative areas, more pressure is placed on managers to understand treatment processes and outcomes, and their relation to the growth of administrative job responsibilities. This separation of critical administrative knowledge and tasks disrupts the perceived progression from clinical service into upper level management. The new requirements of administrative competence and the inherent difficulty in progressing linearly and naturally to a top administrative position is a source of the gap in becoming an administrative leader and decision-maker.

Administrative practice has changed drastically in the last thirty years (Drucker, 2001; Lackey, 2006). Administrative competence at an upper level management level requires not only extensive knowledge in an extremely

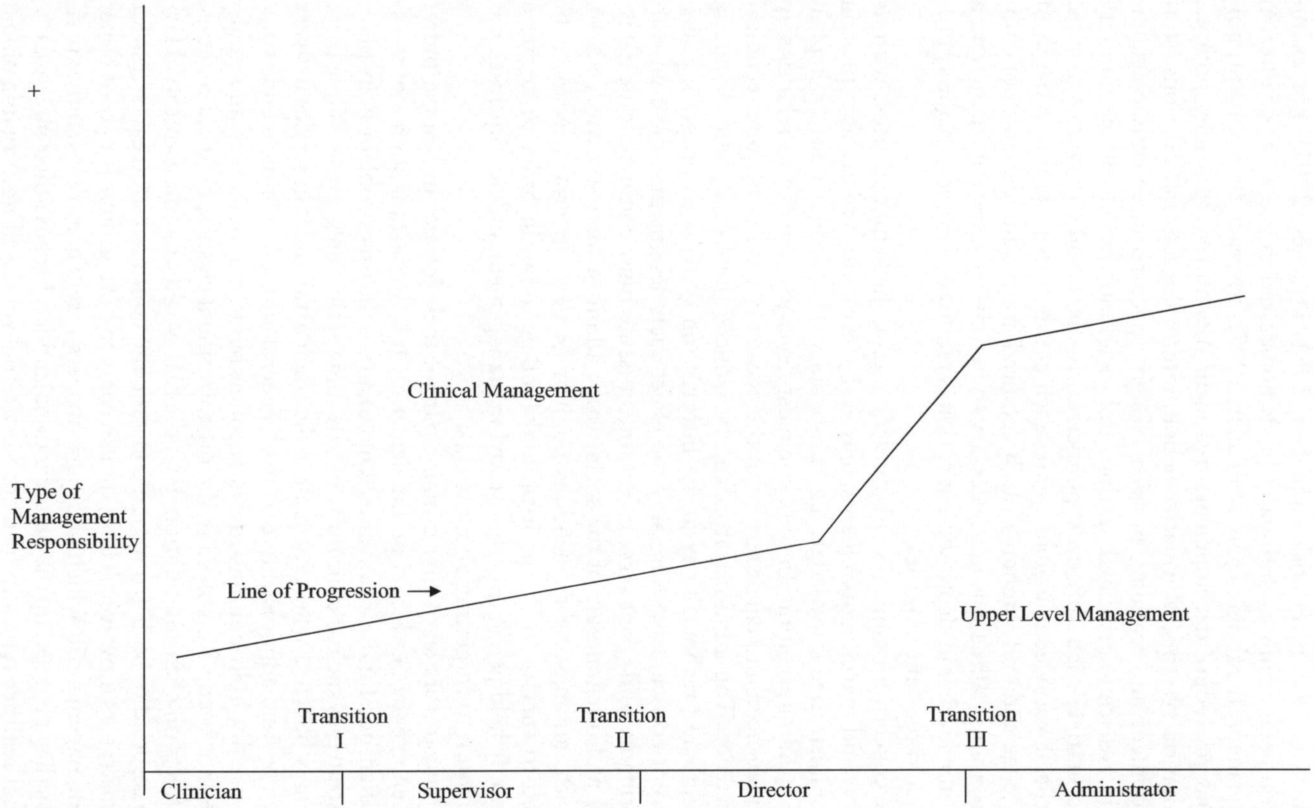

Figure 2.1 Managerial line of progression

wide range of areas but also the ability to apply that knowledge to decision-making action (Holosko and Feit, 1981; Drucker, 2001). For example, competence must continually be demonstrated in the areas of internal management, fiscal management (Tuller, 1997), contract development, policy and procedure development, treatment modalities, personnel policies, information systems, affirmative action, interorganizational relations, staff development and training, physical design, space requirements, consultation, interdisciplinary collaboration, and social interaction with community representatives such as Boards, politicians, funders, and community groups. Superficial knowledge is inadequate; each content area requires a depth of knowledge and understanding rarely required in the administration of clinical programs. While it is not necessary to become an expert in each area, a minimum level of in-depth sophistication is required in order to make appropriate and relevant inquiries.

The concern for clinical work, understanding the helping process with its nuances and special requirements, may easily be overlooked in this explosion of administrative knowledge. The probability of oversight must be kept in focus by administration. In sum, one must never lose sight of its relationship to human need and client service in the necessary rush to acquire technical competence. Top administrators can be seduced quite easily into designing elaborate and technically exquisite information systems or program plans, while not consciously addressing the effect such designs may have on staff performance and client service. Treatment issues must continue to be a necessary and integral part of the social work administrative knowledge base. Notwithstanding, the tremendous amount of new material needed to be learned to survive in the political and funding arena in order to negate a commonly held perception that studying management and administration is tantamount to forgetting about clients.

Administrators learn that a major part of their job lies in being a buffer between agency needs and public demands. It is a constant source of stress and often not totally resolvable. One example of this problem is in planning strategies such as continuity of care and service integration. While these goals may be worthwhile, the issue is that their attainment in service delivery is often beyond administrative control. Federal and state planners and evaluators usually hold administrators accountable to the outcomes and goals, and do not become involved in the organizational clashes, political realities, and effects on client population, e.g., the real world of administrators. Having to respond to both groups is a constant and continual source of stress for administrators, however. The responsiveness to both groups is part of upper level management in which clinical managers rarely gain first-hand experience as they progress up the organizational ladder, because their interorganizational realities typically focus on service delivery, and not organizational accountability.

The increased technical competencies required of current upper level administrators are clearly some of the major differences separating those who manage clinical programs from upper level administrators. The usual evolution or progression up the management ladder, apparent in the first three categories described, does not easily occur at the administrator level. First, as has been noted, the technical knowledge required for upper level management is extensive and complicated. There is much to learn that is new and very different from the knowledge needed for managing treatment programs. Second, the type of management style needed, the manner of dealing with people at this level, and the types of decisions which must be made are also very different.

Some examples would explain these two points. In the technical arena, an administrator is often faced with problems requiring legal advice, establishing and maintaining billing systems, maintaining a cash flow, deciding whether to purchase or rent equipment, understanding the purpose, conducting and using a financial or program audit (Hairston, 1985), allocating resources across diverse work units, having a constant access to vital control information, developing and maintaining a network of people external to the organization who can be relied upon for all kinds of support, taking corrective management action when indicated to keep the organization solvent, etc. While one can never teach or train personnel for these and other contingencies, as new knowledge must be applied on the job to be most effective, it is now possible to provide administrators with basic knowledge for understanding the technical aspects of upper level management, such as financial management and evaluation strategies.

As previously noted, the first three administrative and managerial categories do not adequately prepare one for overall upper level management. The learning needed for upper level management must therefore come from another source such as training or actual experience. Although one may not be well prepared at the level of clinical management to address certain staff problems at the top management level, supervising employees, ensuring that people do their jobs, evaluating worker performance, conducting staff meetings, setting goals and objectives, are previously learned and therefore familiar and transferable.

There are, however, some very important differences. One such difference lies in the power ascribed to the executive level positions. An administrator has the authority and the responsibility to make major decisions and is held accountable by all groups (employees, board, clients, interested community groups, regulatory and funding agencies). A decision scrutinized by all these parties inevitably insures high visibility and an inherent probability of criticism by one or more groups. An administrator must be prepared for such occurrences.

Another difference is the arena where decisions must be made. Upper level administration requires that an administrator has the ability to manage situations where conflict is common. At this level, one must continually negotiate the differences between professional groups and treatment ideologies, between professional and non-professional, between external pressure groups and internal work groups, between external service organizations, and between all components of an organization including maintenance and clerical, in such normal organizational functions as allocating resources, evaluating programs, selecting services to be offered or cut back, determining program objectives, and distributing the work assignments. Nowhere in managing clinical programs does one deal with these common problems on a regular basis where interorganizational and intraorganizational decisions are routinely required.

Problems posed to upper level management are numerous, complex and often the result of a series of related problems. Thus, "problems" defined at the upper level of management are not always the way they appear, as "the problem" is usually the culmination of a series of smaller and related problems at other organizational levels that have percolated to top management. Management of these problems involves an analysis of how "the problem" came to the attention of top administrators and, in turn, how decisions impacting downward must reflect the relative importance of "the problem" and any related problems of the affected workers. For example, a decision to proceed with program evaluation at the administrative level requires an understanding of the different problems likely to emerge at all workers' levels. As there is an inherent strain in the researcher–practitioner relationship (Weiss, 1987), administrators must learn how to minimize potential negative effects arising from their interaction at the organization level. Such an approach would require a thoughtful and carefully planned series of related activities targeted at the concern of workers at the various levels in the organization.

While lower level personnel provide the information without which the upper level manager cannot function, the nature of their primary task and orientation to a clinical focus preclude their major involvement in the overall administrative area. Also, external sanctioning groups, legislature bodies, governing boards, media representatives, and political supporters will only deal with those who have legitimate organizational power. While certain reporting and negotiating functions can be delegated, the essential political operation must be carried on by the top administrator.

In summary, upper level management has been described in the fourth category and shown to be distinct from clinical management. Progression up the organizational ladder from clinical to executive evolves naturally until the executive level is reached when a wide gap is seen to occur. This gap poses the greatest hurdle in making the transition to administrator from clinical and to upper level management from clinical management.

The gap results from several sources. One source is the increased technical competencies required of current administrators; second, the amount of external work required of administrators; and, third, the authority for agency survival goes with the domain of upper level management. Clinical management usually lacks the opportunities for its managers to gain the knowledge and experience required for competent upper level management. Indeed, as the context of such change is realized, its complexity and tension are enhanced by the need to make decisions and demonstrate leadership when one is so highly visible.

3

CURRENT TRENDS INFLUENCING HEALTH AND HUMAN SERVICE ORGANIZATIONS (HSOS)

INTRODUCTION

Although organizational theorists have long espoused the importance of understanding how the organizational environment impacts an organization, it was Hasenfeld (1983) who formally brought prominence to this notion in social work. He conceptualized organizational–environmental relations by identifying this dynamic interactional relationship as both: a) a set of resources that the organization must mobilize to survive and carry out its activities, and b) a set of constraints to which it must adapt when operationalizing service objectives (Hasenfeld, 1983: 51).

Illustrated conceptually as six concentric domains in Figure 3.1, the HSO is nested first in its immediate task environment, in which it constantly interacts and seeks to achieve resources and domain consensus. In turn, the task environment is embedded in a broader general environment composed of economic conditions, political-legal conditions, socio-demographic conditions, cultural conditions, and technological conditions (Hasenfeld, 1983: 51–63).

As indicated in Figure 3.1, this places the HSO in a centralized configuration within the external environment which is rather tenuous and vulnerable, as it will either survive, thrive, or die. This rather blunt outcome is contingent upon the HSO's ability not only to understand these two interrelated domains, which it holds various power and dependency relationships with, but it also requires the HSO to effect ongoing and meaningful transactions or exchange relationships with various stakeholders in this schema.

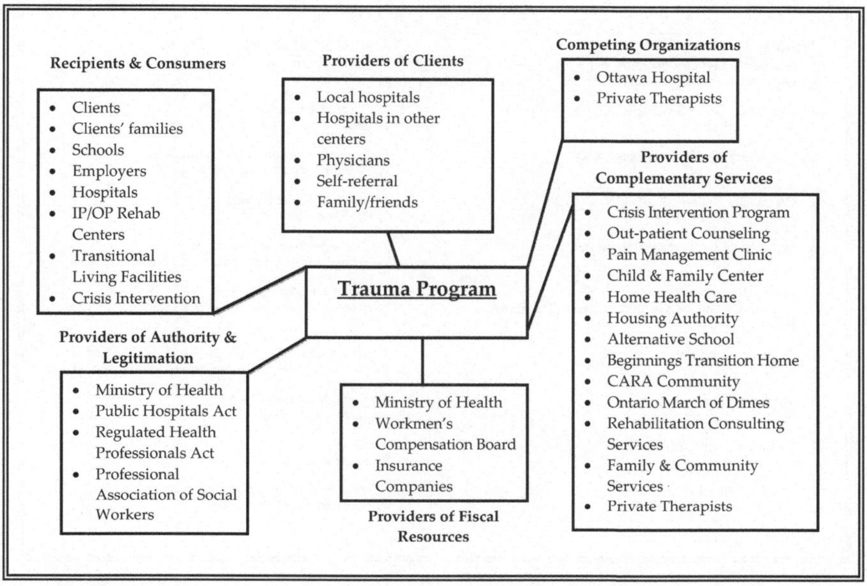

Figure 3.1 The six domains in the task environment – the trauma program

TRENDS IN THE EXTERNAL ORGANIZATIONAL ENVIRONMENT

Any social work supervisor, middle or upper level manager who perceives that their HSO is immune to the environmental milieu is administratively remiss. Denial of this reality is tantamount to administrative negligence at best and a certain death knoll for the organization at worst. Indeed, the days of organizational partitioning and petty turfdom, lack of organizational accountability or effectiveness, and naivety about organizational–environmental transactional relationships are long gone (Mason, 2007).

Figure 3.2 presents ten of these more pervasive trends and then candidly presents the "stories behind the trends."

Increase in service demands → decrease in funding

More and more individuals require more and more social welfare services all over the world. Social welfare defined broadly here is taken to include education, health, housing and social services. Although "real spending" as a percentage of GDP reflected in constant dollars (and adjusted for inflation) has grown in North America, per capita spending for social welfare (actual dollars per person) has not significantly changed in the past 25 years or so (Pati *et al.*, 2004). This is particularly true for the two most vulnerable groups in our society, the very young and the very old (Pati *et al.*, 2004).

Trends	The Story Behind the Trend
1. Increase in Services/Programs ↑ Decrease in Available Funds ↓	1. Do More with Less 2. Think Smarter
2. Community Devolution: Federal→Provincial→Local	1. "Crazy Glue Syndrome" – YTI-YOI 2. More Local Accountability
3. Community "Problem" Reconfiguration	1. Communities Lag Behind the Concept 2. Matching Mandates to Problems
4. Community 'Capacity Building'	1. No Definition of Capacity 2. No Resource to Build
5. Integrative Approaches to Service Delivery	1. Define Partners & Stakeholders 2. Develop Joint Agreements
6. Chaos Theory Prevails: Reversals, Randomness, Sudden Leaps, Paradoxes, Rapid Changes	1. Funding Bodies Perpetuate Chaos 2. Need to Organizationally Adapt
7. Visionary Leadership	1. ULM's & Boards are Windows to External World 2. Need to Play Big "P" and Small "p" Politics Like Never Before
8. Myth of Prevention	1. Body Count Data Prevails 2. Keep the Myths Going
9. Re-Engineering & Re-Imaging	1. How Do We "Unlearn"? 2. Alignment of Organizational Environment
10. "Era of Legitimacy"	1. Evaluation of Program & Services 2. Interventions → Outcomes

Figure 3.2 Current trends in the environment influencing health & human service organizations

At the organizational level, HSOs:

a. compete fiercely for limited funds
b. find supplemental ways to offset their escalating costs through revenue sharing, limiting eligibility criteria, re-prioritization and re-structuring their organization's mandate
c. use more and more non-professional, and/or volunteer staff
d. borrow money against their limited budgets
e. actively seek out more funding avenues, e.g. external grants, private donations, cost-shared arrangements and contractual services.

Heller (2006) referred to these responses as HSOs seeking more "fiscal space," or finding additional resources to service clients in these troubled financial times.

The story behind this trend is bleaker as with such limited resources, and in order to do our allegedly important client-centred work, HSOs are scrambling just trying to survive – let alone thrive. Practitioners, supervisors, and middle and upper level managers are constantly under the gun to "do more with less," as caseloads and waiting lists for service increase daily. Financial uncertainty is both ubiquitous and pervasive in most North American HSO cultures. Indeed, there is not a supervisor or manager in an HSO who would not be elated if their annual funding was re-approved next year with a "zero percent increase" – as they have come to realize that this could be a far worse case scenario.

The HSO climate in which our professional work is conducted creates challenging environments for all, where if we continue to do too much more – with no complementary supports or resources, we may find ourselves compromising the very services we are mandated and ethically bound to deliver to our clients (Allen & Smith, 2008). Finally here, one can only be asked to "think smarter" and "be more efficient" a finite number of times, and the double edged sword of quantity vs. quality is sure to cut someone in an injurious way – most likely our clients.

Community devolution: federal → state → local

Holosko (2009b) recently completed a special edition journal entitled "Global Realities of Social Policy: The Devolution Revolution." In it, he documented the globalization of this devolution-revolution in the countries of Canada, the United States, Great Britain, and Sweden. As such, he demonstrated how:

a. the devolution-revolution is relatively immune to the political ideology of the country
b. it shifts both funding and authority for social welfare service provision from federal → state → local levels
c. when such cascading shifts occur, they almost always shift downward to local levels – never upward
d. often times, local infrastructures or resource allocating systems are inadequately prepared to assume such responsibilities, which are now plunked squarely at the feet of the community (Holosko, 2009b).

The resultant effects of more locally administered but under-resourced care significantly impacts our definitions of "community care."

The story behind this trend includes first more local accountability to the community's system of care – which if re-framed from a strengths-based perspective (a social work framework for practice) may not be such a bad or negative thing for our profession. In his concluding remarks to this edited journal he stated: "the 'devolution-revolution' to local levels, therefore, provides social work with a unique opportunity to build on its history and legacy of providing ethical and humane services to the vulnerable populations in the very communities in which they reside" (2009b: 128).

The second story (see Figure 3.2) has to do with the "Crazy Glue Syndrome" or YTI → YOI! The latter refers to the colloquial North American idiom – "you touch it → you own it!" Here, the reality is that as the responsibility for providing services gets passed along locally, now local community agencies are "on the hook" to provide these essential services. And, when such agencies ask for state, and/or federal help to assist with this mandate, they are frequently reminded that "we don't fund these programs any more" and "it is not our responsibility to do so" (Holosko, 2009). Finally here, it has become very apparent that civic leaders must take a more proactive role in re-defining their communities, as well as their problems or concerns. Over a decade and a half ago, Osborne and Gaebler (1992) called on lead governmental officials to learn to re-invent how they govern by acting as facilitators for their government to function and service the community in ways to strengthen their local economies. These authors stated:

> city government will have to make some adjustments and in some ways redefine its traditional role. I believe the city will more often define its role as a catalyst and facilitator. The city will more often find itself in the role of defining problems and then assembling resources for others to use in addressing those problems . . . City government will have to become even more willing to inter-weave scarce public and private resources in order to achieve our community's goals.
>
> (Osborne and Gaebler, 1992: 27)

Community "problem" reconfiguration

There has been a decided shift in the quiet devolution-revolution to developing social welfare programs and services in communities, not from a population or demographic imperative but from a "problem reconfiguration" one. In this focus, the community's problems are prioritized based on the so-called "problems of individuals in the community." So, depending on "the problems the community has" and the existing infrastructures – if one is fortunate to end up with a problem that this community has "identified" – care can be accessed. Conversely, if one's problems do not match up with "the community problems," clients must travel (if they can) to usually an adjacent community to receive care.

For example, in Canada's universal health care system, smaller towns and cities cannot afford highly specialized health care for all citizens. As a result, Canadians are accustomed to driving to, or being airlifted to, adjacent communities which have the specialized care that they require (Holosko, 1997).

The stories behind this reality are stated in Figure 3.2. Communities clearly lag behind the concept and they have difficulties in matching their infrastructures and mandates to the "problems of the community." To exemplify these stories behind the trends, Brown and Stevens (2006) studied seven U.S. communities aiming to expand health coverage to the uninsured and improve their care.

Funded by the Robert Wood Johnson Foundation's *Communities in Charge* (CIC) program, when these communities (with identified community problems) were evaluated they concluded that: "despite solid leadership and carefully crafted plans, political, economic, and organizational obstacles precluded much expansion of coverage and constrained reforms . . . CIC's record offers little evidence that communities are better equipped than are other sectors of U.S. society to solve the problems of un-insurance" (Brown & Stevens, 2006: W150).

Community capacity-building

Although sounding like a noble idea which is rather difficult to do but indeed still a noble idea none the less, the concept of community capacity-building has seen a renewed interest in the social welfare field. Turner (1998: ix) stated that human service professionals increasingly search for: "the holy grail of community and neighbourhood in an attempt to strengthen the effectiveness of their interventions."

Community capacity-building refers to the ability and will of the people residing in a community to participate in actions based on community interests, both as individuals and group organizations and networks (Williams, 2004: 730). It is not the definition itself that is problematic, but it is fraught with two underpinning questionable assumptions. These tend to undermine the current love affair that the social welfare field has with the concept of capacity-building. The first is that *community based groups are synonymous with capacity-building*. This is the dominant and traditional way that capacity-building is described in the literature. However, Williams (2004) demonstrated how informal one-to-one groups and engagement are a more popular form of community involvement. They are also more characteristic of the participatory culture of less affluent populations – such as the clients whom we routinely see on our social welfare caseloads.

Similarly, Shirlow and Murtagh (2004) concluded their analyses of communities in Ireland stating that if capacity-building is ever to take hold, it will have to change this assumption of affiliation of community members with community groups. They ended their analysis by highlighting the need for capacity-building to reach deeper into the concerns of local citizenry, rather than the priorities of statutory funders, as a basis for meaningful service provision and local planning.

The second rather spurious assumption is that *residing in a community implies a sense of community belonging*. Studies have shown that if one has a sense of community, individuals have a greater sense of viewing the community more positively and will participate in community capacity development through bonds of unity and support and satisfaction (Bowen *et al.*, 2003; Bowen *et al.*, 2000; McMillan & Chavis, 1986).

Residing in any community means to many individuals nothing more than a place to close their door to the external world and a place to sleep at night. To infer that residence involves a sense of inclusive belonging, a willingness to feel connected to one's community, attachment, and some sort of well-being is remiss from a social, and/or psychological perspective. It is no wonder then, why capacity-building indicators are delimited by the variables of: person and family, neighbourhood, one's health status, one's values, the community, demographics, income, county, state, resources, the economy of the community, its civic leadership, and by the will of individuals not to feel connected at all to their respective communities (Robert Wood Foundation, 2007). These assumptions need to be more seriously addressed by community planners if the issue of capacity-building is to ever take hold in any meaningful way.

The stories behind this trend (see Figure 3.2) include first, there is no definition of capacity, so how do we envision building one? The nebulousness around this lack of definition and its potential negative impact for capacity-building has been tabled by Levitas (2000: 196):

> My first worry about "capacity-building" as about "community development", is that it often seems to be a way of expecting groups of people who are poorly resourced to pull themselves up by their collective boot straps. So-called social capital is expected to take the place of economic capital. The imputed absence of social capital is potentially stigmatising and laid at the door of (mainly) poor people themselves. "Capacity-building" may be an alternative to economic regeneration. A large part of the effective resourcing therefore takes the form of unpaid work.

This is just one of many deleterious effects of not being able to clearly define capacity-building.

From a social work strengths perspective, it appears that one's capacity is limitless. However, if community capacity-building is to be effective it must have clear benchmarks delineated for success (Grady, 1995). Further, specific interventions should be marketed and targeted for specific groups, and communities should be allowed to define the community within the nature of the intervention/initiative being implemented in their respective community (Holosko & Feit, 2006). In addition, both an understanding of the community environment itself linked with *source appropriate* information, meaning obtaining the right information from the right people who need to be accessed, is paramount if capacity-building is to ever have any success (Robert Wood Foundation, 2007).

The issue of "resources to build" a community's capacity is almost never considered, but in studies of actual capacity-building efforts, this issue is not trite (Bowen *et al.*, 2003; Shirlow & Murtagh, 2004). We recognize also that capacity-building is a transformative process, and one that is time consuming and vulnerable to the local economy and political reality of any community. In this regard, we temper the well-worn and age old African adage: "it takes a village to raise a child" to "it takes time and money to raise the village to raise a child."

Integrative approaches to service delivery

Due to devolution and agency cutbacks for health and human services in many industrialized countrses of the world, services and providers have become collaboratively bundled together with multiple agencies offering a defined system of care in their respective communities. These are often referred to as cross-sectional collaborations – networks, alliances, or partnerships among public, secular, and faith-based non-profits, and for-profit organizations. They either consist of distinct organizations that develop relationships with each other to meet client needs called self-organizing networks. Or they are community organizations sub-contracted with a lead organization, which is expected to create a mandated community-based network of service providers (Alexander, 1995; Provan & Milward, 2001). The latter (lead organization model) is the more preferred modality, as it is frankly cheaper. But both arrangements are expected to yield the benefits of increased efficiency, innovation, local adaptation, increased flexibility, and enhanced community ties (Graddy & Chen, 2006: 534).

This idea is certainly tenable and required for HSO survival in today's reality, but again the concept is ahead of the community's ability to implement it. Clouds of uncertainty about integrative service approaches loom large over issues of: costs; organizational, programmatic, and community influences; democratic and consensual accountability; efficiency and effectiveness; integrative models that are viable and ones that are not; organizational and community care constraints and contingencies; community capacities; access; outcomes; policy considerations; and network size and scope (Bryson *et al.*, 2006; Dunlop & Holosko, 2004; Graddy & Chen, 2006; Knitzer & Cooper, 2006). Despite such uncertainty, HSOs continue to move forward with this seemingly altruistic community-spirited ideal.

The deficit reduction strategies of federal, state, and local governments has led to a resurgence of interest in collaboration. Increasingly, mandates for collaboration are linked to conditions of funding (Holosko, 2009b). As governments mandate collaborative networks as an implementation mechanism for integrating social welfare services, empirical studies about how inter-organizational collaboration is implemented among community partners is an emerging research, policy and practice problem (Bryson *et al.*, 2006; Dunlop & Holosko, 2004).

Middle and upper level managers need to be mindful of a few issues or the real "stories behind the story of collaboration" (Holosko, 2009b). Here are but a few.

1. *Funding issues require collaboration* – Regardless of the "will" to collaborate such partnerships will be tied to funding. Those HSOs who do so will thrive and those who do not will wither away. Developing relationships with partners in the community, however strained, is integral to organizational survival (Dunlop & Holosko, 2004).
2. Voluntary vs. mandatory collaboration – Although different joint agreements are voluntary and some are mandatory, the nature of the collaborative relationship transcends this distinction (Dunlop & Holosko, 2004). This means that agencies collaborate to ensure funding and typically will do anything they can to make the collaborative relationship work (Holosko & Dunlop, 1992).
3. *All communities are not created equal* – Finally here, communities vary in their demographics, organizational relationships, service networks, pre-existing partnerships, resources, and infrastructures. Collaborations

magnify such inequalities. Thus, some communities are able to develop more effective collaboration networks than others (Dunlop & Angell, 2001; Warner & Hefetz, 2003).

4. *Evaluation complexities* – Evaluating collaborative initiatives has been challenging to say the least (Holosko & Dunlop, 1992). These initiatives are typically multi-site, multi-level, with different programs, goals, objectives, costs, outcomes, services, stakeholders, etc. (Buckingham & Coffman, 1999; Dunlop & Holosko, 2004). The assumption put forward in this global devolution-revolution movement is that complex community-based collaborations are more efficient than singular service delivery models. This has never been empirically determined or validated (Kee, 1999).
5. *Collaborations are more likely to succeed when they have legitimacy* – Human & Provan (2000) cited three necessary conditions for collaborative networks: 1) legitimacy of the *network as a form* that can attract internal and external supports, 2) legitimacy of the *network as an entity* responsible to both insiders and outsiders, and 3) legitimacy of the *network as an interaction* that builds trust among members to freely communicate with one another.

Chaos theory prevails

Chaos theory has a long history in meteorology, physics, mathematics, ecology, and other non-social science fields. Since the early 1980s its application to the social sciences has become more relevant (Gregerson & Sailer, 1993). In simple terms, chaos theory posits that systems are not static but dynamic in nature and as a result, they exhibit patterns of chaotic and unpredictable behaviors.

As such, HSOs are transformational systems which, in order to survive, constantly need to adapt from one moment to the next, subject to internal and external environmental conditions. Watching the different countries of the world in our global village respond to today's current and unpredictable [to the extent projected] financial crises is a prime example of how the ongoing chaos↔seeking stability volatile relationship becomes perpetuated.

Chaos theory contends therefore, that we all live and must learn to survive on the "edge of chaos." It is similar to a large tsunami rising rapidly behind our power boat as we zoom ahead of the wave trying to avoid it, before it swamps us. This leads to a prevailing sense of uncertainty in which sudden leaps, reversals, randomness, paradoxes, and rapid changes in our HSOs and their external environments are the norm, not the exception.

This organizational adaptation to such constant chaos has profound implications for HSOs in areas of: community development and networking (Gilchrist, 2000); policy-making (Hacker, 2008); contracting relationships (Van Slyke, 2006); leadership and organizational viability (Osborn & Hunt, 2007), and research and evaluation (Gregerson & Sailer, 1993).

The story behind this trend is that funding bodies perpetuate this chaos as they themselves are entities of a larger uncertain socio-political arena (see Figure 3.1). It is not unusual in today's tenuous fiscal climate to have programs funded one day and being discontinued the very next day with little concern for the clients, their issues, or their lives. As well, constant cut-backs and reduced budget scenarios resulting in longer waiting lists; fewer staff to serve the needs of clients; the devolving of authority and responsibility to lower level workers and volunteers; and the stretching of organizational mandates to match programs to available funding streams are the norm, not the exception in most North American HSOs.

Organizational adaptation is the prescription for our survival on the "edge of chaos," and it requires a way of "unlearning old ways of doing things in the HSO." This is probably the greatest impediment to organizational change, as not just a few individuals, but an entire organizational governing structure's internal processes require not just re-tooling – but a re-consideration of what the entire organization must do, in order to survive in such turbulent times. Without sounding too gloomy, it is adapt organizationally or die for many HSOs, and some can actually hear the rattling chains of the grim reaper in the not too distant future.

Visionary leadership

In Chapter 4, we articulate the five top core leadership attributes ranked in descending order, from a content analyses of the literature on this transformational and rather elusive concept. It was no surprise to us that vision, both having one and also implementing one, were ranked as number 1 and number 1A, respectively.

This ranking (in Chapter 4) came out of our frustration in teaching numerous courses and providing workshops on supervision, leadership, management and administration etc., in which the concept of leadership is a rather loosely used garbage can term, where many attributes of it are heralded as "essential ingredients" of its broadly interpretive and inclusive definition.

Some administrators can have a vision, or develop one, yet they cannot implement it. Conversely, others may not have a vision but can effectively implement one. We applaud either of these, and fully acknowledge that there is indeed a different skill set involved in "the vision business." And we also realize that it is only the most adeptly skilled administrator, either middle or upper level, who can do both, that is, have one and implement one.

Our contention is that vision is the highest ranked attribute of leadership and should be the foremost calling card of any middle or upper level manager. This requires creativity, futuristic thinking, alignment thinking – with the mission, vision, values, goals, objectives, and services of the HSO, and a resourceful way of developing, presenting, seeking consensus and buy-in from the organization, its board and stakeholders. This then, becomes the operational definition of the term visionary leadership.

So what does visionary leadership require of middle and upper level managers? The first is a re-framing of administration as a "window to the external world." Here, administrators and their boards have their finger on the pulse of external trends, resources, supports, their communities of care, and always filter their enviro-scanning data back to the HSOs. Long gone are the days of a territorial moat being built around the HSO to allegedly safeguard its transparency, access, and services. Today's prevalent chaos theory (see Trend 6) and living on the edge of chaos precludes such limited thinking.

Second, building on this "conduit to the external world" notion, administrators need to play the political game like never before, if they are to survive and move their HSO's goals and agenda forward. As illustrated in Figure 3.3, we offer a set of both big "P" and small "p" politics that may assist middle and upper level administrators with this important task.

We fully realize that there could be more gamesmanship added to Figure 3.3, but we contend that these shake out as being primary concerns that visionary middle and upper level managers need to minimally address in today's climate.

Myth of prevention

Prevention is a word bandied about rather insincerely by both individuals and HSOs. At the individual level, never before in North America have we ever had more ubiquitous information available to us about our: health, diets, lifestyle, stressors, spirituality, relationships, occupations, environments, parenting,

Big "P" Politics

1. Being Aware of the Government's Agenda
   - Knowing funding sources
   - Knowing timely and topical concerns
   - Having access to the corridors of government and officials
2. Playing the "Game"
   - Develop relationships with all stakeholders and networks
   - Tie vision, mission, goals & objectives to the agenda
   - Comply with the government's mandates and develop relationships
   - Develop ongoing relationships with government officials
3. Grantsmanship
   - Develop or acquire a credible grant writer for the HSO
   - Ensure the HSO can deliver on their funded promises
   - All interventions and requests for their fund minimally require: needs assessments, no service duplication in the community, outcomes, strict compliance to protocols, and multidisciplinary initiatives

Small "p" Politics

1. Guide the HSO to learn to work within its numerous contradictions
2. Seek upper level board, administrator and stakeholder support for all initiatives
3. Develop consensual planning and decision-making processes in the HSO
4. Keep your "eyes" always on the ever-changing external organizational environment
5. Keep your "eyes" on the money at all times
6. Build a humane and respectful organizational culture
7. Be flexible and adaptive in processes and internal governance structures

Figure 3.3 Visionary leadership – big "P" and small "p" politics

etc. There indeed seems to be a curious paradox about this readily accessible fingertip prevention information. The more we know about the importance of preventing illness, diseases, or behaviors which can impact us in negative ways, the more we do nothing about preventing their occurrence for the most part.

For example, drinking and drug abuse are occurring at greater levels than ever before (*Alcohol Abuse*, 2004; Dunham, 2008); Type II diabetes and obesity are at epidemic levels in North America (*Fact sheet*, 2008; *Obesity and overweight*, 2008); our air and water quality are at near toxic levels in some settings (Gordon, 2002; *EPA Orders*, 2008); teenage violence is rampant (*Violence in Schools*, 2008; *Youth Violence*, 2007); and our overt stress has been linked to over 64 known diseases including cancer, heart disease, and stroke (*Stress a Major Health Problem*, 2007; Young & Welsh, 2005). So just how are individuals responding or changing their behaviors as a result of their "prevention awareness"? In short, they are not. In fact, empirical data would suggest that we are going in the opposite direction! Thus, the rhetoric of prevention seems much more apparent than its reality (Holosko *et al*., 1998).

Organizationally here, another set of variables gets "tossed in the mix." HSOs are in "the treatment business" and in an ideal world, if people were well and not needing services, they would be out of business. Holosko and Taylor (1992) in their analysis of social work practice in various health care settings in Canada and the United States concluded that "the business of healthcare in North America is illness – not wellness."

Subsequently, Holosko & Feit (2006) pointed to the financing of HSOs as a further disincentive to prevention. They contended, like Hasenfeld (1983: 5–7), that our HSOs are not "people changing" organizations, but rather "people sustaining" or "people processing" ones. Since HSOs are still funded by one pot funding and use body count data to receive funds, the more people you see, the more money you get – so what is the financial incentive to pursue a preventative mandate (Holosko *et al*., 1998)? Until funding allotments change and incentives are built in for prevention in HSOs, the concept is rhetoric at best and disingenuous at worst.

The stories behind this trend are that HSOs need to legitimately target funding and provide real incentives for prevention initiatives. Given the realities of: increased waiting lists, less money per capita per client, financial cutbacks and uncertainty, and living on the edge of chaos (see Trend 6 in Figure 3.2), one would assume that the issue of prevention may be addressed more meaningfully in the future – if not for any other reason than a lack of money to serve clients in minimally ethical and responsibly mandated ways.

We also need to dispel the myths associated with our clients and the way we view and serve them. One of the social work roles we tend to forget is giving voice to clients who are vulnerable, marginalized, and mired in myths (Greene, 1986; Holosko & Holosko, 2004). It is incumbent upon HSOs and all social workers, therefore, to dispel erroneous myths when they arise and confront them in assertive and appropriate ways. Therefore, we need to tell our clients that we are not funded to provide prevention services when appropriate, direct them to those interventions that do have prevention components, and assist them to avail themselves of such initiatives. Our collective job is to stop the rhetoric of prevention, even if we don't actually do it (Holosko *et al.*, 1998).

Re-engineering and re-imaging

It is inevitable that HSOs must re-engineer, re-image, and re-tool how they are currently structured in order to provide services to clients in these volatile and rapidly changing times. Easy to say – hard to do! There is an old joke about the heroic and solo flight of Charles Lindbergh which goes something like this: when Lindbergh flew his plane, the Spirit of St. Louis, in 1927 from New York to Paris, two men in a bar were talking. One said "do you believe what that man just accomplished, crossing the Atlantic all by himself?" The other retorted, "that's no big deal – let him try it with a committee of people."

Since 1951, organizational theorists (c.f. Etzioni, Argyris, Schön, Bettis, Arendt, to note a famous few) have long espoused that pervasive organizational barriers unique to any organization preclude meaningful organizational change and effectiveness. These include:

a. "the way of doing things" prevails pervasively in any HSO – for good or bad
b. leaders do not know how to effect organizational change
c. organizations do not typically seek the active voices of their constituent members to effect change
d. many view organizational change as a product not a process
e. it takes both individual will and collective action to overcome barriers to change
f. governance, action strategies and consequences all need to be addressed to effect organizational change
g. any effective change requires a "buy-in" from all internal and external organizational stakeholders
h. members of the organization must desire actions or change to move the organization to another place, rather than just change for change's sake.

As indicated above, the question of how do we "unlearn ways of doing things" is a challenging one, given that collective energy, as well as many structures and processes in any organization guide and direct our day-to-day behaviors. Our suggestion to this very real and formidable task is twofold. One is to first purge then open up lines of communication in more transparent ways in the organization overall, as this will be required if any change process is ever to unfold. Second, is to have both visionary leadership (see Trend 7) and effective leadership (see Chapter 4) to make such change happen. We know HSOs who have embraced these two cornerstone tenets for change, and they have been far more successful than those who have not.

In addition to the above, creating an organizational change climate is essential. Spreier, Fontaine and Malloy (2006) assessed N=2000 IBM managers including N=300 top leaders, and interviewed them about their motives and leadership styles. From their analyses, they identified six factors which created a strong workplace climate that could influence leadership initiated organizational change. These were: flexibility, responsibility, standards, rewards, clarity and team commitment (p. 81). They concluded that: "a climate with high levels of standards, clarity and team commitment and at most one gap in the other [six] dimensions is very strong" (p. 81). As such, some of these organizational factors are more important and are weighted more significantly than others.

In re-engineering, HSOs need to ensure that they first align their missions to the organizational environment. This means that the external environment is the starting point for the alignment process as indicated in Figure 3.4. This, then, aligns with the next tier below, from goals to outcomes as shown in Figure 3.5.

This process reinforces the visionary leadership trend (7) previously discussed, and positions the HSO within the context of its general and task environment. It also reinforces the point about ULMs and boards acting as conduits filters or windows to their external worlds.

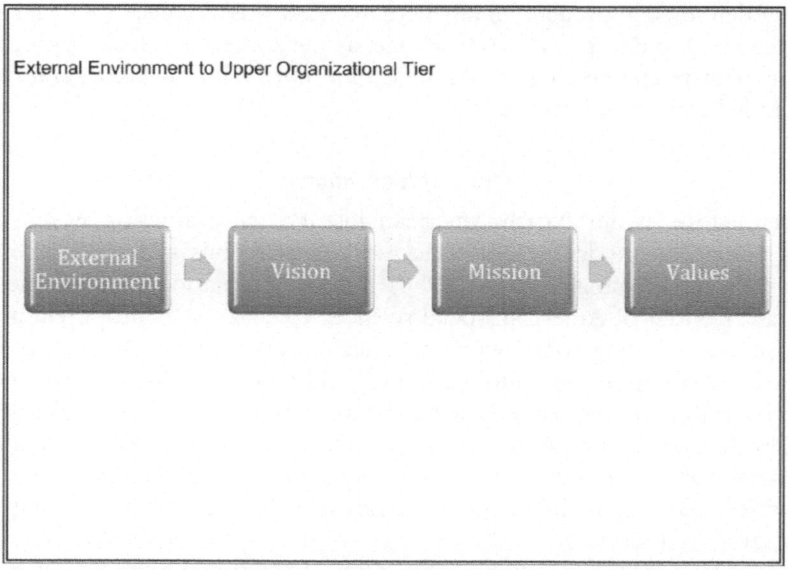

Figure 3.4 Alignment grid 1

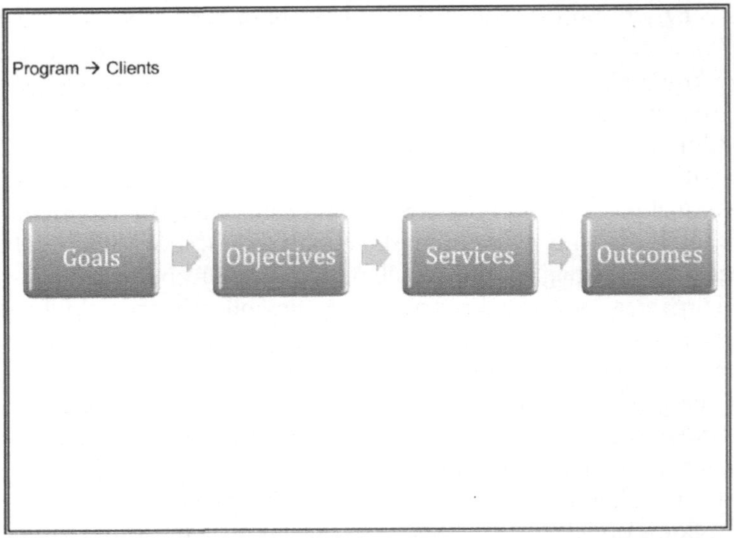

Figure 3.5 Alignment grid 2

We also recommend that each step in this alignment process (in Figures 3.4 and 3.5) be reviewed for continuous accuracy and simplicity on an annual basis by the entire agency. Traditional ways to conduct such HSO alignment typically start at the walls of the agency with the mission and cascade down only to the objectives. This re-framing (in Figures 3.4 and 3.5) expands that rather delimited approach. Finally here, we view this as a necessary first step for the HSO to effect any future change, as the context for such change and subsequent re-engineering is presented in a more realistic, transparent and expanded way to embrace it.

Era of legitimacy

Never before in our North American history has evaluation been "part and parcel" of the delivery of social welfare programs and services. Some 29 years ago Cronbach *et al.* (1980) stated: "evaluation has become the liveliest frontier of American social science" (pp. 12–13). Since then, many disciplines including social work have staked claims to both practice and program evaluation methodologies and published accounts of evaluations occur with great frequency in a variety of social and behavioural science and professional journals. We are no longer on the frontier of program and practice evaluation activity but are in the midst of a groundswell of such activities becoming mainstream in federal and state social welfare initiatives, programs, and services.

In addition, public scrutiny of the administration and financing of social welfare programs is more apparent than it ever was historically. We have evolved from offering social welfare programs directed by the rather noble motives of altruism and case wisdom, or "a need for such services," to much more legitimizing ways of providing educational, health, and social services. These include: the empirical testing of interventions; developing more empirically defined protocols for our interventions; developing pilot projects to justify larger initiatives; ensuring interventions are tied to frameworks (i.e., logic models) and outcomes; developing organizational and community capacities to ensure success of interventions; funding initiatives with the assurance of self-sustainability over a shorter time period; ensuring that funded social welfare initiatives include timely best, and/or promising practices; and ensuring that funded programs/services are both effective and efficient. Indeed, we have clearly evolved from the "era of accountability" to the "era of legitimacy" in the provision of North American social welfare.

We acknowledge that such legitimacy requires middle and upper level managers to be more adept at "showing their programs really do work and make a difference." We also realize that it places the onus on such individuals to also understand the political and organizational realities of such legitimacy. This jettisons certain pre-requisite knowledge and skill elements to the surface that are normally beyond the current knowledge, education and training offered in schools of social work (Holosko, 2009c; Wimpfheimer, 2004). We now require knowledge and skills in areas of: visioning, strategic planning, aligning program goals with policy goals, grantsmanship, politicizing (see Trend 7), marketing, agency advocacy, board governance, re-engineering of existing organizational structures and processes to be more politically responsive (see Trend 9), developing community partners through joint agreements, ventures or contracts, creative financing in lean fiscal times, making timely decisions, and program evaluation.

Such knowledge doesn't just require the middle or upper level manager to "change hats" (Davidson Perlmutter & Crook, 2004) to be effective, but to wear multiple hats often at the same time, in order to render effectively responsible administrative decisions. A middle or upper level manager becomes, for instance: a schmoozer, an advocate, a grant person, a marketer of his/her program, a partner in the community of care and a financial manager – all within the same one-hour meeting with a group of HSO stakeholders. The visionary leader in this meeting then moves comfortably and seamlessly from hat to hat, sometimes wearing two, three, four, or five hats at once, all of which are interrelated and necessary to move the HSOs' agenda forward.

Generally, evaluations serve as both the validation and legitimacy for many social welfare programs and it is almost unconscionable in today's climate to allocate funds to such programs without building in money for evaluation costs.

Outside of the aegis of government, numerous private and charitable foundations have stepped up to the plate here and pushed the national agenda for evaluations of federal and state welfare programs forward. They have also had much success in advancing our evaluative knowledge in areas of: methodology; theoretical applications; using models to evaluate performance contracting; providing more timely programs and service; and linking interventions to outcomes, pilot tests and evidence-based practices. Some of the U.S. foundations, which stress simultaneously both research and evaluation of social welfare programs and service provision, include: the Annie E. Casey Foundation, the MacArthur Foundation, the Carnegie Corporation, the Gerber Foundation, the Foundation for Child Development, the Ruddie Memorial Youth Foundation, the William T. Grant Foundation, the Allen Foundation, the BEA Foundation, the John Hartford Foundation, the Kellogg Foundation, and the Robert Wood Johnson Foundation, to name a prominent few.

It is not just the organization's goals and objectives which must be aligned to conduct an evaluation (see Figure 3.5), but all interventions require not just a traditional focus on inputs and outputs but also (now) on outcomes and impacts. And these must be assessed empirically with a view to what it costs to provide such interventions. Clements, Chianca and Sasaki (2008) said it succinctly when they stated: "evaluations should estimate the total impacts that can be attributed to an intervention and also estimate the intervention's cost effectiveness . . . Also, evaluations of this nature are likely to be more helpful for program managers" (p. 196).

CONCLUDING REMARKS

In this chapter, we selected ten primary trends that HSO middle and upper level managers need to understand if they are to administer their programs or agencies in responsible ways. We also tried to write plainly and candidly about the real stories behind these trends. Astute middle and upper level management need to identify how such trends impact their HSOs and more importantly, develop strategies for dealing with their very real and future impact. This is what visionary leadership is truly about in this day and age of administering responsible social welfare programs.

4

SOCIAL WORK LEADERSHIP: IDENTIFYING CORE ATTRIBUTES

INTRODUCTION

Social work has a rather storied history of not defining core concepts which either direct and inform its practitioners or educate and train its students. For example, despite the fact that professional social work practice (as we know it today) has evolved in North America since about the turn of the century, it was not until 1958 that the profession through the National Association of Social Workers (NASW), and spearheaded by Harriett Bartlett, put forward a clear working definition of practice (Bartlett, 1958). Ironically, up until today, this scaffolding definition is still not widely known or acknowledged (Holosko, 2003).

Continuing to educate, and/or train individuals without defining terms we routinely tout as being germane to social work can be viewed as the "Wallenda Syndrome." This was the legendary family of aerialists and tight rope walkers who refused to ever use a safety net. It has also been referred to as our profession's penchant for circuitously traveling around in "conceptual cul-de-sacs" (Wakefield, 2003).

In a sense, one might argue that defining terms we routinely use in practice may delimit our ability to practice in such altruist, client-driven and malleable ways (Lubove, 1973). That is, one of our profession's greatest strengths has been its ability to respond rapidly to client needs as they arose, without the encumbrance of theories or empirical research to direct practice (Holosko & Holosko, 2004). Indeed, often when we have been both timely and effective, and were one of the first professions "in the door" as it were, to address a social problem (e.g., hospice care, HIV/AIDS, poverty), it has been because our front-line practitioners simply forged ahead and were proactively responsive to those who needed help.

So a case could be made for social work practitioners to not necessarily have things so precisely defined, as their initiatives and efforts extend the very parameters of definitions, guidelines, and concepts that we often use in practice. As we are keenly aware, it has been our practitioners, who through their day-to-day work with clients, are the "profession's eyes and ears" and the "figurer-outers" of many loosely defined practice concepts used differentially, for example: ethical dilemmas, self-determinism, best practices, value conflicts, treatment frameworks, individual capacity, community capacity, time-framed interventions, outcomes, advocacy, case management, clinical significance, practice effectiveness, etc.

Where this conceptual quagmire has potentially a more deleterious effect is in our formal education and training (Nesoff, 2007). However one looks at the issue from this standpoint, we are professionally remiss in this regard, and it appears that we have a rather long and comfortable history of evolving without clearly defining either who we are or how we should practice (c.f., Bartlett, 1970; Boehm, 1958; Flexner, 1915; Gordon, 1962; Germaine & Gitterman, 1980; Reid & Epstein, 1972; Pincas & Minahan, 1973). Educators, accrediting bodies and legitimizing organizations (e.g., licensure boards, NASW) should take it upon themselves to better define the very concepts we promote and use (Holosko, 2006). Indeed, we need to break the Wallenda Syndrome so that our professional competency-based and accredited standards can be more clearly imparted to our students – who will be our future professionals one day.

Just in the past decade for example, numerous evolving and transformational definitions have been put forward for many core practice concepts we take for granted, but use routinely in education and training social work students. Some of these include: critical thinking (Gambrill, 1997); social justice (Wakefield, 2001); multi-cultural social work practice (Sue, 2006); evidence-based practice (Gibbs, 2003; Gibbs & Gambrill, 2002; Pollio, 2006); social work theory and its application (Thyer, 2001b); evaluation research (Donaldson & Scriven, 2003); policy practice (Chapin, 2006); empowerment (Chapin & Cox, 2001; Van Voorhis & Hostetter, 2006); disempowerment (Holosko *et al.*, 2001); clinical social work (Goldstein, 2006); macro social work practice (Brueggmann, 2002); global social work practice (Rowe, 2000); generalist practice (Johnson & Yanca, 2006); advanced generalist practice (Derezotes, 1999); cultural competence (Armour *et al.*, 2006); and direct practice (Franklin, 2001) – to name a few.

SOCIAL WORK LEADERSHIP

The history of North American social work is characterized by many altruistic leaders who, through their compassion for vulnerable individuals, acted humanely and made a difference in their lives. William James' (1906) classic essay on pragmatism makes the point more succinctly, as "seeking the difference that makes the difference."

These early, turn of the century pioneers, led by advocating, reforming, transforming, reflecting, and most importantly giving names, voice, hope, and inspiration to the clients and communities they served. They included the likes of: Jane Addams, Dorthea Dix, Josephine Shaw Lowell, Mary Richmond, Ellen Gates Starr, Frances Perkins, Florence Kelly, Ida Cannon, Grace Abbott, Lillian Wald, and Paul Kellogg – to acknowledge a few.

Our profession's legacy of leaders is much longer than its conceptualization or research about leadership, and this reality is typical of other disciplines who similarly embrace the concept. As Graham (2002) stated:

> Research into leadership is a young and still rather shapeless discipline. While leaders and leadership may provide the stuff of bar-room wisdom and talk-show humor, it is an elusive subject from which to glean analytical insights and prescriptive value at a level approaching normal academic standards. Although some literature exists offering unfalsifiable theories about leadership behavior and personality, there is a dearth of primary empirical information about leaders, the philosophical prisms through which they perceive reality and the principles by which they conduct themselves.
>
> (p. 87)

As indicated by Williams (2003), "leadership" has as many definitions as texts, as the definition itself is constantly evolving (Ciulla, 1998).

Despite the fact that leadership was a core concern of the Council on Social Work Education (CSWE) as indicated in its *Strategic Plan 1998–2000*, and the National Association of Social Workers (NASW) who sponsored the "Leadership Academy" from 1994–1997 and conduct an annual leadership meeting on leadership development, Brilliant (1986) referred to leadership as essentially a "missing ingredient" in social work education and training. After reviewing its sporadic attention in our professional literature, she concluded it was essentially a "non-theme" in social work training and education. Similarly, Stoesz (1997) lamented that social work professionals are often forced to rise to positions of leadership within the profession with little or no mentoring.

Rank and Hutchinson (2000) investigated individuals (N=75) who held leadership positions within CSWE and NASW and concluded that education and training in this area fell short of both the demands for leadership in the field and also our curricula's ability to adequately teach and educate students about the concept. Their comprehensive analyses made a cogent case for the uniqueness of social work leadership and they offered a number of constructive suggestions to direct social work in this regard into the twenty-first century.

It appears that the profession has had better success in "taking the concept forward" when it responded to the leadership needs expressed by clients and practicing professionals in our fields of practice. For example, the National

Network for Social Work Managers (NNSWM) established in the mid-1980s developed a curricula focused on 10 competencies needed to run well-functioning, high quality agencies/organizations. Their Academy grants the Certified Social Work Manager (CSWM) credential to social work managers who meet criteria which minimally include: education, training, experience, demonstrated competency in 12 core areas and approval by the Academy (Wimpfheimer, 2004).

Further, in response to the "national demographic imperative" of becoming an aging society, the John A. Hartford Foundation (www.jhartfound.org) in conjunction with the CSWE has for about 10 years played an integral and proactive large scale leadership role in gerontological social work by:

a. identifying future geriatric education and training needs of the profession
b. infusing content on aging into the social work curricula
c. funding research based initiatives like the Faculty Scholars and Doctoral Fellows programs to established gerontological leaders in research and education
d. advocating about aging issues
e. developing national leadership coalitions
f. assessing work force and employment issues
g. developing best practices and policy initiatives
h. developing social work practicum partnerships
i. promoting evidence-based treatment and research practices
j. developing geriatric enrichment programs
k. attracting additional private funding for gerontological social work
l. creating a cadre of national leaders committed to building on the accomplishments of Hartford initiatives
m. developing collaborations between agencies and social work educational institutions
n. spawning the National Leadership Coalition and the Social Work Leadership Institute.

Since making gerontology a priority from about 1997 onward, between 1998 and 2005, they have spent approximately $41 million dollars on programs for geriatric social work (www.jhartfound.org).

Although not as large sweeping as Hartford's national programs, many other social work leadership initiatives have taken place at the state or agency level in the areas of: child welfare, child care, mental health, family services, education, juvenile justice, community development, and poverty. In each instance above, the needs of clients triggered the need for agencies to take a leadership role and respond to, and address a gap in service, as such, providing ethical, proactive and competent practice for those in need (c.f., Holosko & Feit, 2006).

ON BECOMING A LEADER

Although leaders may certainly have inherent traits or innate talents, studies of leaders who have come to shape history have put to rest a long standing controversy, that leaders are not born – they are made (Rejai & Phillips, 2004). A simple conception which underpins the plethora of leadership definitions is the "3 P"s put forward by Hartley and Allison (2002). These refer to: "the person", "the position", and "the process."

The "person" refers to personal characteristics of an individual. Theories put forth to describe these attributes are commonly referred to as trait theories. The "position" involves the ability to use authority, governance, and guidance with a specific set of skills in order to influence individuals in organizations. The "process" involves how leadership evolves in helping to shape events, motivate and influence people and achieve outcomes (Taylor, 2007). These involve a leader using a set of situational, transactional and transformational processes, learning from their use and developing practice wisdom or leadership intuition along the way. Over time, this defines one's leadership style, and imprints an operational style on the organization. Figure 4.1 shows how these three elements form a triangle which, taken together, define leadership as a synergetic and interactive process.

The corresponding Figure 4.2 breaks down Figure 4.1 and further delineates the more frequently cited (from the literature) elements of each angle in this leadership triangle.

A main difficulty in defining this rather elusive concept is attributed to the inability for the literature to differentiate which aspects of leadership

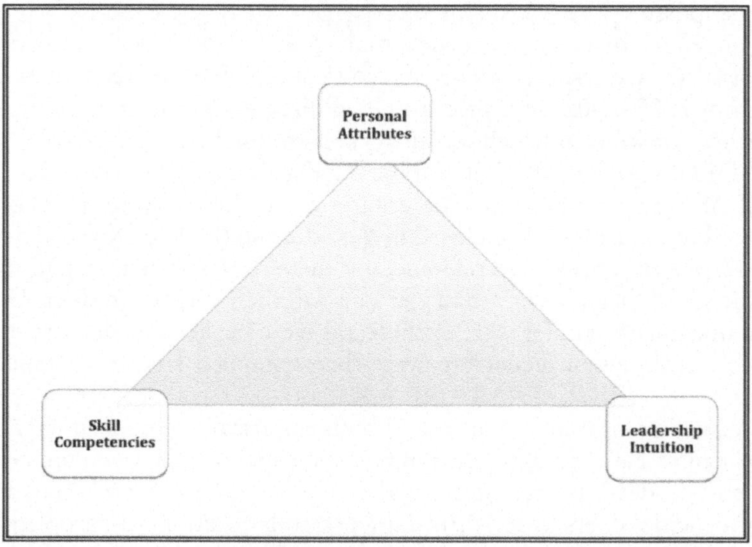

Figure 4.1 The leadership triangle

Main Personal Attributes	Main Skill Competencies	Developing Leadership Intuition
Integrity ➢ Honesty ➢ Ethics ➢ Transparency Decisive ➢ Easy Decisions ➢ Difficult Decisions ➢ Be Assertive Role Modeling ➢ Personal ➢ Professional Physical Presence ➢ Have One ➢ What Would...Do? ➢ Come to Work Charisma ➢ Promote Positive Energy Self-Confidence ➢ Exuding, Not Over-Bearing ➢ Contagion Effect	Communication ➢ Oral & Written ➢ Sender & Receiver ➢ Pleasant ➢ Diplomatic ➢ Appropriate Empowering ➢ Difference Between Empowering and Disempowering ➢ Enabling ➢ Consciousness Raising ➢ Believing in Other Managing Other ➢ Administering ➢ Collaborating ➢ Coordinating ➢ Task Orientation ➢ Respecting Governance ➢ Focusing on the Goal ➢ Personal Issues are Not as Important as Organizational Ones Knowledge Competence ➢ Specialized and also Broad ➢ Develop "$ Eyes" ➢ Factual & Researched ➢ 'I also don't know' is OK ➢ Thinking Smarter Inspiring/Influencing/Persuading ➢ Group vs. Individual Strategies ➢ Motivating ➢ Timing ➢ Negotiating Using Power and Authority Judiciously ➢ Non-Authoritative ➢ Tact & Discretion ➢ Devoid of Personal Agenda ➢ Do Not Apologize for Using Power/Authority ➢ Share Power & Authority	Know When To ➢ Pick your spots for expending resources ➢ Defer Power & Authority ➢ Manage Conflicts ➢ Use Your Strengths ➢ Acknowledge Your Weaknesses ➢ Deal with Troubled Employees ➢ Coach vs. Mentor ➢ Reflect & Process Issues ➢ Lose Gracefully Know How To ➢ Lead vs. Manage ➢ Transform vs. Transact ➢ Say you were wrong ➢ Unlearn Bad Responding Habits ➢ Make Lemonade from Lemons ➢ Provide Feedback ➢ Provide Positive Reinforcement ➢ Avoid Micro-Managing ➢ Be Seen & Always Heard ➢ Always Follow Through

Figure 4.2 Leadership necessities – the three angles of the triangle

are more or less important than others, when surveying the vast leadership landscape. This "mushing" together of numerous attributes (DuBrin, 2000) complexifies and further obfuscates one's ability in getting to the nub of the leadership issue.

In an effort to reach the conceptual core of this leadership abyss, the author (with two research assistants) content analyzed refereed journal articles from 1999–2002 published in the 70 disciplinary journals published in English worldwide, in which social workers routinely publish (Thyer, 2005). In addition, searches of bibliographic databases (e.g., PsychLit, ERIC, and Social Abstracts) were used. The criteria for inclusion were: (a) the word "leadership" must have been listed in the title, and (b) when this occurred, at least 15 percent of the cited references of these retrieved articles had to have had the word "leader" or "manager" also in their respective titles. Unpublished documents/studies were excluded as were master's or doctoral theses. Lists of attributes of leadership were then compiled from each remaining study.

Using a simple content analyses of both empirical and conceptual articles (N=51) and frequency data, the top five cited aggregated attributes, referred to as core leadership attributes, ranked in descending order were: (i) vision, (ii) influencing others to act, (iii) teamwork/collaboration, (iv) problem-solving capacity, and (v) creating positive change. These are now identified in the center of the triangle in Figure 4.3.

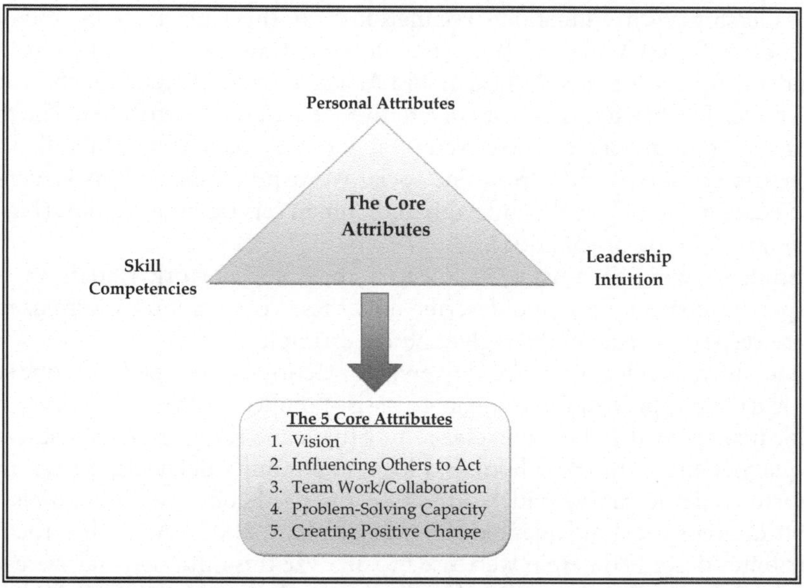

Figure 4.3 Leadership necessities – the five core attributes of leadership

Based on this literature overview and content analyses, some simple definitions for these core terms are now offered:

1. Vision
   a) Having one – *To have a description of a desired condition at some point in the future.*
   b) Implementing one – *To plan and put in place strategic steps to enact the vision.*
2. Influencing others to act – *To inspire and enable others to take initiative, have a belief in a cause and to perform duties and responsibilities.*
3. Teamwork/collaboration – *To work collectively and in partnership with others toward achieving a goal.*
4. Problem-solving capacity – *To both anticipate problems and also act decisively on them when they occur.*
5. Creating positive change – *Moving people in organizations to a better place than where they once were.*

USING THE CORE ATTRIBUTES

Two examples of the use and application of these core attributes will be offered here. Since they are presented as aspirational in nature, other examples of their use and application have yet to be determined. First, for two years, the core leadership attributes were used by the author in a graduate course on

"Leadership with Vulnerable Populations" at the University of Windsor, School of Social Work, in Windsor, Ontario, Canada (www.uwindsor.ca). Students used a pre-tested "Leadership Analysis Grid" (LAG), which was a 5 × 3 table. The five items in rows one to five were the core attributes. The three items in columns one to three were: "upper level managers," "middle-managers/supervisors," and "front-line social work practitioners," as leadership can emanate at any level of a health and human service organization (Jago & Vroom, 1977; Tourish, 2005).

Students were then asked to identify three social work leaders in their respective communities and describe how these core attributes were used by these respective leaders through concrete examples.

Secondly, a colleague at the University of Georgia developed a unique service learning approach for students to assist families in Athens, Georgia who relocated there after being displaced by Hurricane Katrina in August, 2005. In partnership with the school and local community agencies, a responsive disaster relief initiative which addressed the needs of these individuals and their families was implemented (Bliss & Meehan, 2008). After this, the core attributes described herein were used to analyze this initiative and were subsequently presented at a national conference on leadership (Bliss & Holosko, 2007).

Finally here, the core attributes are being used to: (a) examine social work leaders in the U.S. Virgin Islands, through Norfolk State University's School of Social Work's affiliation with the U.S.V.I., and (b) assess international leaders who have provided empowerment approaches through youth volunteering at City University of Hong Kong.

CONCLUDING REMARKS

Although some of our professional associations and bodies such as the Society for Social Work and Research (www.sswr.org), the Institute for the Advancement of Social Work Research (www.iaswresearch.org), and the International Association of Schools of Social Work (www.iassw.soton.ac.uk) have taken proactive roles in promoting various aspects within the profession, recently the Council on Social Work Education (www.cswe.org) has identified leadership as a renewed educational priority. In February, 2007, they sponsored a two-day conference entitled "Building Leaders in Social Work Education: Pathways to Success" in Mesa, Arizona. This entire conference was devoted to social work leadership in areas of teaching, classroom and field education, training, research, and practice. CSWE is also currently surveying the syllabi of programs recently under review by their accreditation office to gather baseline data on the inclusion of leadership content in various schools of social work (J. Holmes, personal communication, July 2007).

Given this reality, it appears that social work is embracing leadership as something that holds legitimate promise for education, training, practice, and professional development. That being the case, the responsibility for defining social work leadership in ways that are simple, clear, timely, and consensually accepted and relevant are not only important, but essential.

5

CLINICAL VS. UPPER LEVEL MANAGEMENT: PROGRAM EVALUATION

INTRODUCTION

Although Crobach and colleagues touted the rather prophetic contention over thirty years ago that "evaluation has become the liveliest frontier of American social science" (Cronbach *et al.*, 1980, pp. 12–13), many of us working in this field never really thought it was so. Today however, from a perusal of the social science and applied professional literature, they were "spot on." A recent content analysis of three core North American empirical social work journals reveled that approximately 25 percent of the published articles across a three year span were about program or practice evaluation (Holosko, 2010a). Indeed, in the past 35 or so years in North America, the ubiquitous trends of increased demands for social and health care services coupled with scarcer resources, have resulted in a burgeoning of program and practice evaluation activities. Generally, these often serve as the validation or legitimacy for many health and social service programs, and well-conceived programs, be they federal, state, or local, now routinely incorporate evaluation requirements and funding formulae for their disbursement of services.

SELECTED DEFINITIONS

Unfortunately, social work has had a rather long and storied history of not precisely defining terms we use frequently in practice (Holosko, 2009a). The differential application of various practice terms, as well as the use/misuse of numerous evolving or transformational terms routinely used in practice (Ramsay, 2003) has stalled our ability to advance knowledge, educate or train students and professionals, and/or conduct research about many important phenomena. Wakefield (2003) aptly referred to this as our profession's penchant for traveling around "in conceptual cul-de-sacs." Rather than cite a number of these niggling terms here (c.f. Holosko), we offer the current topical bandied about social work phrase "evidence-based practice" as just one of many such examples. Enough said!

Normally when the term "evaluation" is used in social work, it refers to: *needs assessments*, *personnel evaluations*, *evaluations of practice*, and *program evaluations*. Simply defined these are:

a. *Needs assessments* – Perceived needs, and/or service use patterns of individuals in order to plan services or interventions.
b. *Personnel assessments* – Structured and systematic evaluations of social welfare employees.
c. *Evaluations of practice* – These have two connotations:
    i. Evaluations *on* practice – Assessments of clients, client systems, interventions, and/or outcomes,
    ii. Practice evaluations – Assessments of practitioner planned interventions, *with* clients as full partners in the process.
d. *Program evaluations* – Systematic appraisals of the merit or worth of programs/interventions/services.

Approximately 80 percent of the remainder of this chapter will focus on (d) above and 20 percent refers to (c) above.

OBSTACLES TO CONDUCTING PROGRAM EVALUATIONS (PE)

There are a number of obstacles inherent in the conduct of any social or health evaluation, which presents very real and formidable challenges to the program evaluator and agency alike. The extent to which these are acknowledged by both the evaluator and the host agency is the extent to which the evaluation may proceed with less potential for problems arising during its conduct (Holosko, 1996).

The "word" evaluation

For a number of reasons, the word evaluation itself scares the heck out of many individuals. From our experience, it appears to be more frightening than the terms "research" or "statistics" – but belongs in the same class of conceptual species. Unfortunately, many evaluators have perpetuated this fear by the ways in which they have conducted evaluations. Such unnecessary anxiety about program evaluations in general has been noted by a number of authors (Deborah, 2010; Guba & Lincoln, 1981; Rossi & Wright, 1967; Schwarz & Struhkamp, 2007; Suchman, 1967; Thomas &

Dahler-Larsen, 2006), and ways of offsetting this have also been offered (Chambers, 1993; Donaldson *et al.*, 2002; Geva-May & Thorngate, 2003; Greene, 1988; Guenther *et al.*, 2010; Holosko, 1988; Patton, 1988; Rossi & Freeman, 1993; Rutman, 1980; Scriven, 2007). The word itself implies the possibility of finding out that there might be something wrong or lacking, or that the program is going to be rated publicly. It is possible that for many stakeholders, evaluation means only fault-finding, and *not* the possibility of glowing discoveries. There is also anxiety about internal or external evaluators (in-house or out-of-house) appraising a helping professionals' world of work. Part of the anxiety of our professionals is motivated historically by their high degrees of altruism (Bulcke, 1994). Further, these well-intended caregivers may perceive that in a few instances, they weren't as effective as they wanted to be (which is the norm for all such employees) with their clients or client systems. The point is, that if conducted properly, a PE can be a most worthwhile, meaningful and positive experience for all stakeholders involved in the process (Hasenfeld *et al.*, 2003; Royse *et al.*, 2011).

THE POLITICS OF EVALUATION

Since its formal early beginnings (about the 1930s onward in the USA), PEs have typically "smacked" of politics. Indeed, the two are often inextricably intertwined. The extent to which politics influence the context, process and outcomes of program evaluations has been well documented in the PE literature for a number of years (Campbell, 1969; Cohen, 1970; Mertens, 2009; Royse *et al.*, 2011; Weiss, 1977). For example, context may include the funding body's agenda, overt or hidden (e.g., to cut a budget to a program). The process can be directly or indirectly influenced by any of the stakeholders (e.g., consumers, community leaders, politicians, etc.). Outcomes may be influenced either by selectively focusing on some PE data to the exclusion of other data, or slanted data interpretations of the data. Rather than deny this reality, agencies and evaluators would do well to forthrightly table the political agenda of the PE early on, in a cooperative planning fashion (Dunlop & Holosko, 2004; Hasenfeld, 1983; Holosko, 1988; Holosko & Dunlop, 1992; Rutman, 1980; Scriven, 2007).

INADEQUATE RESOURCES

Despite the perceived and acknowledged importance of PEs by most funding bodies, policy-makers, and/or administrators, ironically, most are still currently underfunded (Hendricks & Bamberger, 2010; Miller *et al.*, 2006). Coupled with this reality (with the exception of needs assessment planning evaluations), is the fact that many PEs come about as an "after thought" – that is, as a consequence of a funding arrangement (e.g., for public or political accountability, program continuation, termination, program expansion, efficacy, etc.). The implications of these two realities are many and various.

Suffice to say, that if PEs are to be more credible, they should be: 1) funded accordingly, and 2) built in to the overall program, early on in the process (Davis & Auchter, 2010; Holosko & MacCaughelty, 2009; Pizacani *et al.*, 2009; VanLandingham, 2006).

TENDENCY OF ORGANIZATIONS TO RESIST CHANGE

Often times, PEs are perceived as threats to the homeostasis or "way of doing things" in human service organizations (HSOs). Financial or business institutions have shown a far greater capacity to respond quickly to their external and sometimes rather chaotic and unpredictable organizational environments (Judge *et al.*, 2009; Rama *et al.*, 2009). HSOs, however, have historically been more tradition-bound and less willing to adapt their structures as such, via their interorganizational relationships with their environments (Dunlop & Holosko, 2004; Hasenfeld, 1983). In this regard, their capacity to resist change, or change-inducing mechanisms (such as PEs), is often an inherent feature of their character (Holosko & Leslie, 1998). Breaking through such resistance and "re-framing" PEs toward positive change orientations becomes a rather formidable challenge for any responsible evaluator (Hasenfeld *et al.*, 2003).

LACK AN UNDERSTANDING OF THE CONTEXT OF PROGRAM EVALUATIONS

For any number of reasons, many PEs have not been well integrated into the various programs they purport to assess (Holosko & Leslie, 1998). As such, they are conducted for "some reason" (see "inadequate resources" above), and if deemed relevant or appropriate by key decisions-makers, they are used. Conversely, if they are not deemed relevant or appropriate, they are not used in making decisions about a program. For example, if a PE is assessing a practice intervention, its findings should underpin and provide new facts/knowledge to practitioners to drive the continuum of practice knowledge in the agency as illustrated in Figure 5.1.

Thus, responsible program or practice evaluators collect data to direct and inform practice knowledge in order to make decisions. Indeed, this should be the primary reason why an evaluation should be conducted. Other primary purposes are noted in Figure 5.2.

Figure 5.2 reveals that for any given program or practice evaluation, there may be more than one of the purposes listed here, or others. In short here, the evaluation is driven by ongoing empirical data collection continuing to inform better decisions at all times.

The purpose of identifying these obstacles as such is not to unravel them or suggest they can be easily or readily resolved. However, evaluators need to recognize: 1) that they are real and do exist, and 2) that a large part of

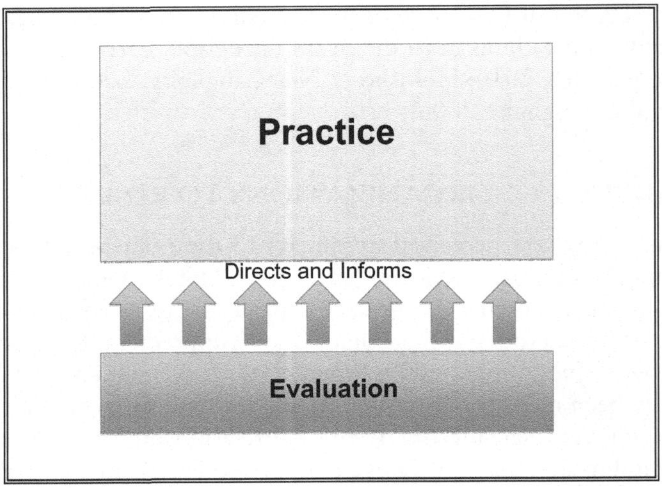

Figure 5.1 Relationship of evaluation to practice

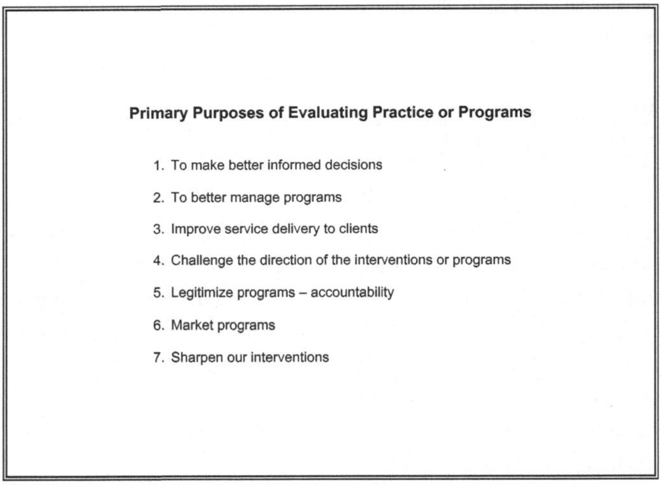

Figure 5.2 Program evaluation

their role is to negotiate successfully around these obstacles. If not, their potential to undermine any evaluation should not be underestimated.

PRE-REQUISITES FOR PLANNING PES

The amount of evaluation activity (previously noted) in the so-called "era of legitimacy" (the era following the previously deemed "era of accountability") has produced some interesting evaluation trends which include:

a. the use of more rigorous designs in evaluation activities (Durning *et al.*, 2007; Weersing, 2005)
b. the use of more mixed methodologies to evaluate programs (Bullet, 2006; Hubball & Bert, 2007)
c. more funding is now available for evaluations today than ever has been offered (Phillips *et al.*, 2003)
d. new service delivery initiatives at federal and state levels typically now include evaluation monies built into their budgets (Kaufman *et al.*, 2006)
e. evaluations now include the use of models (e.g., program logic, etc.) and/or theoretical frameworks to nest the methodologies used within them (http://www.cdc.gov/; http://www.wkkf.org)
f. practice evaluations are included as viable methodologies more so than they ever have been (Powell, 2006; Wade & Neuman, 2007)
g. the use of empirically-based best practices are becoming incorporated more systemically in evaluations (Cramer *et al.*, 2007; Reedy *et al.*, 2005)
h. the voice of clients and consumers is being incorporated more routinely than ever before (Chambers & Connor, 2002; Hasenfeld *et al.*, 2003)
i. information technology (IT) has become meaningfully incorporated in the field (Hardy, 2007; Holosko & MacCaughelty, 2009; Reardon & Hartley, 2007).

This has resulted in a requirement for more meaningful planning to proceed the conduct of any practice evaluation (Holosko *et al.*, 2009a), or PE (Holosko & MacCaughelty, 2009; Scriven, 2007). The discussion here will focus on the latter and the major assumptions underpinning it are: 1) that PEs will be more meaningfully developed, conducted, and disseminated if more time and energy is devoted toward such planning activities; and 2) that the host organization, its personnel, and evaluators should learn to work together more cooperatively in planning PE evaluations. The point of departure for this analysis is that transparency, coupled with open collaboration and dialogue, can and should be effectively used in this important planning process.

The following are construed as essential ingredients for successful PEs, and all must be systematically addressed to some degree at the beginning of the planning process. In another sense, if any one of these is not addressed, subsequent evaluation efforts could be seriously undermined (Holosko, 1988; Holosko & MacCaughelty, 2009). These include:

1. a sincere commitment on behalf of the organization and program to both conduct and support the evaluation
2. answering the *why*, *when* and *how* of the evaluation
3. the goals and objectives of the program, or components of it which are being evaluated, need specification in measurable terms, and
4. information needed to conduct the evaluation should be in retrievable form.

Although these may seem obvious, many organizations and programs continue to conduct evaluations without considering them, and invariably such efforts prove to be unsuccessful. Each of these will be briefly discussed and, where appropriate, the roles and relationship between the host organization, personnel, and evaluators will be highlighted. All of the suggestions offered herein have been successfully "field-tested" for many years by the second author (MJH) and colleagues in conducting program evaluations of small, medium, and large scale health and human service organizations (Leslie *et al.*, 2006).

ORGANIZATIONAL AND PROGRAM COMMITMENT

Any agency embarking on an evaluation without having the support of the administration, managers, and key decision-makers in the respective organization or program is seriously remiss. It does not matter whether the impetus for the evaluation comes from the external organizational environment (e.g., the community, other organizations, funding sources, accrediting bodies etc.), or the internal environment (e.g., clients, line staff, the union, personnel, supervisors, administrators, the board of directors, etc.). In either case, a sincere administrative commitment is critical to the PE's development and conduct.

Administrative support from the organization's upper level administration is the key to influencing and obtaining other levels of support in the organization or program, and as a result, needs to be obtained first. Consistent with the so-called "domino theory," other levels of support (e.g., supervisors, front-line workers) quickly follow the administrative lead, although their motivation for desiring the PE may be very different from others in the domino chain. Thus, gaining support for the PE is an area in which much reciprocal learning, dialogue, and cooperation between managers of the host organizations' personnel, program administrators, and evaluators (whether in or out-of-house evaluators) needs to come about. For example, administrators or key decision-makers can learn to provide input to the evaluation and its activities and support them in more effective ways, and program evaluators can learn how to tailor their efforts to meet the needs of the respective organization or program which they are evaluating (Hasenfield *et al.*, 2003). This essential first level of support solidifies the purpose of the evaluation and shapes its subsequent assumptions, design, conduct and ultimate dissemination.

Additionally, a quick surf of the Internet can locate websites providing helpful information about evaluation consultation, examples of PEs, and access to clearing houses providing previously tested and validated evaluation instruments. Time spent in reviewing such material and entering into exchange of information situations can enhance significantly the knowledge and understanding required to develop third generation information systems appropriate for ongoing PE requirements. This formative process can only lead to the establishment of collaborative relationships which can enhance the PE planning process by providing sources of comparative program data, information about experiences from similar program endeavors, best practices, and helpful hints for both program implementation and evaluation.

ANSWERING THE WHY, WHEN, AND HOW OF THE PE PRIOR TO ITS CONDUCT

These three apparently simple and straightforward questions seem harmless enough, yet if they are not satisfactorily answered prior to conducting the PE a veritable "Pandora's Box" of problems may unfold. They are best answered in sequence – in that *why* needs to be answered before *when* and *how*. It matters less whether the latter two (*when* and *how*) are out of sequence here because they are usually addressed simultaneously, as the answer(s) to one usually influences the answer(s) to the other, and vice versa. However, it is imperative that *why* be answered first.

Programs should not be too concerned if their answers to the question – *why* conduct an evaluation – seem as frivolous or obvious as some of the standard responses. These may include:

1. it was mandated (e.g., by a funding source)
2. it was recommended (e.g., by personnel, an accrediting body, the host organization, the union, etc.)
3. the program may be having some difficulties, and would like to assess them
4. other programs have conducted evaluations which have influenced this organization or program to want to conduct one
5. it may be "politically astute" for the organization or program to conduct a PE at this time (e.g., for program justification)
6. "it seemed like a good idea at the time" – as we had some funds to do it.

Regardless of the reason, which could be any one of these (or combinations of them), the point is that at the onset of the PE, the host organization and program coordinator must agree in an open and honest way to answer *why* they are conducting the evaluation which in turn, directly influences *where* and *how*.

When the evaluation should be conducted is an important issue which program administrations and evaluators need to be sensitive to. The general preference is the earlier the better, as programs may build the potential for subsequent evaluations into their overall planning and operational frameworks and avoid certain obstacles early on. Examples of this may include: addressing issues of confidentiality; establishing baseline data for comparison at some point in the future; recording information which can be updated or elaborated on in the future; formatting records, files, or forms for subsequent retrievability; and, commencing the process of socializing the organization or program toward the evaluative process and its implications.

Without question, *when* the evaluation occurs determines both the nature and outcomes of the actual evaluation.

Ironically, the least favorable yet most frequent situations which occur are *post hoc* PEs conducted after the program has been operational for some time. These PEs face a host of inevitable problems such as: contending with staff turnover, and contending with missing, lost, misplaced or forgotten information or data which inevitably occurred over time. Such difficulties may be avoided by commencing the evaluation process at the onset of the program implementation (Holosko, 1988; Holosko & Dunlop, 1992; Royse *et al.*, 2011).

Finally, *how* to do the PE is best resolved by those who are conducting it. More specifically, *how* clearly implies issues which may be beyond the scope of those not directly involved with the evaluation (e.g., resource utilization, research methodology, cost involved, etc.), and one should leave such matters for those who are best trained to do them, namely, program evaluators. Thus, administrators, managers, and coordinators should defer judgment to such expertise, and work with the evaluator (or evaluation team) ensuring that the evaluation does not consume the operational aspects of their program which may in turn, influence service delivery. This model suggests a cooperative approach which allows for the evaluators to do what they do best, yet at the same time ensures that they are accountable to the host organization and program for planning and conducting the evaluation.

Again, as discussed above, the use of the Internet for collection and exchange of information can be an important means of understanding and formulating answers to these *why*, *when*, and *how* questions. However, this is the point where enquiries and collaborative activities can be made more specific, in terms of content, sources, and resources. In our evaluation practice experience, this is an appropriate time for the evaluator(s) to establish a website accessible only to agency personnel. This encourages feedback on ideas and design issues discussed in meetings, and also to accept expressions of concern, anxiety, and criticism. Further, in our experiences, this somewhat less personalized medium can facilitate honest inquiry from members of the agency at all levels, which might otherwise go unvoiced. This personal feedback can be addressed subsequently in the ongoing planning process by both the evaluators and administrators. Since an important aspect of any evaluation is building trust, confidence, and working relationships among all the participants, the importance of this opportunity should not be underestimated (Chambers & Wedel, 2005; Patton, 2002; Lehoux, Sicotte & Dennis, 1999). Such ongoing exchanges promote relationship building between the evaluation team and members of the agency and allow for more open transparency and accountabilities by all partners in the PE.

ALL GOALS AND OBJECTIVES REQUIRE SPECIFICATION

Evaluators have a justifiable "hang-up" about goals and objectives, because they cannot evaluate programs without them. Goals and objectives when operationalized in evaluation terms eventually become efficiency and effectiveness criteria, and are the lifeblood of any evaluation. In fact, evaluation research is distinguished from basic or applied social science research in that it always assesses the merit or worth of program processes, efficiency, and/or service effectiveness (Holosko, 1996; Holosko *et al.*, 2009a; Scriven, 2007).

In order for program evaluations to evolve, goals and objectives require: 1) specification, 2) consensual agreement about what they are, and 3) operationalization in measurable terms. This process (of determining goals and objectives) is both deductive and reductionistic in nature. In simpler terms, one proceeds from general goals to specific goals and objectives, and during this process, breaks the program down into component parts, each having different (or similar) goals and objectives.

The logical place to commence this process is the operations/policy manual or planning documents of the agency or program, as most specify such criteria in the mandates, proposals, operational aspects, guidelines, letters patent, or requirements. Thus, these criteria constitute the first level goals or mission statements, which guide the program and its components. Although it may seem surprising to some (in this day and age of scarce resources and higher accountability), it would be remiss not to reveal that in some instances, many funding bodies are negligent in holding programs accountable for the outcomes of the service they deliver. Further, some programs operate on the basis of informal, loose, or ill-defined body count output criteria (Holosko *et al.*, 1998). In organizations or programs such as these, skilled evaluators through the process of determining measurable goals and objectives may inadvertently assist the program in clarifying its relationship to the host organization and clients it purports to serve.

In regard to having consensual agreement about goals and objectives, the operative word here is *consensual*. Certainly in some instances, front-line workers, supervisors, managers, coordinators, and/or board members may have differing perceptions about goals and objectives that guide their programs. Thus, this process may further help articulate and clarify what the goals and objectives are to all these respective parties. As well, asking a variety of organization personnel to define their goals and objectives may be a meaningful human relations exercise in getting those involved directly or indirectly in the evaluation to begin communicating more openly, toward achieving consensual and measurable goals and objectives. Through ongoing and continued open dialogue between the evaluator(s), organizational members and program personnel, consensual agreement about this issue usually emerges.

Finally, the specification of goals and objectives in measurable terms is once again a task best left to those conducting the PE. This involves the operationalization of concepts into measurable and attainable terms which are usually: 1) time-framed (i.e., occurred, or will occur over specified periods of times); and 2) quantifiably specified, usually based on units of service delivered (outputs) and the outcomes of those services. Recently, the literature in the field of evaluation has focused attention on better ways of measuring goals and objectives at both micro practice levels (Bloom *et al.*, 2003; Conboy *et al.*, 2000; Drumm *et al.*, 2003; Moses *et al.*, 2003), as well as macro levels (Royse *et al.*, 2011; Thyer, 2001a; Usher & Wildfire, 2003).

INFORMATION RETREVIABILITY

Agencies and programs have a peculiar relationship about collecting information for purposes of planning, evaluating, and decision-making. This relationship is peculiar for a number of reasons. First, most organizations are "information short" when it comes to having meaningful and retrievable information available for program evaluations, yet they perceive of themselves as having information overload. Second, most programs have a disproportionate amount of background information about their clients (too much), and very little about what services or activities these clients received (too little). Holosko & Leslie (1998) noted that for instance, the current way services are delivered delimit the ability for practice or program effectiveness data to be collected or utilized in most agencies. Third, most programs collect information for the wrong reasons. For example, three main ones are: 1) because they have to (it is a requirement); 2) because they have always collected information this way; or 3) so they can better internally manage themselves. The latter reason is the only one that remotely resembles a rationale, which applies to PE.

Information must also be in accessible and retrievable form if any evaluative effort is to occur. Astute evaluators will usually appraise the "state-of-the-art" of the information, files, or data, prior to conducting an evaluation due to its critical importance in this process. Again, the significance of having the PE commence early on in the program planning development stage ensures that, at least, data will be formatted in retrievable form at some point for future use. Another point to be made about information retrievability is that most evaluations, through the actual process of their conduct, will inevitably assist a program organize and systematize its information for subsequent evaluations, program planning, monitoring, and service delivery. For example, formatting or monitoring files or cases, establishing data sources, and developing protocols for subsequent data collection are all part of any comprehensive evaluative effort, and should be construed as a positive organizational spin-off effect, or benefit of the evaluation. As a result, the process of the overall evaluation effort will yield a benefit for any subsequent effort, if done correctly and collaboratively.

The process of ensuring such data retrievability necessitates close collaboration among program personnel, evaluators, data entry personnel, computer specialists, and analysts. It is important that the nature and form of data being collected be understood by all. Evaluators need to ensure that the data collected provide clear and sufficient information for both summative and formative evaluation activities. It is also recommended that analyses should be both statistical and qualitative in nature, but all data need to be:

1. pre-determined
2. easily accessed
3. easily recorded
4. easily entered
5. retrievable.

The advent of numerous software computer analysis programs make it possible for organizations and evaluators to mix and match a wide range of variables and methodologies, without adding significantly to cost or personnel commitment.

In addition, for all to understand the nature and forms of data being collected, it is necessary to be aware of and knowledgeable about the types of data, confidentiality safeguards, storage, and back-up that exist. The orientation and training of personnel who will be involved in data collection or input need to be addressed. Once again, there is no replacement for face-to-face interactions in these processes, but they can be augmented through the provision of on-line guidelines and updates. As well, providing ongoing reports of results as they are acquired can allow staff a role in monitoring the evaluation process and can more quickly identify any areas of difficulty. This process can enhance greatly the ability to make the evaluation adaptable and flexible, and truly reflective of the program and its outcome. It also reinforces the necessity of confidentiality being transparent in this process.

Finally here, these essential planning pre-requisites have evolved from such simple but important questions, to answer various planning issues to address (Holosko, 1988), into what is termed "evaluability assessment" (Rutman, 1980), which are more formal, detailed, and elaborate more so than previously presented (Scriven, 2007; Thurston *et al.*, 2003; Trevisan, 2007). They include the likes of: glossaries of terms used in the PE, check lists, methodological rigor appraisals, instrumentation scrutiny, fidelity checks and dissemination plans, and ethical standards for conduct (American Evaluation Association, 2009). Many agencies are spending wisely used time and resources, in doing such important pre-evaluation assessments today than ever before.

CONCLUDING REMARKS

These are but a few of the many so-called important common ground issues that either clinical and/or upper level managers need to table prior to conducting an evaluation. Without question, time spent by organizations, agencies and evaluators in forthrightly tabling such issues results in better quality evaluations, overall. Being focused on how important it is to develop and plan a good evaluation design, nested in a good evaluation question, which develops a collaborative process, which shapes the organization's culture to being more receptive, open and willing to proceed with the evaluation, is what these common ground issues are really all about.

LEVEL 1 EVALUATION REQUIREMENTS – CLINICAL MANAGEMENT

This second sub-section describes the various minimal evaluation requirements of agencies, and/or units that are administered by clinical managers (CMs). The latter can be very small programs/units (i.e., less than 4 employees), or much larger (i.e., more than 10 employees). As indicated earlier in the text, we make the assumption such organizations are also only health and human service ones, including a broad array of social services, healthcare, social welfare, and/or educational settings.

As mentioned previously, it is our professional responsibility to evaluate our clients and services/interventions (Holosko *et al.*, 2009a), as reflected in our Code of Ethics (NASW, 2008). Also, well-conceived evaluations provide timely data from which we make informed decisions about the services we provide. Holosko (2010a) referred to using such data as "practice-based evidence" – a twist on the rather well-worn social work research and evaluation phrase "evidence-based practice."

This is referred to as Level 1 evaluation (in the sub-title), as it lays the foundation stone for any subsequent, and/or more complex evaluations (Level 2 evaluations will be presented later). CMs need to be always mindful that their primary business of client-centered work is their only business – and evaluation activity is just that, one supplementary activity which helps us provide better service to clients. If it evolves to anything else, then we have missed the point of what evaluation truly is. The important issues of time/resources/expertise, etc., all come to the fore in implementing such evaluations, and they are legitimate concerns that are very real. However, any baccalaureate (BSW) or master's level social worker (MSW) can implement these activities, as we have both simplified and field tested them for many years in a variety of social welfare agencies. Figure 5.3 illustrates these basic and minimally expected and core Level 1 evaluation activities.

As indicated in Figure 5.3, these are deemed typically as process evaluation activities, as they collect and use primarily qualitative data (Holosko, 2011). The main themes of their qualitative inquiry include: naturalistic inquiry, inductive analysis, holistic perspectives, personal contracts and insights, case studies, contextual sensitivity, and design flexibility. Overall, process evaluations basically answer the sequentially related questions: a) *"what happened to who?"* and b) *"how, when and where did it happen?"* Once such data are systematically collected on an annual basis, programs/units become seemingly more legitimized almost overnight to all of their stakeholders, including their clients. These types of evaluation activities were referred to colloquially many years ago as "everyday evaluations on-the-run" by Wadsworth (1991).

PRIMARY ACTIVITIES	PURPOSE AND USE	MAIN TOOLS/FORM(S) USED
1. Evaluation Housekeeping	To get the "house in order" for evaluation	Brochures, websites, ethics forms, policy manuals, glossary of terms
2. Administrative Chronology	To chart administrative/ program activities	The Administrative Chronology (TAC)
3. a) Aligning EE→V→M→G	To identify external stakeholders	External Environment Map (EEM) (Hasenfeld Chart)
b) Aligning EE→V→M	To align external environment to vision to mission	Alignment Grid – Figure 5.6
b) Aligning G→Ob→S→Ou	To align goals to objectives to services to outcomes	Alignment Grid – Figure 5.7
4. Treatment Process Defined	To illustrate how clients come into care, receive care and exit care	Treatment Process Diagram (TPD)
5. Annual Client Data	To describe services offered to clients and their problems	a) Demographics Chart (DC) b) Presenting Problems Chart (PPC) c) Services Received Chart (SRC)

Figure 5.3 Level 1 minimal evaluation activities for clinical managers (CMs)

Figure 5.3 presents the 5 core annual evaluation activities recommended and deemed as minimally essential for CMs to administer annually in their programs/units. Indeed, many others could be added to this list, once these are fully in place, and "up and running." Programs/units and agencies are encouraged to determine which other annual requirements their programs would require based on their unique funding requirements and program needs. In any such discussions, the notion of the easiest, and "the simpler the better" should underpin their consideration.

EVALUATION HOUSEKEEPING

CMs need to take a leadership role in ensuring that evaluation becomes "part and parcel" of day-to-day service delivery. Thus, the linking of routine evaluation data to client services, and/or overall program decision-making becomes part of the normative organizational/unit culture. For those programs/units where evaluation currently receives minimal consideration, CMs need to have preliminary and focused discussions with their administrators, funding bodies, and/or staff which address at least the following five key planning questions:

a. What are the purposes of evaluating our clients, and/or programs?
b. How will these evaluation activities be done?
c. Who will carry them out?

d. Who will it involve?
e. What will be done with these data?

Once these essential questions are reasonably answered, getting the house (unit) in order now for evaluation requires some basic housekeeping tasks.

First, all brochures, promotional materials, policy manuals, websites, descriptions of programs/services, etc., need to include a commitment, or rather a re-commitment in writing, to client and program evaluation. Thus, all of these need to be reviewed and "freshened-up" to bring evaluation more to the program's forefront.

After this, one effective tool we recommend for building this renewed organizational culture is to develop a simple glossary of program services, interventions, research and evaluation terms that reflect your own unit's programmatic language information, and also it needs to include all terms that will be used in the evaluation itself. These should not only be crafted from the program up, but they should be consciously written in 5¢ not 10¢ terminology/language. Some terms we recommend for this 3–5 page glossary include: stakeholders, vision, mission, core values, goals, objectives, outputs, outcomes, best/promising practices, qualitative methods, quantitative methods, theory, frameworks, anecdotal data, baseline data, service satisfaction data, interventions offered, and benchmarks for success and failure for clients and programs. An excellent starting point for this is the research and evaluation *Pocket Glossary for Commonly Used Research Terms* (Holosko & Thyer, 2011). Developing this initial glossary for our in-house evaluation(s) will save considerable time and resources later on. It is also a nice organizational development tool for the unit to have, and helps staff input and share their opinions about important program/unit concepts used in the evaluation(s).

The second thing that needs to be tended to in this first evaluation housekeeping step is to ensure that all ethical protocols (for research and evaluation) are in place. This requires writing or amending all of the unit's ethics forms. Our position here is that clients come to the agency for services/treatment foremost, and if they choose not to participate in evaluation activities, so be it. That right should be emphasized fully respected and safeguarded. Also, services/treatment should never be leveraged (implicitly or explicitly) for a client's right not to participate or participate in any research or evaluation activity. Consent forms for actual treatment or services also need to be uncoupled from program/unit consent forms for research evaluation purposes (Holosko *et al.*, 2009a). Similarly, single system practice consent forms and agreements are different than program evaluation ones (Holosko *et al.*, 2009a). Finally here, CMs should double check with their funding bodies or larger unit which houses them (e.g., hospitals, mental health centers, school boards, etc.), and/or their boards of directors, when these various research and evaluation ethics forms are developed for use in the unit, as these larger organizational entities may have their own ethical protocols.

ADMINISTRATIVE CHRONOLOGY

It is important for CMs to keep an administrative log book on a weekly and monthly basis of activities conducted in the unit, highlighting minimally: date, events which transpired, policies/procedures, service delivery, personnel/budget, and comments. The focus of these entries should be written from the lens that the CMs use to view their units/programs. Indeed, programs have an organizational life to them – and staff, clients, and funding comes and goes, over this life. It becomes often difficult to track (or even remember) all the nuances and details of our evolving programs. Having these data systematically recorded for subsequent aggregation, annual reports, funding bodies, etc., becomes an important documentation and record of the unit/program's administrative life.

A helpful tool developed by the second author (MJH) to use here is the administrative chronology (AC) (see Figure 5.4). CMs can add/amend or modify their ACs to meet their own unique program/unit's needs, as needed.

As indicated in Figure 5.4, AC should be:

a. administratively focused
b. simple
c. chronological
d. directed toward major events occurring in the program/unit (Holosko, 1987).

	Month	Major Events	Policies/ Procedures	Service Delivery	Personnel/ Budget	Comments
Week 1						
Week 2						
Week 3						
Week 4						

Figure 5.4 Administrative chronology (AC)

ALIGNMENT, ALIGNMENT, ALIGNMENT!

All over the world, health and human service organizations are encouraged to align the various elements of their programs from the external worlds in which the program is housed or nested, down to the clients who receive services. As indicated in Figure 5.3, this can be achieved in three sequential related steps.

First, CMs need to define their organizational domains in the communities in which they are located. These then become the identified stakeholders that the host organization holds numerous ongoing exchange relationships with. The majority of these identified stakeholders collaborate regularly with the organization/program/unit, others may move in, and/or out of the domain on an annual basis, as exchange relationships come/go, or change. Many are also not mutually exclusive of one another, and may exist in more than one area. Hasenfeld (1983) was one of the first theorists to describe and illustrate these exchange relationships in an organization's domain. In Figure 5.5, the External Environment Map (EEM) based on his (prophetic) task environment conceptualization (1983) is presented as an example of a one such agency domain evaluated in Canada.

The second step in this process (see Figure 5.6) involves linking the external environment via the upper administrative strata of the program/unit. This involves linking the External Environment → Vision → Mission → Values.

This requires programs/units to annually re-visit their Vision, Mission, and Values statements, to ensure that their alignment terminology is in place

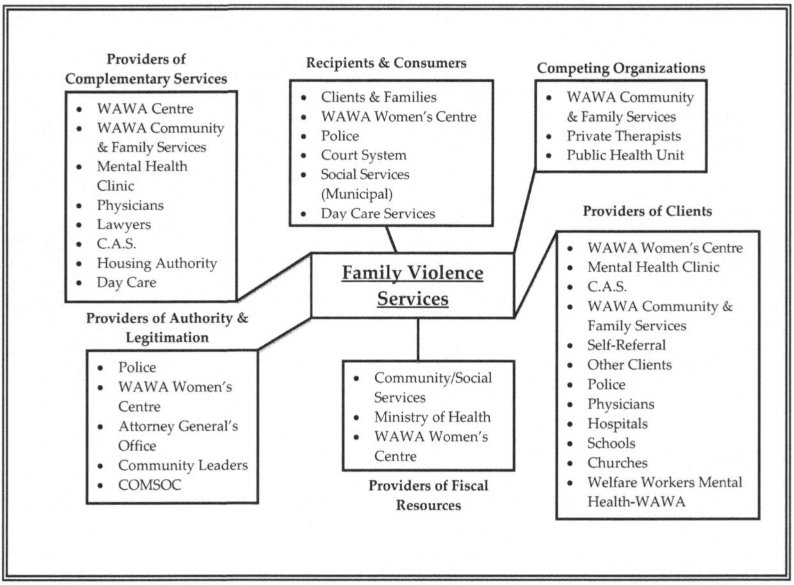

Figure 5.5 Example of External Environment Map (EEM) – WAWA Family Violence Services

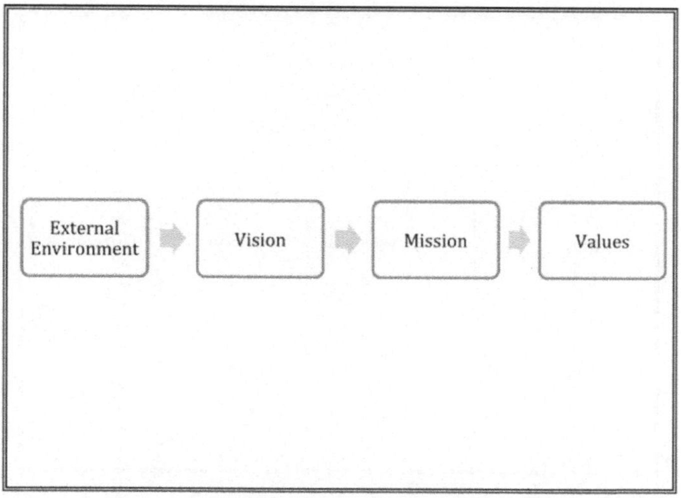

Figure 5.6 Alignment grid 1: external environment to upper organizational tier

and all of these are indeed aligned. For the Values statements, programs/units are encouraged to identify no more than 7–10 agreed upon core values, which underpin the present Vision and Mission.

Today, the use of numerous simple software programs, Internet surveys (e.g. Survey Monkey, etc.), have facilitated the ability for agencies to collaborate consensually in conducting this alignment step, in rather short order. However a program conducts this, it is critical that all agency employees, and key stakeholders e.g., board members, volunteers, etc., participate as their "buy-in" to the defining process is integral here. Our experience has shown that they also feel organizationally included in this formative alignment step, and they perceive that have had "their voice heard." Any subsequent evaluation(s) involving staff, administration, etc., and/or will inevitably proceed much smoother, as their input to the agency's Mission and Vision have been tabled, with them as full partners in the process.

The final sequentially related alignment step funnels this process down to clients and the services they receive. This includes aligning program/unit's Goals → Objectives → Services → Outcomes, as illustrated in alignment grid 2, Figure 5.7.

This step is best achieved by the paid employees and volunteers of the unit, as they are the ones who directly deliver its day-to-day programs and services. This step is also recommended to be also done annually, as a routine organizational development evaluation exercise, as well as re-visiting the goals/objectives/services/outcomes which may have been amended, or have migrated throughout the year, for a variety of unforeseen reasons.

The current North American popularity with outcomes seems rather well justified in the social work evaluation literature (c.f. Thyer & Myers, 2007)

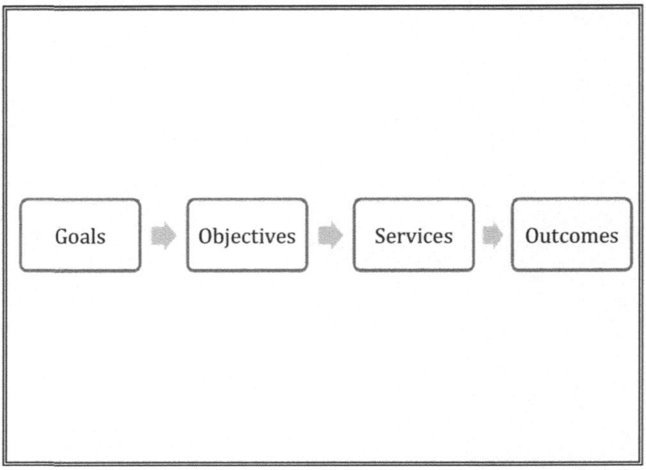

Figure 5.7 Alignment grid 2: program goals → client outcomes

for two reasons above all others. Well-articulated outcomes help sharpen the services/interventions we offer our clients as they are offered in more systematically aligned ways. Second, all outcomes (ideally) require measureable empirical indicators which both help us to ethically evaluate our practice (Holosko *et al.*, 2009b), and also make us more accountable to all stakeholders, including our clients.

TREATMENT PROCESS DEFINED

Annually, a chart illustrating the process steps of how clients come into care and the programs or services they receive should be written and visibly posted in the program/unit. This helps programs/units describe their own treatment processes and makes them more accountable to their funding bodies, stakeholders, as well as their units. An example of one is presented in the Treatment Process Diagram (TPD), depicted in Figure 5.8.

In this simple TPD example, one could embellish it by adding a time line on the bottom of the page depicting how long each intervention process actually took, and/or add the numbers of clients who entered and exited each process step. The TPD should always flow from left to right, and should be written as simply as possible. The idea is to seek a visually clean, uncluttered diagram.

We also recommend embellishing the TPD with a "typical case scenario" and conversely, an "atypical case scenario" charts illustrating how these clients typically receive their services, and also what the outliers to a typical case looks like. These typical/atypical case scenarios should be a footnote at the bottom of the TPD, or written as a separate addendum chart to the TPD.

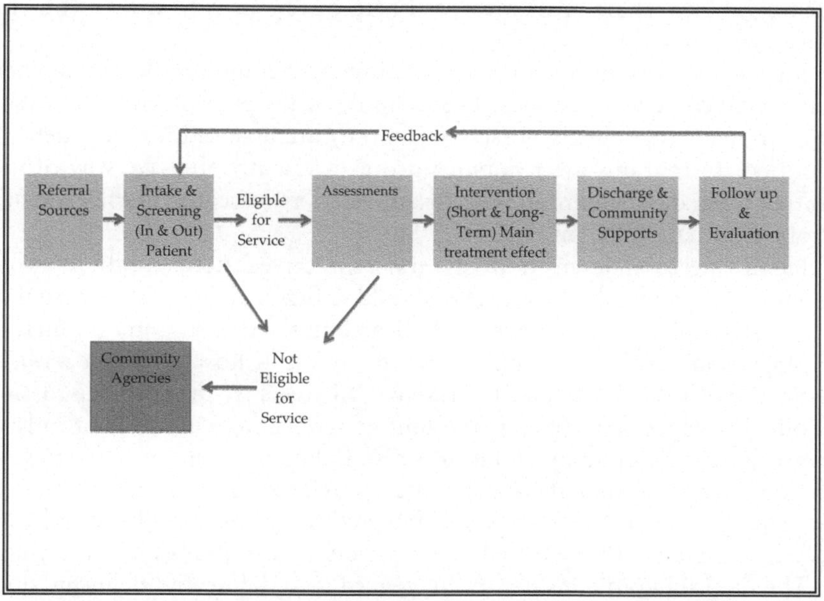

Figure 5.8 Example of the Treatment Process Diagram (TPD): the trauma program

ANNUAL CLIENT DATA

The final task to this Level 1 evaluation activity (for CMs) is to present annual client data, as simply as possible. These data are underpinned by the two coupled questions: a) *who are the people we serve?* and b) *what services did they receive?* Data collected in most health and social service organizations are primarily used for monitoring clients, not evaluating them. As such, the irony is that social workers and allied professionals spend countless hours filling out tedious data forms that once submitted – are lost in the bureaucracy, and/or cyberspace. So, practitioners never really get a read on their organization or program's effectiveness, or even their own effectiveness. This reality serves as a formidable obstacle to collecting new information for evaluative purposes (Holosko & Leslie, 1998), as it shifts the existing data collection process to including data that can be used for different evaluative purposes.

Three types of descriptive data that need to be collected and aggregated monthly here include: a) client demographic data, b) presenting problems, and c) number of services offered. In regard to the former, many health and human service organizations are positioned strategically in their communities to serve a certain proximal geographic area, as well as a certain targeted demographic group. The systematic collection of these data both monthly and annually serve to verify/corroborate the program's/unit's assumptions about who it is, they actually serve. As an example, the monthly

Demographics Chart (DC) presented here can be used to achieve this purpose (see Figure 5.9).

It is also important to describe the actual presenting problems that clients have, who come in for service. These should be the primary or main presenting problems that clients possess when they are assessed for treatment. Pie charts or histograms are recommended as a visually effective way of illustrating these data either monthly or annually, as indicated in the Presenting Problems Chart (PPC) in Figure 5.10.

Finally here, a description of services received needs to be compiled monthly and annually. Here, CMs should define their program's actual single (costed out) unit of service. As indicated in the next chapter on financial management, the issue is neither trite or moot, as how a unit of *service* is defined, positions it for a cost variable. CMs need to "have the discussion" about this important issue, as the unit of service definition is not only the cornerstone of cost analysis, but it is also linked to program outcomes. For example, the question then begs, after providing these units of service to our clients . . . *what difference did they make?* The Services Received Chart (SRC) in Figure 5.11 presented here provides an example of this variable.

The final thing to consider in this regard is to define and delineate duplicated from unduplicated services. Duplicated refers to multiple services given to the same client unit e.g., individual or family. Unduplicated refers to

Client Demographics	$\bar{x}$	Range	Number (+)	Category	% in Categories	Comments
Age						
Marital Status						
Gender						
Race						
Housing						
Socio Economic Status						
Referral Source to Agency						
Residence Distance from Agency						
Client's Perception of Presenting Problem						

Figure 5.9 The Demographics Chart (DC)

Clients to Trauma Program – Post Assessment 2009, N=161

Memory Loss	31%
Depression	20%
Lifestyle Adjustment	14%
Home Support	10%
Emotional	8%
Lack of Social Skills	7%
Stress	6%
Pain	4%

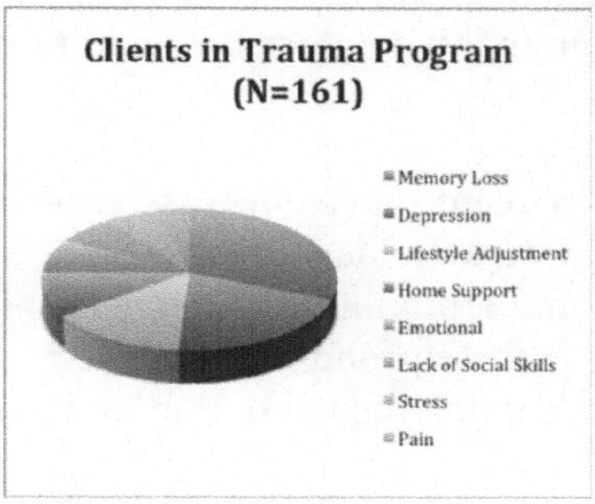

Figure 5.10 Presenting Problems Chart (PPC)

Services Received in Trauma Program – 2008, N=100

Types of Services Provided	Frequency (f)	Percent (%)
Direct Treatment	28	
Residential Services	18	
Psychological Assessment	8	
Social Work	7	
Psychotherapy	6	
Counseling & Rehabilitation	5	
Alcohol/Drug Abuse	7	
Speech Therapy	4	
Crisis Intervention	5	
Service Coordination	4	
Advocacy	3	
Attendant Care	2	
Accident Benefits	3	

Figure 5.11 Services Received Chart (SRC)

singular services provided to one client unit. A careful partitioning of these will also take some time, but similar to defining the units of service above, this has important implications about how such data gets eventually costed out, and eventually funded.

LEVEL 2 EVALUATION REQUIREMENTS FOR UPPER LEVEL MANAGEMENT

ULMs must ensure that all of the aforementioned Level 1 activities have been conducted in their programs/units, and as indicated in Figure 5.12, they need to minimally conduct four additional activities, on an annual basis. These are:

a. a client satisfaction assessment
b. a stakeholder survey
c. underpinning all interventions and outcomes with evidence-based literature/promising practices
d. framing their program/unit's using a program logic model.

Again, as indicated previously, these are considered as minimal annual evaluation activities, and ULMs should certainly add to them as they see fit.

CLIENT SATISFACTION ASSESSMENT

In the past decade or so, consumers in a variety of health and human service organizations have received much airplay about how their voices/opinions are important, and need to be solicited to plan for better quality services. Although client voices have not been as effectively used as they could be (Holosko *et al.*, 2001), there has been certainly much more attention given to their inclusion and input into our existing service delivery systems.

PRIMARY ACTIVITIES	PURPOSE AND USE	MAIN TOOLS/FORM(S) USED
1. Client Satisfaction Assessment	To survey clients about service satisfaction	CSQ-8 Plus [+]
2. Stakeholder Survey	To assess how stakeholders related to the program/unit	Custom Designed
3. Evidence-Based Interventions and Outcomes	To underpin all main interventions and outcomes with evidence-based literature	a) Best Practice and Promising Practice Literature b) COPES Question Grid
4. Frame Program/Unit in Program Logic Model	To establish a framework for: inputs, activities, outputs, outcome, impact	Basic Program Logic Model

Figure 5.12 Level 2 minimal evaluation activities for upper level managers (ULMs)

Typically, upon exit or discharge from an intervention, clients are asked to briefly comment on their overall satisfaction with various aspects of the services they received, while in care. Although these data are important (and often mandated), they are typically conducted rather haphazardly, anecdotally, idiosyncratically, and/or with no systematic measuring tool. Our advice is for ULMs to continue with this process – as they may be bound by their mandates to do so – but while collecting these data, ask existing clients to sign a separate consent form, requesting that they may be sampled 4–6 weeks later, for a quick telephone/internet survey about service satisfaction. This gives clients time to reflect about the program in retrospect, voluntarily and after they have left the program for some time.

Although it has come under some recent methodological scrutiny for its non-differential weighting of items (Hseih, 2006; 2009), the most frequently normed and standardized tool used all over the world in 30 different languages for assessing client satisfaction is the Client Satisfaction Questionnaire (CSQ-8) by Larsen, Attkinsson, Hargreaves and Nguyen (1979). It is brief, has excellent norms and is very easy to administer (http://www.CSQscales.com). As noted in Figure 5.12 (row 1, column 3), the tools we recommend to achieve this activity are the previously mentioned CSQ-8 "plus." The "plus" (+) refers here to a recommended additional 5–6 questions, and an additional 2–3 open ended questions which are unique to your particular program/unit, and which you feel are important to collect data on for decision-making purposes.

STAKEHOLDER SURVEY

It is important to canvas/survey all of your stakeholders, and/or a sample of them annually, about how they partner/collaborate with your program/unit. Since their funding and mandates change (like yours), and since they hold important exchange relationships with you, it is important to assess these systematically. From an organizational "community of care" standpoint, such data could not only be used for program planning and decision-making, but also for a variety of venues such as public relations, marketing, funding bodies, consumer, annual reports, brochures, and the like. The External Environment Map (EEM), mentioned previously in Level 1 activities, Figure 5.5, is a good place to start this process.

As indicated in Figure 5.12 (row 2, column 3), we recommend that you "custom design" this (recommended) internet survey, as per your program's/unit's annual programmatic needs. ULMs again need to "have the discussion", about who, why, and what data they need to collect, in order to craft this survey diligently.

EVIDENCE-BASED INTERVENTIONS AND OUTCOMES

The social welfare field has matured empirically from case wisdom → empirically-based practice → evidence-based practice (Thyer & Kazi, 2004). The extent to which the latter two of these have been actually achieved and incorporated into day-to-day practice has been the subject of much debate in our field (Green, 2008; Holosko, 2009a). Nonetheless, a fairly convincing national and international case has been promoted, primarily by both philanthropic and governmental social welfare funding bodies for the required inclusion of evidence-based practices and promising practices to underpin our interventions and outcomes.[1] This recent paradigm shift is particularly promoted in health, mental health and the addictions field.

Obviously, this first requires that all of the main interventions offered to clients be defined in precise terms minimally including:

a. purpose
b. goals
c. objectives
d. time frames
e. formats typically offered
f. how the intervention relates to the overall program's treatment goals
g. training to offer the intervention.

These should then be summarized on a so-called "one-pager" – with the previously mentioned criteria used as sub-headings for this (on a single page).

Second, a systematic review of all the best practices, theories, practice frameworks, assumptions, and promising practices – all of which (or the majority) should be empirically-based data – should also be conducted and summarized in 2–3 succinct paragraphs appended to the aforementioned "one-pager." Here 7–10 current references should be cited, main variables articulated, and the evidence assembled in a concerted way that addresses: a) the purpose of this intervention, b) why you are using it, c) its empirical justification, and d) how you are currently using it in your program/unit.

Similarly, for outcomes, an intervention may have more than one outcome, and all need to be defined and more *importantly measured*. Indeed, more and more funders are requiring that all outcomes need to be measured or they cannot be used. A current trend in this regard is the further delineation between short-term outcomes and long-term outcomes, or as they are now referred to, "sustainable outcomes" (over time). All of these outcomes should include minimally:

a. how they are measuring proposed change?
b. are they standardized, and how?
c. how they can be used so clients can visibly see clinical changes?
d. specifications of whether they are short- or longer-term outcomes?
e. how does the outcome relate to the overall program's goals?

Again, a systematic review of best practices etc., as mentioned above (for interventions) should be conducted and summarized accordingly. A rather pragmatic approach to linking evidence to interventions and outcomes is by using the COPES question grid developed by Gibbs in 2002. COPES is an acronym for Client Oriented Practice Evidence Search which helps practitioners anchor their daily practice in evidence, which shapes the focus of the questions posed (http://www.evidence.brookscole.com/copse.html). An example of this rather creative approach to connect evidence to questions and outcomes is presented in Figure 5.13.

Element Types	Client Type and Problem	What Might You Do	Alternate Course of Action	What You Want to Accomplish
Example 3: Assessment	If aged residents of a nursing home who may be depressed or may have Alzheimer's Disease or Dementia	Are administered Depression Screening Tests	Or Short Mental Status Examination Tests	Which measure will be the briefest most inexpensive valid and reliable screening test to discriminate between Depression and Dementia?
Example 4: Description	If family members of persons diagnosed with Aphasia meet in a support group	And receive a Short Client Satisfaction Questionnaire of all support group participants	Or we rely on practical judgment unaided by a risk assessment scale	Which will the clients list as their area of Areas of Greatest and Least Satisfaction?
Example 5: Risk	If crisis line callers to a battered women shelter	Are administered a risk assessment scale by telephone		Then will the Risk Assessment Scale have higher reliability and predictive validity regarding future violence?

Note(*):Used with personal permission of L.Gibbs

Figure 5.13 Five COPES question types

The COPES grid has been used effectively by BSW and MSW students in research internships and in agencies for over a decade in North America. It is simple, pragmatic, and helps braid the practitioner's need for answering an agency-based client question in the best available evidence.

FRAME THE PROGRAM/UNIT IN PROGRAM LOGIC MODEL

Many private charitable funding organizations in North America have had a significant impact in the area of program evaluation our health and human service organizations. Indeed, their overall mandates in the past decade have become more: stringent, rigorous, uniform in their specification of requirements, evidence-based, and national in their scope. They also have come to incorporate comparative data, embrace more mixed methodologies, promote more practice-based and policy-based dissemination of findings, and require the use of standardized models/approaches to evaluate their programs and service delivery structures.

In regard to the latter, the W.K. Kellogg Foundation in Battle Creek Michigan (www.wkkf.org) developed the Program Logic Model (available on their website for free). As stated in their 71-page downloadable manual:

> A program logic model is a picture of how your program works – the theory and assumptions underlying the program . . . This model provides a roadmap of your program highlighting how it is expected to work, what activities needed to come before others and how desired outcomes are achieved. (W.K. Kellogg Foundation, nd: 35)

As such, program logic models provide a systematic and visual way to represent and share the understanding of the resources a program has, the activities they plan, and the intents, changes or results they hope to achieve. It is a learning and management tool that facilitates ULMs to effectively plan, implement and evaluate their programs/units. The types of models (as noted in their website) include:

a) Theory approach logic models
b) Outcome approach logic models
c) Activities approach logic models
d) Research performance logic models.

The basic model recommended for programs/units is presented in Figure 5.14.

Programs who use this basic model need to read the very simple manual online and complete the planning exercises in this well-crafted manuscript. As an aside, we have noted that many programs use simpler versions of this approach, e.g., INPUTS → THROUGHPUTS → OUTPUTS, or INPUTS →

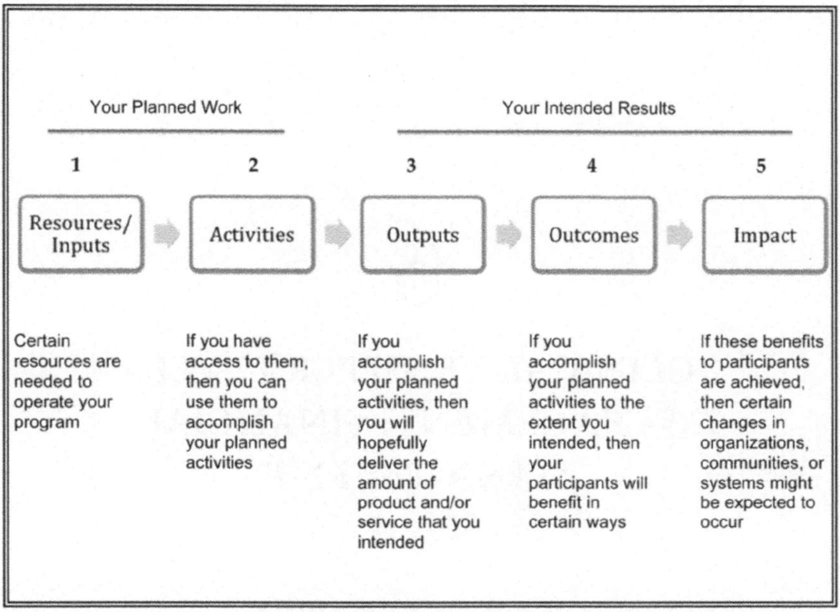

Figure 5.14 Basic program logic model explained

RESEARCH ACTIVITIES → OUTPUTS → OUTCOMES (back to INPUTS, etc.,) which although are "a start," do not do justice to the Basic Model, and its overall intents and purposes. We recommend, therefore, that all ULMs use at least the basic model and perhaps CMs (Level 1) could embrace a simpler model. In short, any logic model is better than no logic model!

In sum here, CMs and ULMs have numerous evaluation activities (noted in this chapter) that require tending to, if program evaluation is to be seriously considered in the agency. We acknowledge that it may take time to move an agency to accepting that evaluation is part and parcel of day-to-day practice. However, if not conducted, a program/unit renders itself more fiscally vulnerable than ever before, to budget cuts or reductions in our very uncertain fiscal times.

NOTE

1. See, for example, http://www.samhsa.gov/Federalactionagenda/NFC_FMHAA.aspx, http://www.scotland.gov.uk/Publications/2004/05/19394/37560, http://www.omh.state.ny.us/omhweb/2004/5070408Chapter10.htm.

6

CLINICAL VS. UPPER LEVEL MANAGEMENT: FINANCIAL MANAGEMENT

OPENING STATEMENT

It is critical to distinguish between the aspects of a clinical manager (CM) compared with the task and activities combined with the upper level manager (ULM). While each area has some common ground issues, there are several very important distinctions which need to be made so that managers at each level have a clear understanding of what to expect and what skills are needed.

Several common ground issues have to do with such things as agreement on the organizational purpose, identifying a specific marker appropriate to the mission of the organization, determining how many clients can effectively be served in the course of a year, and how to appropriately evaluate the effectiveness of the services. Based on a fiscal perspective, all managers have a concern for the overall budget and particularly the budget in their unit. A reason is that they want to stay within their budget so that they can carry out their functions without much difficulty. The budget picture for CMs center on just their unit whereas the ULM has to focus on all units of the organization including those that comprise a significant portion, such as fiscal maintenance, building resources, secretarial and staff, support, and information technology. Therefore, the fiscal management task record for both levels while being somewhat related are quite different and requiring a different set of skills.

Financial management is the most important component of any organization. The obvious reason is that it centers on the entire money system upon which all decisions must be based. Financial management for social service agencies can be defined as administrative activities that can be represented by four administrative subsystems normally: budget and accounting;

service coordination and management control; program planning; and program evaluation. Each of these subsystems are critical in that they provide the upper level manager (ULM) with important information relative to making a decision affecting client services offered and the money used to underwrite them in an organization.

Previously, Feit and Chei Li (1998) viewed the fiscal budgeting and accounting activities as those such as record processing, document and report monies received, monies committed, expenditures committed, services provided, and the number of clients served. Service coordination was seen as those that would determine case management, the transfer of case management activities, staff supervision, orientation and timeline period. Program planning defines goals and directions of an organization, establishes standards for organizational performance, management of people based on the results and coordination of services and programs with other organizations (Drucker, 2001).

Program evaluation covers utilization of programs in meeting the objectives in an efficient manner (Holosko and Feit, 1981). In this area, one is examining issues related to increase or decrease, maintain or eliminate a service. Clinical and upper level managers at the outset need to understand what is occurring in existing programs and what is likely to be happening or needed in a new program. A reasonable question is whether one is serving or likely to serve the optimum type of clients for each program area.

CLINICAL LEVEL FISCAL MANAGEMENT

As one continues to clarify the differences between fiscal management at the clinical and upper level management, it is important to note that the former is likely to have many considerations not usually understood. However, many of the tasks, while often not very difficult, are generally not done on a regular basis. Thus, CMs often need assistance in understanding some of the minimum requirements necessary to do an effective fiscal projection in their units. This section addresses those concerns and provides an illustration of what CMs need to know in order to be effective.

There are a full range of fiscal tasks which can be seen as integral to clinical management. For example, clinical personnel often provide direct services to clients and requires them to determine the best and appropriate services for their clients. Management requires and considers the relationship between the types of services offered and those most utilized. In this service context, such tasks include the services offered or proposed to be offered, the types of workers needed, the type of supervision required, the documentation needed for services, the effect of the services on clients, the costs of the services on the agency, and the need to continually evaluate practice. These tasks will be described in more detail.

In the services already being offered, one must consider the relation of the services to the overall purpose of an agency. The services must also meet the different needs of the clients, including the types of problems likely to surface in the treatment process. The supervisor would also be expected to examine the utilization of each service in an effort to determine the cost reimbursement needed and its appropriateness for that service.

The CM and direct service personnel are also aware of developing new services as determined by the needs of the clients. This task becomes more difficult to project because one must determine an expected use of the type of problems to be addressed, as important as the type of worker needed to address the anticipated problems. The CM, when proposing new services, is minimally required to provide the costs necessary to start and continue a new program. Such costs at the clinical level are related directly to personnel and to outcome or performance measures. It would minimally include the type and number of workers needed, their level of competence and projected wages, a projection of basic operating costs, an understanding of the need to evaluate the program on a regular basis, and how many clients are projected to be served on a monthly/yearly basis.

Often overlooked is the effect of any programs, particularly those being proposed, on the rest of the agency. Typical questions include adequate staff needs, such as salary, benefits, and so forth. It should also project some possible reimbursement issues, as well as the expected income, the requirement for incorporating or developing technical needs and the overall supervision requirements for the type of services, such as new supervisors would be needed or the additional workload could be assigned to existing supervisory personnel. In other words, when service programs are developed, integrated, or adjusted, one must pay attention to the adjustments that may be likely to be felt throughout the agency and be able to address them as they are implemented.

When a new service is proposed its cost has to be calculated in the overall cost, utilization of service, the workload effect on others in the agency. With new programs, the question becomes what evidence is being provided to document the need for the service. In effect, this begins a major fiscal feasibility study which is necessary to assist in making a decision to start a new program or to make adjustments in an existing program. For example, it may become practical to reassign a direct service worker or add new workers to start a program. Such a reassignment makes it possible to control costs and determine the extent to which it is practical to offer a new service. Thus, documentation is very critical to making fiscal decisions based on reasonable actual data on existing as well as new services.

The type of work that the CM would project is very important because personnel costs normally account for 80–90 percent of service delivery. First, one must determine how many workers are needed and their degree level, such as whether a bachelor's or graduate degree is needed. This is important to determine the wage for such workers leading to reimbursement from insurers and health plans. A CM would probably need to inquire about existing market prices both in the agency and in the community. If reimbursement is going to be needed, then probably one with a graduate degree is needed for the funding sources. Should certain clerical, secretarial and/or administrative staff be needed to support the program, then these costs may be projected in the same way as service personnel.

A CM may need to provide some projected costs of evaluating the program and its practice. While this task is not thought to be in the development of a service or in determining the basis of an existing service, it is important to include because judgments need to be made, about making adjustments or taking corrective management action periodically, throughout the program. It helps if a clinical manager has had experience in assisting and or designing an evaluation effort.

In summary, the CM is an integral part in helping to determine the relationship between program service costs and utilization. Paying attention to these basic requirements of good fiscal management would provide the basis for a clinical manager to lay the foundation for determining the unit cost per service.

UPPER LEVEL FISCAL MANAGEMENT (ULM)

In upper level management, the focus of financial management is on very different issues. In effect, this type of manager has to make decisions for new and ongoing service programs, prepare and submit reports on a regular and/or annual basis, determine evaluation strategies and review evaluation results for services, and is fiscally responsible for acquiring money, spending/expenses, and accounting/auditing concerns. These concerns will now be addressed.

One of the most important aspects of the ULM deals with fiscal accountability. Costs breakdown depends on an analysis of the delivery and utilization of services, overall income and expenditures, and outcome measures. The ULM must be able to determine the cost benefit and cost effectiveness of each service offered by the agency in an effort to assure fiscal reliability. For example, one area of concern would be whether expenses at certain times in the year are 10 percent over or under where they are expected to be. When the factor is more than 10 percent in either direction, the ULM needs to make an appropriate decision related to whether corrective action is needed.

The manager has to relate to the funding source such that the agency is meeting liability requirements and deliverables. For example, it may be possible to increase reimbursement relating to the type of personnel and the specific problems addressed in the services delivered. The level of indirect costs allowed by the funding source would be another area of discussion and possible negotiation.

The ULM must be able to inform the Board of Directors and other external constituents of the fiscal health of the organization, the types of services they offer, and likely specify the unit cost for providing each service. The

ULM must be able to indicate the extent to which costs are being controlled and that the cash flow is doing well. The awareness of fiscal responsibility and fiscal determination of costs is a managerial responsibility of the ULM and must not be left to another people, such as an accountant, bookkeeper, auditor, and so forth. The upper level manager must be able to understand and ask the questions needed to prepare, understand, and interpret a financial report and other reports that he or she may receive.

In the same context, a ULM must be able to determine a unit cost for providing each service and whether that unit cost is reasonable and competitive. In all programs, and particularly in new programs, projections have to be reasonable and provide an appearance of being successful most likely within a year or so. Existing programs provide actual information because they are providing up-to-date service data and evaluative data can more factually be determined.

One of the areas where more difficult questions arise is with the implementation of a new service. A manager at the upper level receives recommendations and service proposals from a unit supervisor or other executive personnel. Such proposals need to be reviewed based on the relationship between anticipated utilization, and evidence that expected cost return on investment, the program would be successful. In this regard, additional issues have to do with determining the optimum maximum of the type of personnel, where the income for providing income is likely to come from, what are the data needs of the service, how would it be incorporated in the existing data bases, what would be the service outcome, and how will the program be promoted or advertised as well as any potential difficulty in implementing the service. When determining the values of a new service, this is where the need of understanding of evaluative data and insight is critical.

In summary, the types of fiscal related and fiscal decisions are different at the CM level and ULM. It is obviously important to know and be aware of this difference and how one can learn the skills needed to prevail and be effective in each area. It should also be clear that being effective at one level does not automatically lead to being effective at the other level without additional experience and training.

The major responsibility of an ULM is fiscal. This responsibility should not be relegated to other people in the organization nor to certain members on the board, such as accountants. These personnel are very helpful, but they should be seen as providing important data and/or offering suggestions leading to a final decision. The ULM needs to be comfortable with asking others for suggestions and reasons leading to a decision. The point here is that the knowledge and content of financial management must include a sense of risk in detailing the outcome. Thus a manager must recognize that an apparent understanding of content needs should be enhanced by the manager's leadership ability and undertaking of risks.

In order to determine unit cost, it is imperative that one defines a unit of service for which it can be charged. The two main components are the length of the services offered and the type of services provided. For example, one has to decide the length of time for providing a counseling session which could be 15, 30, 45 or so minutes in direct contact with a practitioner. The second aspect for the type of services is just what will be provided? In that example, counseling is the specific service provided. Thus a unit of services could be a 30 minute counseling session with a practitioner which would meet the definition of a unit of services for which the cost could be determined. The other and last component in dealing and moving from a unit of services to the actual cost is the qualifications of the practitioner such as one with no degree, an associate degree, bachelor's degree, master's degree and/or a doctoral degree. The cost of profit based on qualifications is a significant determining factor in determining the unit cost. If one wanted to lower unit costs, then the qualification of the practitioner would need to be lowered or one with a higher professional degree who has many more clients such as counseling will determine the unit of services and the unit of cost for the services provided for an upper level manager.

Unit cost for providing a service is very important because it has to include all costs, such as direct and indirect, which are related to each part of the overall service, and whether that cost is competitive in the market place. For example, if the unit cost is too high, other community groups and agencies can compete with the funding source to take over that service. On the other hand, if a particular task is not included in the unit cost, then it places a financial hardship on the agency personnel since they will have to complete the task.

A good example of the importance of the inclusion of unit cost has to do with the fundamental difference between grants and contracts. A grant normally includes all of the activities and personnel, and usually projects an equal distribution of funds over a given time period such as a year. A contract, which may outline the services a grant covers, provides reimbursement when specific services, i.e. deliverables, are completed in a shorter time period such as a month or two. Thus, a contract calls for reimbursement of specific services, when provided over a given time, and the reimbursement is likely to be uneven due to the range and type of service being provided. In any event, a manager cannot exceed the overall cost of either the grant or the contract.

An ULM must realize that financial management goes beyond accounting. A budget is a useful tool and is an organizational plan of financial action (GAO, 1999). A budget performs two basic functions. First, it identifies in normal terms the direction of the program and is based on clear objectives emerging from the planning process. Second, budgets are excellent tools to monitor the financial activities throughout the year.

Financial review for both basic functions should be done each month. If problems arise, they can more easily be dealt with on the monthly or bi-monthly plan of action rather than near the end of the program year. A manager needs to be making sure that there is a regular cash flow, that cost overruns are in check, thus monitoring program income and expenditures frequently and regularly. One must remember that generally one will not be able to add staff or increase cost during the program year since the entire budget and fiscal arrangement will need to be revised and recalculated.

Another component of monitoring a budget is to examine the relationship of service utilization with expenditures. In other words, is the program reaching the client for which it is intended, are the services being provided by appropriate personnel, and is utilization meeting expectations? Availability of such information is critical to maintain a good fiscal management system. One of the areas of fiscal management that ULMs have virtually no knowledge of is when they get to the top level in financial accounting and auditing.

DIFFERENT ASPECTS OF UPPER LEVEL FINANCIAL MANAGEMENT

There are some areas of fiscal management which are very important for ULM. These areas are necessary primarily to ULM and not to clinical managers. Generally, ULM have virtually no knowledge when they get to the top level, such as in the area of financial auditing, but also in contributions, dividends, the different types of contributions, and ledgers in understanding financial balance (Feit *et al.*, 1995).

Financial auditing is one of the more difficult aspects of financial management for an ULM to learn (GAO, 1999). This is due to many factors, such as no experience in moving to the management level in an organization, lack of adequate support in graduate and doctoral programs, and lack of accounting knowledge if one is promoted, which are essential to more management level responsibilities. Thus, this is the new experience for upper level managers when they move into that position.

Financial auditing is useful to an organization since it provides an outside and objective assessment of the current operation of the organization and its processes and mission (Tuller, 1997). An audit is normally done on an annual basis and can include or suggest forms of corrective action which need to be taken with the goals and accomplished tasks.

An audit usually addresses compliance of the direction of the agency with its existing policies, mission, and work activities. Thus, expenditures must be related to specific tasks of the agency, such as operating costs. It is critical in financial auditing to verify that fund allocations are well documented and can be authenticated properly. It is not generally understood by ULM that in an organization people who receive funds need to be differentiated from those who document expenditures so as to minimize possible embezzlement and missing allocations of funds.

It is for these reasons that an ULM needs to learn about finances and accountability and the different effects of financial auditing. These perspectives will make the manager much more effective in understanding the fiscal picture of an organization and enable one to make more appropriate decisions. Contributions are one of the areas an ULM should understand fully. One needs to make certain that the nonprofit organization is registered with IRS for tax exempt status so as to appeal to particular contributors. At times a manager may ask for general contributions or for funds to be targeted to specific programs.

Part of the overall income, the manager needs to keep track of this money source and it will need to be recorded accordingly (Tuller, 1997), perhaps as an expenditure item. The same advice is for the need to receive consultation which would be when certain contributions are made. For example, one who provides funds for a specific activity which may occur at a later date will need to be recorded separately as that constitutes an investment which is the completion of a task. Another type of contribution which requires close scrutiny occurs when it is made for a specific purpose. A good example is when donations are made to provide subsidies for children to come to a program at a significantly reduced rate.

In summary, financial information provides limits on which services can be provided. It gives the ULM an excellent idea of the financial flow of funds acquired and spent at each phase of the organization. It sets a tone for how much could be spent for each service and whether those expenditures are within reason. In addition, it allows these managers to be accountable to directors and other constituents for services provided and for related expenditures. It certainly sets a tone for determining the unit cost for each service provided and gives a very good understanding of the organization's ability to compete and be effective in the market place.

This picture is critical to the upper level manager since it is valuable in determining an organization's survival, particularly in severe economic times. Evaluative information becomes crucial because it can provide the determination of whether to spend, maintain, reduce, or eliminate services. This is one reason for a manager to also have a good grasp and knowledge of evaluation as both areas are essential to good and effective administrative practice. This is the core of these two areas. From the core is making administrative decisions regarding clients served and purchases provided.

ESSENTIAL COMPONENTS OF FINANCIAL MANAGEMENT

This section of the chapter discusses the essential components of an internal financial management system and builds on the work of Holosko and Feit (1981).

Financial management is probably the most important aspect of every agency administrator's job because it concerns money – for without money one cannot provide services. Therefore, every administrator must understand:

1. How to obtain money.
2. How to allocate money wisely.
3. How to spend money appropriately, i.e., according to budget.
4. How to report or account for each dollar.
5. How to monitor or track each dollar and make budget revisions when indicated.

Financial management covers a lot of administrative ground. It means the allocation of funds according to a set of services while making the best use of funds in the most cost-effective manner.

It includes:

1. Identifying a funding source.
2. Preparing a grant and/or a resubmission for funds.
3. Determining a unit cost for each service.
4. Keeping financial records for *every* business transaction.
5. Preparing and writing regular financial reports.
6. Completing forms on time for the funding agency or agencies and sometimes the regulatory agency (e.g., federal, state or local agency).

UPPER LEVEL FISCAL MANAGEMENT

Differences between profit and non-profit organizations

A non-profit funding account is the basic system used. For example, any time money is to be transferred from any operating expense category to another category, it has to be formally moved from one category to another category. It must follow accounting principles which means that you have to debit one account and credit another account. Likewise, personnel cost and all of the operating expense costs cannot be massed or combined except under one condition. This occurs when there is a full- or part-time vacancy and thus there will be a specific dollar amount available as one moves towards the end of the fiscal year. In this case, one may ask for special approval to use the money for a one time only cost such as furniture, technical equipment, or another one time only fund use.

There are at least five areas of accounting differences between profit and non-profit organizations (GAO, 1999). They are as follows:

1. Cash versus accrual accounting – accrual-keeping records so that in addition to recording transactions resulting from the receipt and disbursement of cash. This allows one to also record the amounts payable (owe others) and receivable (owed to the agency or organization).
2. Fund and accounting – assets are segregated into categories according to the restrictions that donors place on their use.
3. Treatment of fixed assets – fixed assets may or may not be recorded. There is no single generally accepted principle or practice to follow.

4. Transfers and appropriations – transfers are frequently made between "funds," and unless carefully disclosed, such transfers tend to confuse the reader of the financial statements (Norvelle, 1989).
5. Contributions, pledges, and noncash contributions – a pledge may or may not be legally enforceable; it is difficult to record them as accounts receivable. Noncash contributions include donations of securities, equipment, supplies and services.

(Adapted from Gross and Jablonksy, 1979)

PLANNING AND PROCESS

In planning, a distinction must be made immediately between a *plan* and a *planning process*. A plan is the final completed document submitted to an individual organization, donor, foundation, or government agency for the purpose of securing funds (either a new grant or a grant renewal). A grant application is one example of a plan and its planning process.

A planning process includes all activities that an agency staff performs in relation to completing the plan. Each of the tasks completed in the workbook section of this chapter, when done in an orderly and systematic time frame, with the submission of a grant application or plan being the last step, constitutes a planning process.

To summarize, a *plan is the final product of a planning process*, or, to say it another way, the end product of any planning process is a plan.

A typical planning process has the following minimum steps:

1. Identify the goal of an agency and define problems in the community.
2. Determine which problems the agency wants to address in a given year.
3. Determine the existing situation including needs assessment and other data. Translate these problems or the existing situation into identifiable services for the target population.
4. Determine specific objectives for each problem.
5. Consider at least two or three ways to meet the specified objectives including a financial analysis, a budget and manpower preparations, etc.
6. Evaluate these alternatives, analyze the predictable positive outcomes and possible side effects or negative outcomes.
7. Decide which alternative or alternatives are best.
8. Prepare a first draft which includes record keeping, evaluation, client services, etc. according to the guidelines in the grant application kit.
9. Have the first draft reviewed by the appropriate individuals such as other staff, clients, funding agency personnel and Board members. Obtain their comments and suggested revisions.
10. Review commends and revise the first draft making important recommended changes by staff, if they can be revised or justified.

11. Revise first draft and produce a final draft after proofreading and completing all the submission requirements.
12. Submit final draft to Board for approval.
13. Obtain other approvals as required by the local government of other local agencies.
14. Submit plan or grant application to funding agency.
15. If the application looks as if it will be accepted, prepare the Board members and staff for implementation.

Please remember that each step in the planning process has a product. Each product is normally completed by staff. For example, steps one through three result from needs assessment, population data, and the funds available from potential funding sources. The outcomes of steps one through three are clear statements of the problems communities face and the services agencies will establish to deal effectively with them. For example, to deal with the isolation of seniors, one might establish or continue a telephone reassurance and/or friendly visiting service.

Step four, which determines objectives with regard to each service, has been completed in preparing the agency mission worksheet. So have all the other products of each step, such as budget preparation and needed manpower, needs assessment, organizational charts, etc. Therefore, several key personnel have successfully completed all the parts for a grant application or written proposal.

Evidence of the actual writing of a grant or proposal is but one step in the overall planning process. All steps and their products must be completed and put together according to funding agency guidelines before this actually becomes a grant or proposal. To insure effectiveness of each step in the planning process, one must allow the proper amount of time. Although there are variations in some instances, one should allow a minimum of four months for grant applications to be properly completed for submission.

There may be instances where a new proposal or grant has to be submitted quickly because ULMs are notified a grant deadline only when they inquire about funds. ULMs must still go through all the steps in a much shorter time frame, however. As a result, some steps may be curtailed. For example, one may have to rely on other data, such as census data, to identify need rather than conduct a community needs assessment in order to obtain documentation for the range of services one wishes to provide. Each step and product in the planning process must still be completed, however.

When time is short, a ULM must communicate with staff and other constituents about the truncated time and share the plan with all as soon as possible. When time is short, there is time for feedback and an opportunity to make changes during implementation. Effective use of time is of paramount importance to avoid becoming overwhelmed by approaching deadlines for grants or proposals.

One way to avoid mounting pressure as submission deadlines loom is to design a planning process and adhere to it. The planning process outlined earlier in this chapter can be used to create such a design. Identifying each step and the time it would take to complete each over a four-month period would be beneficial. The four-month chart shown in Table 6.1 may be useful.

After submission of the grant or proposal, implementation is the next step. To organize the various tasks in preparing a grant or proposal, one may also list the products and the names of persons responsible for completing the products in relation to each step. This technique helps to divide the work and to keep track of the proposal while the problems of daily agency administration are occurring. Table 6.2 shows a suggested form to achieve the goal of implementation.

In summary, a plan is a document which details the goals and objectives of an organization and its staff and the proposed method of accomplishment. A plan over a period of time results from a process or a series of orderly steps through which the needs of people, services to be offered, objectives, budget

Step	Time Frame for Completed Work
1	One week
2	One week
3	One week
4	Three days
5	Two weeks
6	Two weeks
7	One week
8	Three weeks
9	Two weeks
10	One week
11	One week
12	One week
13	One week
14	Four days

Table 6.1 A four-month chart

Step	Time Frame for Completed Work	Product	Person Responsible

Table 6.2 Implementation plan

and other financial considerations, personpower, record keeping and evaluation procedures are considered, and the best methods selected on the basis of quality service at a reasonable unit cost.

Types of financial forms

Every ULM must complete a series of financial forms to stay in business. Table 6.3 summarizes several key forms which must be completed, the frequency of completion and the time frame for completion (Tuller, 1997).

The grant application or resubmission package which is usually obtained from the funding agency contains a series of forms to be completed. Each package usually comes with a series of instructions on properly completing each section of the application, including the budget.

In any application one is projecting the amount of money which will be needed to operate the program for the following year. While the figures may not be entirely accurate, projections are based on known facts such as the number of people served in all agency programs the previous year or a "guesstimate" of the number of people who will use a new service.

It must be remembered in a grant application that one is preparing a proposal to secure funds for services to be provided at a later date; therefore, changes will have to be made during implementation and throughout the year to keep the funding accurate and current. Such changes are monitored through the quarterly financial report forms that are required by the federal and/or state agencies.

Each quarterly report summarizes the amount of money spent or disbursed over a three-month period in each of several line-time budget categories such as personnel, travel, building space, communications, utilities, printing and supplies, equipment, contracts, etc. Some forms also require computation of

Type of Form	Number to be completed	When due	Purpose of Form
Grant Application or Resubmission	1	Before the start of the funding by cycle or fiscal year	To obtain from a funding source
Federal Financial Report (if applicable)	4	At end of each quarter of the funded year	To report your financial status to the funding agency
State Financial Report or Foundation report	4	At the end of the quarter of the funded year	To report your financial status to the funding agency
Request for Payment	Up to 12	Prior to the start of the period for which funds are being requested	To secure operating money for agency

Table 6.3 Various financial forms

cash balance and earnings of project funds. This part of the form accounts for money received and disbursed, and the cash balance on hand for use by the administrator.

The request for payment form is used by the operating agency to request operating funds from the funding agency for each month or for a specific period of time. The information requested on this form is intended to arrive at a dollar figure needed to cover all expenses incurred during the month funds are being requested.

Financial forms have been developed by agencies outside of the local agency for their own purposes and often do not help a ULM effectively monitor and manage his or her own program. This is what *financial management* is all about – learning how to use financial and budget information to make the best possible administrative decisions.

MONITORING

Once a dollar amount has been set or awarded, a budget has different uses. Its best and most effective use is monitoring expenditures of money to see if one is on target. Monitoring is accomplished through financial reporting at regular intervals, usually monthly, for maximum internal decision making or quarterly when completing the federal and/or state forms. ULMs must also monitor their program internally according to their own needs and purposes. Internal monitoring is a means of evaluating one's agency financially as well as assisting administrators in taking management action when indicated, making decisions requiring the use of funds and reporting to the advisory or Board of Directors.

DETERMINING UNIT COST

In financial management most administrators seem to have the most confidence in preparing grant applications or resubmissions (projecting costs) and completing necessary financial information to monitor and control their programs effectively. *Monitoring* usually means being able to account for and control costs to see whether money is being spent according to plan and at a proper rate (to avoid overspending and indebtedness or under spending). This part of the program concerns the monitoring aspect of financial management.

Three forms can be used for the internal management and monitoring of each service. Each form is listed in Table 6.4 which also shows the purpose of each form and the date each form is due. These forms provide the basis of an internal management financial system which is compatible to the need of an administrative agency to manage effectively and the requirement of a funding agency to report externally. A ULM must be able to understand and to interpret the data from all these forms to make effective decisions. These forms must be completed in order to understand the total financial management process and to read key fiscal data so as to make timely, informative management decisions.

The lead form is a summary of four financial forms which provide a ULM with specific types of financial information and an overall picture of internal fiscal health. The four forms are:

1. the statement of all income and expense (Table 6.5) – totals income and expenditures from all sources for all services and provides an overall fiscal picture of the organization

TYPE OF FORM	ACCOUNT TO BE COMPLETED	DUE DATE?	PURPOSE	PREPARER
STATEMENT OF INCOME AND EXPENSES			This form totals income and expenditures from all sources for all services and provides an overall fiscal picture of the organization.	
INCOME STATEMENT BY SERVICE			This form collects data regarding income from all sources by month, year to date, and so forth by service. Once then compares the income by the yearly budgeted and projected to end of year so that one can determine whether the balance is more or less than anticipated.	
DISBURSEMENTS/ OPERATING STATEMENT BY SERVICE			This form organizes disbursement to expenditures by month, year to date, and so forth by service.	
COST BREAKDOWN BY SERVICE			This form assembles cost expenditures according to each service.	

Table 6.4 Types of business forms

2. the income statement by service (Table 6.6) – collects data regarding income from all source by month, year, etc. by service and then compares the income by the yearly budgeted and projected figures to the end of year – so that one can determine whether the balance is more or less than anticipated
3. the disbursements/operating statement by service (Table 6.7) – organizes disbursements or expenditures by month, year, etc. by service.
4. the cost breakdown by service (Table 6.8) – assembles cost expenditures according to each service.

The lead form identifies the four major financial forms and indicates the number of times each should be completed. Best practice recommends that each form should be completed monthly in order to take corrective management action.

These forms are internally driven, both individually and collectively and form the basis of making administrative decisions. Additionally, these forms assist the agency in completing requirement(s) for external funding sources.

PROGRAM OR SERVICE CATEGORY	INCOME IN CURRENT MONTH	YEAR TO CURRENT DATE MONTH	YEARLY BUDGETED FIGURE	PROJECTED BUDGET TO END OF YEAR	+ – BALANCE
1. COUNSELING					
2.					
3.					
4.					
5.					

Table 6.5 Statement of all income and expenses

PROGRAM OR SERVICE CATEGORY	DISBURSEMENTS IN MONTH	YEAR TO DATE DISBURSEMENTS	YEARLY BUDGETED FIGURE	PROJECTED BUDGET TO END OF YEAR	+ –BALANCE
1. COUNSELING					
2.					
3.					
4.					
5.					

Table 6.6 Income statement by service

CASH EXPENDITURES	PROGRAM OR SERVICE OBJECTIVES					
	1.	2.	3.	4.	5.	
Personnel Travel Building Space Communications Utilities Printing Supplies Equipment Contracts Other	Counseling					
Total Cash Expenditures						
In-Kind Cash Personnel Building Space						
Total Expenditures						
Output Measure (Objectives)						
Unit Cost						

Table 6.7 Disbursements/operating statement by service

The *statement of income and expense* form summarizes the income and expense of an agency for a specific time period. In agencies with small budgets, it is recommended that this form be completed each month as "small" budget deviations can often have disastrous effects on an overall budget. The form is shown in Table 6.9.

The information to be completed in the first column, "monthly," is obtained from the agency ledger. It shows the amount of money obtained month by month, the amount spent and the balance, if any. The second column is a cumulative figure of each line item in income and expenses at the end of the reported month. Thus, ULMs can clearly see the amount money they have obtained from all sources up to the end of the reporting period and the balance remaining. The column contains the budget figures for each category as obtained from the grant application. When the second

Type of Form	Number to be Completed	When Due	Purpose of Form
Statement of Income and Expense	12	At end of each month	Summarizes income and expenses of your agency for a specific time period, and also shows whether agency is on target with budget.
Operating Statement	12	At end of each month	Summarizes funds obtained and disbursed according to service category, also used to show whether agency is on target with budget.
Cost Breakdown by Service	4	One to be submitted in the grant application. Four to be completed at the end of each quarter four per quarter or one per quarter = 4	Summarizes disbursements of major services by cash expenditures according to each budget line item, used to prepare federal and state monitoring reports and determining unit cost.

Table 6.8 Cost breakdown by service

	Month	Year to Date	Budgeted Figure	+/– Balance
Income				
Grant				
Cash				
In-Kind				
Total				
Expenses				
Personnel				
Travel				
Bldg. Space				
Communication				
Utilities				
Supplies				
Equipment				
Contracts				
Other				
Total				
Net				

Table 6.9 Statement of income and expenditures

and third columns are compared, the percentage figure obtained shows the ULM whether the budgeted or projected figures were met.

For example, if $350,000 was spent on personnel through a certain date and $400,000 was budgeted for the entire year, 75 percent of the budgeted funds have been spent and 25 percent non-expended funds remain. A ULM then needs to determine whether this balance is sufficient for the remaining months in the fiscal year. If these figures were reported for the end of the third quarter, there would be no need to worry because 25 percent is equal to one quarter of the fiscal year – and the agency would be on target financially. If the report period fell at the end of the second quarter, however, an administrator should be quite concerned. At that rate of expense for personnel, the ULM would probably need $60,000 to cover costs for the whole year and would have overspent this line item by $20,000 ($60,000 less $40,000). It should be clear that each column contains information vital to the financial health of the agency. In particular, the last column must be interpreted meaningfully by the administrator.

The second form, the *operating statement by service*, summarizes funds disbursed by each service category to provide an assessment of whether the funds spent for each service are on target with the budgeted or projected figure. This form appears as Table 6.10.

The computations for each column in this form are preformed exactly as in the statement of income and expense except that the column figures are organized by service. For example, all disbursements for I & R are recorded in the first column; this figure may be obtained from the ledger. These are costs for personnel, travel, building space, etc. as they are related specifically to that service. When one examines the balance column for each service, a clear picture of the financial health of each service as well as the entire agency (bottom line) can be obtained.

These two forms, the income and expense statements and the operating statement by services provide any administrator with an awareness of whether there is a need for any corrective financial changes. These forms also pinpoint service categories that are on target, those that are not on target, and indicate the stability of the agency. These forms should assist administers in making monetary decisions because they will know *beforehand* whether cost can be afforded.

The third form is the *cost breakdown by services* which summarizes disbursements of major services by cash expenditures according to each budget

Service Category	Disbursements in Month	Year to Date Disbursements	Yearly Budget Figure	+/ – Balance
I & R				
Outreach				
Transportation				
Friendly Visiting				
Telephone Reassurance				
Center Activities				
Total–Entire Agency				

Table 6.10 Service form

line time. The information on this form can be used to complete federal and state quarterly report forms and is therefore most useful in monitoring all aspects of an entire agency and computing unit cost for the agency.

Following is the procedure used to compute line item costs. For example, the first line item is the costs to commute personnel:

1. List each person.
2. Determine a percentage of time spent by *each* staff member in *each* service. If no time is spent in a particular service, then the column is left blank. An example is shown in Table 6.11.

Staff	I & R	Outreach	Handyman	Telephone Reassurance	Friendly Visiting	Center Operations
V.M.	10	10	10			70
J.B.	5	25	10	2.5	2.5	55

Table 6.11 Cost breakdown by services

3. To arrive at a personnel cost per month, multiply the obtained percentages by the monthly wage of the respective staff member. Total the percentage cost of each person to arrive at the personnel budget line-time figure entered in the Disbursements by Major Services form. For example, if a staff person spent 10 percent of time in one service and the wage was $25,000 then the $2,500 would be charged to that service.

The figures and cash expenditures for each service are obtained from ledger and added together to obtain totals. This part of the form specifies where funds were expended by each line time in the budget according to each major service.

These are two additional steps to be completed in *computing unit cost.* First, insert the annual output measure for each identified service. Then divided the output measure into the total expenditures and enter that figure on the unit cost line. For example, the objective figure for outreach is $479, which is divided into the total expenditures for outreach: $3,558, resulting in the unit cost of $8.48 per unit of outreach service. The formula for the computing unit cost is:

Total Expenditures for Service = Unit Cost
Output Measure (Objective)
$3,588= Unit Cost
479
$8.49= Unit Cost

To be most helpful, this form should be completed five times throughout the fiscal year. It should be first completed in its entirety using annual figures and included in the grant application. This information will provide an estimate of the expenses needed to provide the service and to create an awareness of budget items which could be changed to provide a more efficient service or simply to reduce costs. The form should also be completed at the end of each quarter and actually quarterly service utilization numbers should also be checked for any variation in unit cost which would require administrative action.

In summary, these three internal management forms help ULMs fiscally monitor and control their programs. Each form summarizes ledger information in a manner useful to administrators and promotes a better understanding of making monetary decisions, completing the federal and state report forms in-house, and requesting budget revisions when indicated.

THE IMPORTANCE OF A BUDGET

A budget is an organizational plan of financial action. It tells 1) the number of people necessary to provide a specific service or set of services and the amount to be paid to each person and 2) the cost to support the services such as travel, supplies, utilities, etc.

Thus, in preparing a budget and determining unit cost, the following steps should be taken:

Step 1. Determine the number of services being provided or to be provided in the next fiscal period. Determine an objective for each service. Complete the agency mission worksheet.

Step 2. Determine the number and type of people needed to provide the services identified and meet the objective stated in Step 1. Also, determine their employment status as full time or part time. Make certain that the number of people (person power) and the type of people (job classification, i.e., volunteer, social worker, aide) match the outcome for the service.

Step 3. Determine the cost for each budget item needed to support the delivery of each service.

Step 4. Once each budget line item, including personnel for each service, has been determined; add all the figures for each service to determine the total amount needed to run the program.

Step 5. Divide the total dollar figure for each service by its outcome measure to determine the unit cost for each service.

In each step, use the guidelines prepared by the funding agency to be consistent with their requirements in the grant application. These guidelines usually detail the method to compute or determine the cost for each budget item.

ASSIGNMENT

1. Complete a cost breakdown by service form in relation to your annual grant application.
2. Complete a monthly income and expenses form using last month's ledger information.
3. Complete a monthly operating statement by services form using last month's ledger information.
4. Complete your agency's request for funds form supplied by your funding agency.

Disbursements by Major Services and Funding Source

Federal Funding					State Funding		
Cash Expenditures	I & R	Outreach	Transportation	Tel. Reass.	Friendly Visit	Center	Center Activities
Personnel	7,212	2,483				5,289	800
Travel	492	454					152
Building Space							118
Communications	483						
Utilities							
Printing Supplies	454	87					274
Equipment						15,656	
Contracts							
Other	870		1,121				33
Total Cash Expenditures	9,511	3,024				20,945	1,377
In-Kind Cash Personnel Building Space	778 990	534	198			3,696	
Total Expenditures	10,279	3,558	1,319			24,641	
Output Measure (Objectives)	225 I&R 1,001 FR 888 Tel	419 Visit Reass.	735			7,408	7,408
Unit Cost Per Unit of Service	$5.27	$8.49	$1.79			$3.33	$.34

July – Disbursements by Major Services
Federal Funding

Cash Expenditures I & R Outreach Handyman Tele Friendly **Center State Total** **Reassur** **Visiting Operations**								
Personnel	79	84	90	6	6	636		901
Travel		47				51		98
Building Space		1	1			33		35
Communications	9	4	7	4	4	58		88
Utilities	7	4	7	4	4	50		76
Printing & Supplies								
Equipment								
Contracts								
Insurance								
Other	49	24	48	24	24	316		486
In-Kind Total	146	163	156	38	38	1,144		1,684
Cash								
Personnel				101	101	51		
Building Space	8	8	8	8	8	746		
TOTAL EXPENDITURES	154	171	164	147	147	1,941		
Output Measures	21		11	35	49	1,124		
Unit Cost Per Person Per Unit of Service	$7.33		$15.00	$4.20	$3.00	$1.73		

Worksheets for Determining Unit Cost

In this task, you are to compute a unit cost per service, choosing at least one service from your or another agency. A series of forms are to be used in order to calculate a unit cost and these forms may be used for any service you choose.

Financial Management

Name of Agency: ____________________

A. Mission

B. Major Goals of Agency

C. Agency Service Objectives

1.
2.
3.
4.

D. Agency Performance Measures for each Service Objective

1.
2.
3.
4.

Worksheet for Computing Line Item Costs by Service

A. Personnel

	Service Category			Total (100%)	
Staff			1	2	
1.	( )	( )	( )	( )	
2.	( )	( )	( )	( )	
3.	( )	( )	( )	( )	
4.	( )	( )	( )	( )	
Total					

Personnel Cost by Service Category

B. Travel

Travel	Service Category					Total (100%) Annual
Local	( )	( )	( )	( )		
National	( )	( )	( )	( )		
Total						

Travel Cost by Service Category

C. Building Space

Building Space	Service Category				Total (100%) Annual
Square Feet	( )	( )	( )	( )	

7

WHERE DATA MEETS DOLLARS: DECISION-MAKING EPILOGUE

Decision making occurs at all levels in an organization. When managers of an organization must decide how to solve a problem, two basic types of decisions are made in organizations: programmed and non-programmed (Alkin *et al*, 1985). In programmed decision making, managers respond to issues or problems that are routine or recurring. For example, the clinical managers have to make certain decisions including supervising and evaluating personnel while the upper level managers have to decide about all different components of an organization. However, the upper level manager makes decisions which obviously are more public and have greater consequences on the life and sustainability of an organization. Non-programmed decision making, however, involves searching for the extra information needed to make the right choice because the problem or opportunity has not been experienced before, or the degree of uncertainty about how managers should respond is critical. In this chapter we will look at services that emphasize the critical nature of decision making.

A major distinction in decision making is that one must rely on a combination of the knowledge learned and the evaluation and the financial management chapters, but then incorporate what is occurring in the external environment. For example, one must understand the political context, the availability of dollars and/or funds, the support of certain organizations and the competition of other organizations and key stakeholders that one can rely or not rely upon is the ability of key personnel/staff to develop or implement a project. Decision making in this context is directly connected to the chapter on leadership because it is the factoring in under judgment combined with one's knowledge base which is how one in the upper level management is judged. In short, decision making is a critical factor in determining leadership.

Decision making at the upper level will be stressed because it is critical to the life of an organization. Making decisions is essential to the components at all organizational levels, i.e. that which is personal and those which are organizational in context. Both are dependent on each other, but can be understood separately. Many personal decisions are easy to identify, such as buying a car, buying a house, and so forth (Rudzitis, 1985). Organizational decisions are much more complex because they involve higher investment and many more actors in the process. The outcome may not often be as clear. It is also critical to understand that decision making is dependent on the person and his/her ability to make decisions as well as their leadership ability (Jungermann, 1980).

While knowledge of content has been delineated in previous chapters on financial management and evaluation procedures, a basis for acquiring reasonable good and adequate information for an organizational decision will likely have additional data sources which are likely not to be very detailed. Such information is usually referred to as "soft data" which requires an understanding of an assessment from which a personal determination will have to be made (Berg, 2010).

As previously noted, Mele (2010) could point to decision making being straight forward and complex. Straight-forward decisions may be those in an organization which seem perfectly clear and easy to understand. For example, a straight-forward decision may be the desire for a new service. However, for such a decision to proceed is likely to become complex should it not be clear how the program will pay for itself, whether external or grant funds can be secured, and it may depend on the economy. Ariel (2009) indicates that the end of rational economics is upon us. In short, it may seem like a reasonable amount of funds or grant money is available at one time which may not likely be available in a few months or next year. In short, the reading of the environment often mitigates the knowledge obtained through one's understanding of financial management and evaluation.

In another context, Mele (2010) indicates that practical wisdom is a strong component of decision making. In his concept, practical wisdom involves a decision based on its contribution to the human good. This is very hard to define since it seems to depend on one's experience with the human good. It also involves one's thoroughness and preparedness in understanding the complexity of a decision and the extent to which it will both benefit people and be economically viable. Another key factor for a decision maker to understand is when faced with having to make a decision which is new to him or her and/or different from previous decisions. For example, such decisions may affect responses such as the decision was too complicated, too difficult or too serious. These responses indicate that individual decision makers are likely to have a high degree of indecisions since they will have to bear the consequences of their actions.

Nolan and Johnson (2011) note that self-reflection and self-insight is a very important component of decision making. It is critical to do a self-appraisal and/or assessment when key decisions are made among alternative outcomes (management) to better understand what elements went well and should be stressed, as well as what elements could be improved. For example, were staff, practitioners, stakeholders, Board people, and political people appropriately involved and did they respond as one thought they might? Was the proposal process on target as well as each step being clearly identified?

One typical component often overlooked is the flow of information. In today's environment there is an ever-increasing reliance on information being obtained through technology and the social media. However, information learned via supervisors, clinical and upper level managers is that listening, establishing, and maintaining quality relationships is paramount. This means that decision making and leadership depend much more on personality and communication in establishing and keeping relationships than on a primary knowledge base (Lewis *et al.*, 2007).

Smith *et al.* (2008) notes that power changes not only a person's responsibilities but also the way a person thinks. They suggests that people with powerful positions can make good decisions even when they consciously think they are not, because they may not understand all of the aspects in a situation and may focus directly on components that they understand relative to the outcome. One of the most important aspects of leadership and decision making is the ability of the decision maker to detail and be relatively comfortable with risk assessment. It has been mentioned that practically every decision is likely to have some effects which are more difficult and complex and not easy to understand, thus there is a certain element of risk. This is an area for which one may not have much self-confidence, confidence in detailing with participatory management and much practical experience. Risk often is likely to also involve an understanding of a vision for an organization and its direction under a period of a few years down the road. For example, can the program continue to attract, enroll and sustain clients, or revise service programs, and are they able to be innovative?

When dealing with risk assessment, Martin (2007) notes one should have an understanding of preparing alternatives to a potential problem in a new or existing program. If group input is needed however, the manager should avoid the potential of groupthink by not accurately processing important information relevant to this decision. For example, in the meantime, one should be following a new program throughout the entire process and see how it is moving along or if a problem arises which needs to be addressed. This is an important component of decision making because since one cannot predict what will happen throughout a project, each step of a new project or for regular projects, a decision maker needs to consider alternative steps for action which can be taken should problems arise.

It seems clear that decision making on both the personal and organizational level is more an art than a science according to Ariel (2009), while one can study components of leadership and decision making. As Rudizitis

(1985) indicates, decision making can best be obtained through practical experiences. In other words, one needs to learn decision making by actually doing it and then analyzing and understanding one's behavior. Since it involves taking responsibility for every decision, for considering risk, and for having an understanding of "soft data," that the decision process may be more complex and complicated as one imagines, an understanding which includes a mix and blending of actual financial and evaluation data.

ASSIGNMENTS

In order to operationalize how decisions get made in human service agencies, five core concerns must be addressed:

1. Distinguish between simple/straight-forward and complex decisions.
2. List and describe several aspects of complex decisions.
3. Identify the personal art of decision-making as you understand it.
4. How would you connect leadership with decision-making?
5. Explain how you would integrate/include financial management and evaluation with leadership and decision-making.

REFERENCES

Alcohol abuse up, alcoholism down. (2004, June 11). Retrieved October 23, 2008, from CBS News website: http://www.cbsnews.com/stories/2004/06/11/health/main622706.shtml?tag=mncol;lst;1.

Alexander, E. (1995). *How organizations act together: Interorganizational coordination in theory and practice.* Luxembourg: Gordon and Breach.

Alkin, Marvin C. and Associates. (1985). *A guide for decision makers.* Beverly Hills, CA: Sage Publications.

Allen, B. & Smith, A. (2008). Special report: Reduced funding cripples Head Start from reaching its potential. Alexandria, VA: National Head Start for America Press (www.nhsa.org).

American Evaluation Association. (2009). American Evaluation Association: Guiding principles for evaluators. *American Journal of Evaluation, 30,* 273–274.

Ariel, D. (2009). The end of rational economics. *Harvard Business Review 87* (7/8), 78–85.

Armour, M. P., Bain, B., & Rubio, R. J. (2006). *Educating for cultural competency: Tools for training field instructors.* Alexandria, VA: Council on Social Work Education.

Austin, D. A. (1985). Administrative practice in human services: Future directions for curriculum development. In S. Slavin (ed.), *An introduction to human services management,* 2nd edn (pp.14–27). New York: Haworth Press.

Bartlett, H. (1958). Working definition of practice. *Social Work, 3* (2), 5–8.

Bartlett, H. (1970). *The common base of social work practice.* Silver Spring, MD: National Association of Social Workers.

Berg, R. W. (2010). Competition and cooperation: The wisdom to know when, *Business Communication Quarterly* 73 (2), 176–189.

Bliss, D. & Holosko, M. J. (2007). *Out of the closet and into the fray: Proactive social work leadership in the time of need.* Paper presented at the *Celebrating a Tradition of Caring: Social Work Practice, Today and Tomorrow* conference, Wurzweiler School of Social Work, Yeshiva University, New York.

Bliss, D. & Meehan, J. (2008). Blueprint for creating a social work-centered disaster relief initiative. *Journal of Social Service Research 34* (3), 73–85.

Bloom, M., Fischer, J., & Orme, L. (2003). *Evaluating practice: Guidelines for an accountable professional,* 4th edn. Boston, MA: Allyn & Bacon.

Boehm, W. (1958). The nature of social work. *Social Work*, *3*, 10–18.

Bowen, G. L., Mancini, J. A., Martin, J. A., Ware, W. B., & Nelson, J. P. (2003). An empirical test of a community practice model for promoting family adaptation. *Family Relations*, 52, 33–52.

Bowen, G. L., Martin, J. A., Mancini, J. A., & Nelson, J. P. (2000). Community capacity: Antecedents and consequences. *Journal of Community Practice*, *8(2)*, 1–21.

Brent, R. J. (2006). *Applied cost-benefit analysis,* 2nd edn. MA: Edward Elgar Publishing, Inc.

Brilliant, E. (1986). Social work leadership: A missing ingredient? *Social Work, 31* (5), 325–331.

Brown, L. & Stevens, B. (2006). Market watch: Charge of the right brigade? Communities, coverage, and care for the uninsured. *Health Affairs*, *25* (3): w150–w161.

Brueggmann, W. D. (2002). *The practice of macro practice*, 2nd edn. Belmont, CA: Brooks/Cole.

Bryson, J., Crosby, B., & Stone, M. (2006). The design and implementation of cross-sector collaborations: Proposals from the literature. *Public Administration Review*, *66*, 44–55.

Buckingham, M. & Coffman, C. (1999). *First, break all the rules.* New York, NY: Simon & Schuster.

Bulcke, G. (1994). *An exploration of factors that motivate career choice in social work among a sample of undergraduate social work studies.* Unpublished master's thesis, University of Windsor, Ontario.

Bullet, S. S. (2006). Evaluating the senior companion program: A mixed-method approach. *Journal of Gerontological Social Work*, *47* (1/2), 45–70.

Campbell, D. T. (1969). Reforms as experiments. *American Psychologist*, *24* (4), 409–429.

Chambers, D. (1993). *Social policy and social paradigms: A method for the practical public analyst,* 2nd edn. New York, NY: Macmillan Publishing.

Chambers, D. E. and Wedel, K.R. (2005). *Evaluating social programs.* Needham Heights, MA: Allyn & Bacon.

Chambers, M. & Connor, S. L. (2002). User-friendly technology to help family carers cope. *Journal of Advanced Nursing*, *40* (5), 568–577.

Chapin, R. K. (2006). *Social policy for effective practice.* Boston, MA: McGraw Hill.

Chapin, R. K. & Cox, E. (2001). Changing the paradigm: Strengths-based and empowerment-oriented social work with frail elders. *Journal of Gerontological Social Work*, *36* (3/4), 165–179.

Chess, W. A., Norlin, J. M., and Jayaratne, S. D. (1987). Social work administration 1981–1985: Alive, happy and prospering. *Administration in Social Work*, *11* (2), 67–77.

Ciulla, J. B. (ed.) (1998). *Ethics, the heart of leadership*. Westport, CT: Praeger.

Clements, P., Chianca, T., & Sasaki, R. (2008). Reducing world poverty by improving evaluation of developmental aid. *American Journal of Evaluation*, *29*, 195.

Cohen, D. (1970). Politics and research: Evaluation of social action programs in education. *Review of Educational Research*, *40* (2), 213–238.
Conboy, A., Auerbach, C., Beckerman, A., Schnall, D., & LaPorte, H. H. (2000). MSW student satisfaction with using single system design computer software to evaluate social work practice. *Research on Social Work Practice*, *10* (1), 127–138.
Cramer, A., Roberts, S., & Liyan, X. (2007). Evaluating community-based programs for eliminating secondhand smoke using evidence-based research for best practices. *Family and Community Health*, *30* (2), 129–143.
Cronbach, L. J. & Associates. (1980). *Toward reform of program evaluation.* San Francisco: Jossey-Bass.
Davidson Perlmutter, F. and Crook, W. (2004). *Changing hats while managing change: From social work to administration,* 2nd edn. Washington, D.C.: NASW Press.
Davis, R. C. & Auchter, B. (2010). National institute of justice funding of experimental studies of violence against women: A critical look at implementation issues and policy implications. *Journal of Experimental Criminology*, *6* (4), 377–395.
Deborah, L. W. (2010). Using a systems orientation and foundational theory to enhance theory-driven human service program evaluations. *Evaluation and Program Planning*, *33* (2), 67–80.
Derezotes, B. (1999). *Advanced generalist social work practice.* Thousand Oaks, CA: Sage Publication.
Donaldson, S. & Scriven, M. (eds) (2003). *Evaluating social programs and problems: Visions for the new millennium.* Mahwah, NJ: Lawrence Erlbaum Associates.
Donaldson, S. I., Gooler, L. E., & Scriven, M. (2002). Strategies for managing evaluation anxiety: Toward a psychology of program evaluation. *American Journal of Evaluation*, 23(3), 261–273. doi:10.1016/S1098-2140(02)00209-6.
Drucker, P. F. (2001). *The essential Drucker.* New York: HarperCollins Publishers.
Drumm, R. D., McCoy, H. V., & Lemon, A. (2003). Technology trauma: Barriers to increasing technology utilization. *Journal of Social Work in Health Care*, *37* (4), 39–56.
DuBrin, A. (2000). *The complete idiot's guide to leadership.* Madison, WI: Alpha Books and CWL Publishers.
Dunham, W. (2008). Prescription drug abuse seen up, cocaine down. September 4. Retrieved October 23, 2008, from Reuters website: http://www.reuters.com/article/healthNews/idUSN0331471920080904.
Dunlop, J. & Angell, G.B. (2001). Inside-outside: Boundary-spanning challenges in building rural health coalitions. *Professional-Development*, *4(1)*, 40–48.
Dunlop, J. & Holosko, M. (2004). The story behind the story of collaborative networks – relationships do matter! *Journal of Health and Social Policy*, *19(3)*, 1–18.
Durning, S. J., Hemmer, P., & Pangaro, L. N. (2007). The structure of program evaluation: An approach for evaluating a course, clerkship, or components of a residency or fellowship training program. *Teaching and Learning in Medicine*, *19* (3), 308–318.
EPA orders the lead out of our air: Activists move to slash emissions by 90 percent, but have concerns. (2008, October 16). Retrieved October 23, 2008, from MSNBC website: http://www.msnbc.msn.com/id/27216428/,http://water.usgs.gov/nawqa/Rosen.trends.09262008.pdf.

Fact sheet: Type 2 diabetes. (2008). Retrieved October 23, 2008, from National Institute of Health website: http://www.nih.gov/about/researchresultsforthepublic/Type2Diabetes.pdf.

Feit, M. D. (1979). *Management and administration of drug and alcohol programs.* Springfield, IL: Charles C. Thomas.

Feit, M. D. (1982). Management and administration of alcohol programs, in E. M. Pattison and E. Kaufman (eds), *The encyclopedia handbook of alcoholism.* New York: Gardner Press, Chapter 97.

Feit, M. D. (1987). *Clinician to executive: Steps along the way.* Paper presented at the Second Annual NASW Virginia Conference, Williamsburg, VA.

Feit, M. D. and Chei Li, P. K. (1998). *Financial management in human services.* New York: The Haworth Press.

Feit, M. D. and Landon, P. S. (1982). *Management and administration of social work programs: A model for understanding what it's all about.* Paper presented at the Administration Symposium, CSWE Annual Program Meeting, New York.

Feit, M. D., Paik, Sook Ja, and Wodarski, J. S. (1995). Becoming an administrator: Are current educational practices adequate? *The Journal of Applied Social Sciences 19* (1), 9.37–45.

Flexner, A. (1915). Is social work a profession? *Proceedings of the National Conference of Charities and Corrections.* Chicago, IL: Hildmann Printing.

Franklin, C. (2001). Coming to terms with the business of direct practice social work. *Research on Social Work Practice, 11* (2), 235–244.

Gambrill, E. (1997). *Social work practice: A critical thinker's guide.* New York: Oxford University.

GAO. (May 1999). *Government auditing standards: Amendment No. 1 documentation requirements when assessing control risk at maximum for controls significantly dependent upon computerized information systems.* Washington, D.C., United States General Accounting Office.

Germaine, C. & Gitterman, A. (1980). *The life model of social work practice: Advances in theory and practice.* New York: Columbia University Press.

Geva-May, I. & Thorngate, W. (2003). Reducing anxiety and resistance in policy and programme evaluations: A socio-psychological analysis. *Evaluation: The International Journal of Theory, Research and Practice*, 9(2), 205–227. doi:10.1177/1356389003009002006.

Gibbs, L. (2002). *COPES Evidence-based approach to helping practitioners connect evidence to practice.* Available online at: http://www.evidence.brookscole.com/copse.html (last accessed September 6, 2012).

Gibbs, L. (2003). *Evidence-based practice for the helping professions. A practical guide with integrated multi-media.* Pacific Grove, CA: Brooks/Cole.

Gibbs, L. & Gambrill, E. (2002). Evidence-based practice: Counter arguments to objections. *Research on Social Work Practice, 12*, 452–476.

Gilchrist, A. (2000). The well connected community: Networking to the edge of chaos. *Community Development Journal, 35(3)*, 264–275.

Goldstein, E. G. (2006). Social work education and clinical learning: Yesterday, today and tomorrow. *Clinical Social Work Journal, 35* (1), 15–23.

Gordon, J. (2002). *Our air, their air: Most of it is bad*, November 10. Retrieved October 23, 2008, from New York Times website: http://query.nytimes.com/gst/fullpage.html?res=980DE6D7113EF933A25752C1A9649C8B63.

Gordon, W. (1962). A critique of the working definition. *Social Work*, *7* (4), 3–13.

Graddy, E. & Chen, B. (2006). Influences on the size and scope of networks for social delivery. *Journal of Public Administration Research and Theory, 16*, 533–552.

Grady, A. (1995). Building inclusive community: A challenge for occupational therapy. *American Journal of Occupational Therapy, 49*, 300–310.

Graham, K. (2002). *Studies in vision and management: Interviews with UN leaders.* Unpublished paper, Amman: UN Leadership Academy.

Green, L. (2008). Making research relevant: If it is an evidence-based practice, where's the practice-based evidence? *Family Practice 2008, 25*, i20–24.

Greene, J. (1988). Stakeholder participation and utilization in program evaluation. *Evaluation Review, 12* (2), 91–116.

Greene, R. (1986). *Social work with the aged and their families.* New York: Hawthorne, Aldine de Gruyter.

Gregerson, H. & Sailer, L. (1993). Chaos theory and its implications for social science research. *Human Relations, 46(7)*, 777–803.

Gross, Malvern J. and Jablonsky, S. (1979). *Principles of accounting and financial reporting for nonprofit organizations.* New York: John Wiley and Son.

Guba, E. & Lincoln, Y. (1981). *Effective evaluation: Improving the usefulness of evaluation results through responsive and naturalistic approaches.* San Francisco, CA: Jossey-Bass.

Guenther, J., Arnott, A., Bartjen-Westermann, C., Haynes, L., Howard, R., Kalender, L., & Watkinson, J. (2010, September). Working with non-government organizations: Dropping the defenses and building bridges. AES conference, *Reflecting on evaluation*, Wellington, NZ.

Gummer, B. (1990) *The politics of social administration: managing organizational politics in social agencies.* Englewood Cliffs, NJ: Prentice Hall Publishing Co.

Hacker, J. (2008). Perspective: Putting politics first. *Health Affairs*, May/June, 27(3), 718–723.

Hairston, C. F. (1985). *Costing nonprofit services: Developments, problems, and issues. Administration in Social Work*, 9(1), 47–55.

Hardy, J. (2007). Technology and program evaluation. *American School Board Journal*, 25 (4), 29–31.

Hartley, J. & Allison, M. (2002). The role of leadership on the modernization and improvement in public services. In J. Reynolds, J. Henderson, J. Sedan, J. Charlesworth, & A. Bullman (eds), *The managing care reader* (pp. 296–305). Buckingham, UK: Open University Press.

Hasenfeld, Y. (1983). *Human service organizations.* Englewood Cliffs, N.J.: Prentice-Hall, Inc.

Hasenfeld, Y. Z., Hill, K., & Weaver, D. (2003). *A participatory model for evaluating social programs.* San Francisco, CA: The James Irvine Foundation.

Heller, P. (2006). *The prospects of creating 'fiscal space' for the health sector.* International Monetary Fund, Washington, DC.

Hendricks, M. & Bamberger, M. (2010). The ethical implications of underfunding development evaluations. *American Journal of Evaluation, 31* (4), 549–556.

Holloway, S. (1980). Up the hierarchy: From clinician to administrator. *Administration in Social Work*, 4(4), 1–14.

Holosko, D. A. & Holosko, M. J. (2004). What is unique about social work practice with the elderly? In M. J. Holosko & M. D. Feit (eds), *Social work practice with the elderly*, 3rd edn. Toronto, ON: Canadian Scholar's Press Inc.

Holosko, M. J. (1987). A model for evaluating rehabilitation programs: The case example of the St. John's Job Generation Project. In R. I. Brown (ed.), *Special Edition, Vocational Counseling in Rehavilitation, NATCON, 14*, Minister of Supply and Services, Ottawa, ONT Canada.

Holosko, M. (1988). Prerequisites for EAP evaluations: A case for more thoughtful evaluation planning. In M. Holosko & M. D. Feit (eds), *Evaluation of employee assistance programs* (pp. 59–68). New York, NY: The Haworth Press, Inc.

Holosko, M. J. (1996). Obstacles to conducting program evaluations: Implications for public health evaluators. *Journal of Health and Social Policy, 8* (1), 91–101.

Holosko, M. J. (1997). Service user input: Fact or fiction? The evaluation of the trauma program, Department of Rehabilitation, Sault Ste. Marie, Ontario. *The Canadian Journal of Program Evaluation, 11(2)*, 111–126.

Holosko, M. (2000). The churchs' response to welfare reform in America: Focus on the southeastern states. In L. Nackerud and M. Robinson (eds), *Early Implications of Welfare Reform in the Southeast.* Huntington, New York: Nova Sciences Publishers, Inc.

Holosko, M. J. (2003). The history of the working definition of practice. *Research on Social Work Practice, 13* (3), 271–283.

Holosko, M. J. (2006). A suggested authors' checklist for submitting manuscripts to Research on Social Work Practice. *Research on Social Work Practice, 16* (4), 449–454.

Holosko, M. J. (2009a). Becoming an evidence-based practitioner. *International Conference on Social Work and Counseling Practice: Promoting Harmony and Justice in a World of Conflict.* Invited Keynote Address, Hong Kong, SAR, PRC.

Holosko, M. J. (2009b). Global realities of social policy: The devolution revolution. *Journal of Social Work in Public Health, 24(3)*, May-June..

Holosko, M. J. (2009c). Social work leadership: Identifying core attributes. *Journal of Human Behavior in the Social Environment, 19*, 448–459.

Holosko, M. J. (2010a). Challenges of becoming an evidence-based practitioner: The need for a new knowledge-based model. *Joint World Conference on Social Work and Social Development*, Invited Address, Hong Kong, SAR, PRC.

Holosko, M. J. (2010b). What types of designs are we using in social work research and evaluation? *Research on Social Work Practice, 20*, 665–673.

Holosko, M. J. (2011). Evaluating quantitative research studies. In R. Grinnell, Jr. and Y. Unrau (eds), *Social work research and evaluation* (9th edn). New York: Oxford University Press

Holosko, M. J. & Dunlop, J. (1992). Evaluating interorganizational approaches to service delivery: A case example of the Family Violence Service Project in Kent county, Ontario. *The Canadian Journal of Program Evaluation, 7(2)*, 115–129.

Holosko, M. J. & Feit, M. D. (1981) *Workbook for internal management.* Knoxsville, TN: The University of Tennessee School of Social Work, pp. 71–86.

Holosko, M. J. & Feit, M. D. (2006). Living in poverty in America today. *Journal of Health and Social Policy, 21* (1), 119–131.

Holosko, M. & Holosko, D. (2004). What's unique about social work practice with the elderly. In M. J. Holosko and M. D. Feit (eds), *Social work practice with the elderly,* 3rd edn. Toronto, Ont.: The Canadian Scholar's Press Inc.

Holosko, M. & Leslie, D. (1998). Obstacles to conducting empirically-based practice. In J. Wodarski & B. Thyer (eds), *Handbook of empirical social work, Volume 2: Social problems and practice issues.* New York, NY: Wiley and Sons, Inc.

Holosko, M. J. & MacCaughelty, C. (2009). Planning evaluations of employee assistance programs using information technology. In M. A. Richard, W. G. Emener, & W.S. Hutchison, Jr., *Employee Assistance Programs: Wellness/Enhancement Programming* (4th edn). Springfield, IL: Charles C. Thomas Publisher.

Holosko, M. & Taylor, P. (eds) (1992). *Social work practice in health care settings,* 2nd edn. Toronto, Ontario: The Canadian Scholar's Press Inc.

Holosko, M. J. & Thyer, B. (2011). *A Pocket Glossary for Commonly Used Research Terms*. Thousand Oaks, CA: Sage Publications.

Holosko, M. J., Feit, M., & Bulcke, G. (1998). Health care prevention: Real or rhetoric. *Journal of Health and Social Policy, 10(1)*, 101–104.

Holosko, M. J., Leslie, D. R., & Cassano, D. R. (2001). How service users become empowered in human service organization: The empowerment model. *International Journal of Health Care Quality Assurance, 14* (2), 126–132.

Holosko, M. J., Thyer, B., & Danner, E. (2009a). Ethical guidelines for designing and conducting evaluations of social work practice. *Journal of Evidence-Based Practice, 6*, 348–360.

Holosko, M. J., Thyer, B. A., & Danner, E. (2009b). Ethical guidelines for designing and conducting evaluations of social work practice. *Journal of Human Behavior in the Social Environment, 19*, 448–459.

Hseih, Chang-ming (2006). Using client satisfaction to improve case management services for the RI elderly. *Research on Social Work Practice, 16*, 605–612.

Hseih, Chang-ming (2009). Importance counts: The role of relative importance of service elements in client satisfaction measures. *Journal of Social Service Resarch, 35*, 23–31.

Hubball, H. & Bert, H. (2007). Learning outcomes and program-level evaluation in a four-year undergraduate pharmacy curriculum. *American Journal of Pharmaceutical Education, 71* (5), 1–8.

Human, S. & Provan, K. (2000). Legitimacy building in the evolution of small-firm multi-lateral networks: A comparative study of success and demise. *Administrative Science Quarterly, 45(2)*, 327–365.

Jago, A. G. & Vroom, V. H. (1977). Hierarchical level and leadership style. *Organizational Behavior and Human Performance, 18*, 131–145.

James, W. (1906). What pragmatism means. In *Pragmatism and other essays* (pp. 22–28). New York: Washington Square Press.

Johnson, L. & Yanca, S. (2006). *Social work practice: A generalist approach,* 9th edn. Boston, MA: Allyn and Bacon.

Judge, W. Q., Naoumova, I., & Douglas, T. (2009). Organizational capacity for change and firm performance in a transition economy. *The International Journal of Human Resource Management, 20* (8), 1737–1752.

Jungermann, Helmut (1980) Speculation about decision-theoretic aids for personal decision-making, *Aeta Psychological 45*, 7–34.

Kaufman, J. S., Crusto, C. A., Quan, M., Ross, E., Friedman, S., O'Reilly, K., & Call, S. (2006). Utilizing program evaluation as a strategy to promote community change: Evaluation of comprehensive, community-based, family-violence initiative. *American Journal of Community Psychology, 38* (3/4), 191–200.

Kee, J. (1999). At what price? Benefit-cost analysis and cost-effectiveness analysis in program evaluation. *The Evaluation Exchange, V(2/3)*, 1–4.

Knitzer, J. & Cooper, J. (2006). Beyond integration: Challenges for children's mental health. *Health Affairs*, May/June, *25(3)*, 670–679.

Lackey, J. F. (2006). *Accountability in social service: The culture of the paper program*. New York: The Haworth Press.

Larsen, D. L., Attkinsson, C. C., Hargreaves, W. A., & Nguyen, T. D. (1979). Assessment of client/patient satisfaction: Development of a general scale. *Evaluation and Program Planning*, 2, 197–202.

Lehoux, P., Sicotte, C., & Denis, J. L. (1999). Assessment of a computerized medical record system: Disclosing scripts of use. *Evaluation and Program Planning*, 22, 439–453.

Leslie, D., Holosko, M. J., & Dunlop, J. (2006). Using information technology in planning program evaluation. In J. Dunlop & M. J. Holosko (eds) *Information technology and evidence-based social work practice*, pp. 73–91. Binghampton, NewYork, NY: The Haworth Press Inc.

Levitas, R. (2000). Community, utopia and new labour. *Local Economy*, *15*, 188–197.

Lewis, J. A., Lewis, M. D., and Packard, T. S. F., Jr. (2007) *Management of human service programs*, 4th edn. Belmont, CA: Brooks/Cole.

Lewis, J.A., Lewis, M.D., and Souflee, Jr., F. (1991) *Management of human service Programs*. Belmont, CA: Brooks/Cole Publishing Co.

Lubove, R. (1973). *The professional altruist*. New York: Harvard University Press.

Martin, R. (2007) How successful leaders think, *Harvard Business Review 85* (6), 60–67.

Mason, R. (2007). The external environment's effect on management and strategy: A complexity theory approach. *Management Decision*, *25(1)*, 10–28.

McMillan, D. W. & Chavis, D. M. (1986). Sense of community: A definition and theory. *American Journal of Community Psychology*, *14(1)*, 6–23.

Mele, D. (2010). Practical wisdom in managerial decision making, *Journal of Management Development 29* (7/8), 637–645.

Mertens, D. M. (2009). *Research and evaluation in education and psychology: Integrating diversity with quantitative, qualitative, and mixed methods*, 3rd edn. Thousand Oaks, CA: Sage Publications.

Miller, T. I., Kobayashi, M. M., & Noble, P. M. (2006). Insourcing, not capacity building, a better model for sustained program evaluation. *American Journal of Evaluation*, *27* (1), 83–94. doi: 10.1177/1098214005283185.

Moses, T., Weaver, D., Furman, W., & Lindsey, D. (2003). Computerization and job attitudes in child welfare. *Administration in Social Work*, *27* (1), 47–67.

NASW (National Association of Social Workers). (2008). *Code of ethics*. Available online at http://www.naswdc.org/pubs/code/default.asp (last accessed September 6, 2012).

Nesoff, I. (2007). The importance of revitalizing management education for social workers. *Social Work*, *52* (3), 283–285.

Nolan, T. & Johnson, K. (2011) *The essential handbook for human service leaders*. Indianapolis, IN: Dog Ear Publishing.

Norvelle, J. W. (1989) *Introduction to fund accounting*, 3rd edn. Tucson, AZ: Thoth Books.

Obesity and overweight: U.S. obesity trends 1985–2007. (2008). Retrieved October 23, 2008, from Department for Health and Human Services Center for Disease Control and Prevention website: http://www.cdc.gov/nccdphp/dnpa/obesity/trend/maps/.

Osborn, R. & Hunt, J. (2007). Leadership and the choice of order: Complexity and hierarchical perspectives near the edge of chaos. *Leadership Quarterly*, *18*, 319–340.

Osborne, D. & Gaebler, T. (1992). *Reinventing government.* Reading, MA: Addison-Wesley, Inc.

Pati, S., Keren, R., Alessandrini, E., & Schwarz, D. (2004). Investing in children: Generational differences in U.S. public spending, 1980–200. *Health Affairs*, *23(5)*, 131–141.

Patti, R. J. (1983) *Social welfare administration: Managing social programs in a developmental context.* Englewood, NJ: Prentice-Hall, Inc.

Patti, R. J. & Austin, M. J. (1987). Socializing the direct service practitioner in the ways of supervisory management. *Administration in Social Work 1*, 267–280.

Patti, R. J., Diedrick, E., Olson, D., & Crowell, J. (1979) From direct service to administration: A study of social workers' transition from clinical to management roles. *Administration in Social Work*, *3*, 131–151.

Patton, M. Q. (1988). *Qualitative evaluation methods.* Newbury Park, CA: Sage Publications.

Patton, M. Q. (2002). *Qualitative research and evaluation methods.* Thousand Oaks, CA: Sage Publications.

Perlmutter, F. D. (1990). *Changing hats: From social work practice to administration.* Silver Spring MD: NASW Press.

Phillips, R., Gregory, P., & Nelson, M. (2003). Moving toward collaboration: Using funding streams to advance partnerships in child welfare practice. *Journal of Human Behavior in the Social Environment*, *7* (1/2), 115–124.

Pincus, A. & Minahan, A. (1973). *Social work practice: Model and method.* Itasca, IL: F.E. Peacock.

Pizacani, B. A., Dent, C. W., Maher, J. E., Rohde, K., Stark, M. J., Biglan, A., & Thompson, J. (2009) Smoking patterns in Oregon youth: Effects of funding and defunding of a comprehensive state tobacco control program. *Journal of Adolescent Health*, *44*, 229–236.

Pollio, D. (2006). The art of evidence-based practice. *Research on Social Work Practice*, *16* (2), 224–232.

Provan, K. & Milward, H. (2001). A preliminary theory of interorganization network effectiveness: A comparative study of four community mental health systems. *Administrative Science Quarterly*, *40*, 1–33.

Powell, R. R. (2006). Program evaluation: An overview. *Library Trends, 55* (1), 102–120.

Rama, D., Milano, B., Salas, S., & Liu, C. (2009). CSR implementation: Developing the capacity for collective action. *Journal of Business Ethics*, *85*, 463–477.

Ramsay, R. (2003). Transforming the working definition of social work into the 21st century. *Research on Social Work Practice*, *13*, 324–338.

Rank, M. & Hutchinson, W. (2000). An analysis of leadership with the profession. *Journal of Social Work Education*, *36* (3), 487–502.

Rapp, C. A. & Poertner, J. (1992). *Social administration: A client-centered approach.* NJ: Longman Publishing Co.

Reardon, R. C. & Hartley, S. (2007). Program evaluation of e-portfolios. *New Directions for Student Services*, Autumn (Fall), 119, 83–97.

Reedy, A., Luna, M., Rocio, G., Olivas, G. S., & Sujeer, A. (2005). Local public health performance measurement: Implementation strategies and lessons learned from aligning program evaluation indicators with the 10 essential public health services. *Journal of Public Health Management and Practice, 11* (4), 317–325.

Reid, W. & Epstein, L. (1972). *Task-centered casework*. New York: Columbia University Press.

Rejai, M. & Phillips, K. (2004). Leadership theory and human nature. *Journal of Political and Military Sociology, 32* (2), 185–192.

Robert Wood Foundation (2007) *Elder friendly communities*. Available online at: http://pweb1.rwjf.org/reports/grr/044682.htm (last accessed September 12, 2012).

Rossi, P. & Freeman, H. (1993). *Evaluation: A systematic approach*. Newbury Park, CA: Sage Publications.

Rossi, P. & Wright, S. (1967). Evaluation research: An assessment of theory, practice & politics. *Evaluation Quarterly, 1* (1), 5–52.

Rowe, W. (2000). Social work and globalization. *Canadian Social Work, Special Issue, 2* (1).

Royse, D., Thyer, B. A., Padgett, D. K., & Logan, T. (2011). *Program evaluation: An introduction*. Belmont, CA: Thomson Brooks/Cole.

Rudzitis, Inese (1985) *The art of effective decision making*. New York, NY: The Research Institute of America, Inc.

Rutman, L. (1980). *Planning useful evaluations: Evaluability assessment*. Beverly Hills, CA: Sage Publications.

Schwarz, C. & Struhkamp, G. (2007). Does evaluation build or destroy trust?: Insights from case studies on evaluation in higher education reform. *Evaluation, 13* (3), 323–339. doi: 10.1177/1356389007007862 5.

Scriven, M. (2007). Key evaluation checklist. *Western Michigan University*. Available online at: www.wmich.edu/evalctr/checklists (last accessed September 6, 2012).

Scurfield, R.M. (1981). Clinical to administrator: Difficult role transition?, *Social Work 26*, 6, 495–502.

Shirlow, P. & Murtagh, B. (2004). Capacity-building, representation and intracommunity conflict. *Urban Studies, 41(1)*, 57–70.

Smith, P. K., Dijksterhuis, Ap. and Wigboldus, Daniel, H.J. (2008) Powerful people making good decisions even when they consciously think, *Psychological Science 19* (12), 1258–1259.

Spreier, S., Fontaine, M., & Malloy, R. (2006). Leadership run amok: The destructive potential of overachievers. *Harvard Business Review*, June, 72–82.

Stoesz, B. (1997). The end of social work. In M. Reisch and E. Gambrill (eds), *Social Work in the 21st Century* (pp. 368–375). Thousand Oaks, CA: Pine Forge.

Stress a major health problem in the U.S., warns A.P.A. (2007). Retrieved October 23, 2008, from APA Online: Media Information website: http://www.apa.org/releases/stressproblem.html.

Suchman, E. (1967). *Evaluative research*. New York, NY: Russell Sage.

Sue, D. W. (2006). *Multi-cultural social work practice*. Hoboken, NJ: J. Wiley and Sons.

Taylor, V. (2007). Leadership for service improvement. *Nursing Management, 13* (9), 30–34.

Thomas, S. & Dahler-Larsen, P. (2006). When evaluation meets the rough ground in communities. *Evaluation, 12* (4), 496–505. doi: 10.1177/1356389006073745.

Thurston, W. E., Graham, J., & Hatfield, J. (2003). Evaluability assessment: A catalyst for program change and improvement. *Evaluation & the Health Professions, 26*, 206–221.

Thyer, B. (2001a). *The handbook of social work research methods.* Thousand Oaks, CA: Sage Publications.

Thyer, B. A. (2001b). What is the role of theory in research on social work practice? *Journal of Social Work Education, 38*,101–113.

Thyer, B. (2005). *The potentially harmful effects of theory in social work.* Paper presented at the Evaluation for Practice International Conference, Huddersfield, UK.

Thyer, B. & Kazi, M. (2004) *International perspectives: Evidence-based practice in social work.* London, UK: Venture Press Inc.

Thyer, B.A. & Myers, L. (2007). *A Social Worker's Guide to Evaluating Practice Outcomes.* Washington, DC: CSWE Press Inc.

Tourish, D. (2005). Critical upward communication: Ten commandments for improving strategy and decision making. *Long Range Planning, 38*, 485–503.

Trevisan, M. S. (2007). Evaluability assessment from 1986–2006. *American Journal of Evaluation, 28*, 290–303.

Tuller, L. W. (1997). *Finance for Non-Financial Managers and Small Business Owners.* Holbrook, MS: Adams Media Corporation.

Turner, J. B. (1998). Foreword. In P. L. Ewalt, E. M. Freeman, & D. L. Poole (eds), *Community building: Renewal, well-being, and shared responsibility.* Washington, DC: National Association of Social Workers Press.

Usher, C. L. & Wildfire, J. B. (2003). Evidence-based practice in community-based child welfare systems. *Child Welfare, 82*, 597–614.

Van Slyke, D. M. (2006) Agents or stewards: Using theory to understand the government–non-profit social service contracting relationship. *Journal of Public Administration Research and Theory*, electronic advance access, Oxford Press.

Van Voorhis, R. M. & Hostetter, C. (2006). The impact of MSW education on social worker empowerment and commitment to client empowerment through justice advocacy. *Journal of Social Work Education, 41* (1), 105–121.

VanLandingham, G. R. (2006). A voice crying in the wilderness: Legislative oversight agencies' efforts to achieve utilization. *New Directions for Evaluation, 112*, 25–39. doi: 10.1002/ev.20.

Violence in schools. (2008). Retrieved October 23, 2008, from Virginia Youth Violence Project website: http://youthviolence.edschool.virginia.edu/violence-in-schools/national-statistics.html.

Wade, K. & Neuman, K. (2007). Practice-based research: Changing the professional culture and language of social work. *Social Work in Health Care, 44* (4), 49–64.

Wadsworth, Y. (1991). *Everyday Evaluation On-The-Run.* Melbourne, Australia: Action Research Issues Association INC

Wakefield, J. (2001). *Social work as the pursuit of minimal distributive.* Paper presented at the Kentucky Conference on the Working Definition of Social Work Practice, Lexington, KY.

Wakefield, J. (2003). Gordon vs. the working definition: Lessons learned from a classic critique. *Research on Social Work Practice, 13* (2), 284–298.

Warner, M. & Hefetz, A. (2003). Rural-urban differences in privatization: Limits to the competitive state. *Environment and Planning Government and Policy, 21(5)*, 703–718.

Weersing, V. R. (2005). Benchmarking the effectiveness of psychotherapy: Program evaluation as a component of evidence-based practice. *American Academy of Child and Adolescent Psychiatry*, *44* (10), 1058–1062.

Weiss, C. (1977). The politicization of evaluation research. In C. Weiss (ed.), *Evaluating action programs: Readings in social action and education* (pp. 327–338). Boston, MA: Allyn & Bacon.

Weiss, C. H. (1987). Where politics and evaluation research meet. In D. J. Palumbo (ed.), *The politics of program evaluation* (pp. 47–70). Newbury Park, CA: Sage.

Williams, C. (2003). Global leadership, education, and human survival. *World Futures*, *59*, 301–313.

Williams, C. (2004). Community capacity-building: A critical evaluation of the third sector approach. *Review of Social Policy Research*, *21(5)*, 729–739.

Wimpfheimer, S. (2004). Leadership and management competencies defined by practice social work managers: An overview of standards developed by the National Network for Social Work Managers. *Administration in Social Work*, *28* (1), 45–56.

W. K. Kellog Foundation (nd). *W. K Kellogg Foundation evaluation handbook*. Available online at: http://www.wkkf.org/knowledge-center/resources/2006/02/WK-Kellogg-Foundation-Evaluation-Handbook.aspx (last accessed September 12, 2012).

Young, C. & Welsh, C. (2005). Stress, health and disease. *Cellscience Reviews*, *2(2)*. Retrieved October 23, 2008, from http://www.cellscience.com/reviews6/Stress_Health_Disease.html.

Youth violence: Fact sheet. (2007). Retrieved October 23, 2008, from Department of Health and Human Services Centers for Disease Control and Prevention website: http://www.cdc.gov/ncipc/factsheets/yvfacts.htm.

INDEX

References to tables are shown in bold and italics indicate figures.

ROOF CONSTRUCTION AND REPAIR

By E Molloy

With an introduction by Richard Jordan and Tim Ratcliffe

Routledge
Taylor & Francis Group
LONDON AND NEW YORK

First edition published in 1941 by George Newnes Limited, London.
Second edition published in 1945 by George Newnes Limited.

Published by Donhead Publishing Ltd 2009

Published 2015 by Routledge
2 Park Square, Milton Park, Abingdon, Oxon OX14 4RN
711 Third Avenue, New York, NY 10017, USA

Routledge is an imprint of the Taylor & Francis Group, an informa business

ISBN 13: 978-1-873394-88-5 (hbk)

British Library Cataloguing in Publication Data

Molloy, E.
Roof construction and repair.
1. Roofs--Design and construction. 2. Tiles, Roofing.
I. Title
690.1'5-dc22
ISBN-13: 9781873394885

Introduction to the 2009 edition

Roof Construction and Repair was first published in 1942, during the Second World War, and republished in a second slightly enlarged edition in 1945. The publication of new books was limited in wartime, and the fact that this was considered 'worth the paper' illustrates the practical concerns of the period. As so many skilled roofers had been sent off to fight in the war, the book was needed to give its readers a clear and practical understanding of roofing, even with limited prior knowledge.

Although the text contains simple explanations, and 'step by step' guidance, it is clear that Mr Molloy is a craftsman with considerable knowledge and a real passion for his subject. His real skill is in communicating the complexities of good roofing in ways that are easy to understand. This is the reason his writing is so useful for today's reader.

Anyone stimulated to absorb the level and depth of knowledge of a traditional roofer, who learned his trade before the last world war, will benefit from reading this book. About three quarters of the content relates to traditional roofing materials and techniques, and will be of direct interest and use to those involved with repairing old buildings. The remaining quarter describes materials and techniques that were prevalent at the time. Although these sections may not seem so immediately relevant, the fact that asbestos was used in some roofing felts during this period, as well as in cement tiles, is worth highlighting.

It is no surprise that there is a whole chapter on patching roofs and emergency repair methods. Although the concern was with damage caused by air raids, the methods advocated are relevant to anyone trying to patch a roof to prevent water ingress. Indeed, some of the suggestions highlight the possibilities for repairing roofs, rather than stripping and re-laying them. This is an issue that deserves further thought, as roof coverings are sometimes replaced before it is actually necessary.

This reprint of *Roof Construction and Repair* is of the second edition. This includes additional information on the use of asphalt shingles and also new materials for flat roofs plus, more significantly, further diagrams and illustrations.

The first four chapters of the book describe the timber construction of roofs, covering everything from basic joints through to the differences in the design of traditional and trussed roofs. There is a substantial amount of practical information on the design of pitched and flat roofs, the design of jointing around roof lanterns, fixing lay boards up the pitch of the roofs and the setting out of steps in horizontal gutters. The calculations in Chapter IV on the sizing of roof timbers are quite complicated, and are partially superseded by the 'Roof Tables' in the last chapter, added into the second edition.

Chapter V describes slates and slating, and is illustrated with some good photos. The examples are generally from Delabole and have a West Country emphasis. It explains the principles relating to the 'coverage' of slates, and how to calculate the quantities required. It also includes descriptions of how to sort and grade slates, how to work out of the position of the nail holes in slates and then how to hole them. The chapter ends with random slating and notes 'the gradual decrease in the gauge to give a 3-inch lap throughout should be noted'. This should really emphasize that a *minimum* lap of 3-inches is required.

Chapter VI explores the tiling of roofs, and begins with a very useful description of the different types and variations of tile used historically. This includes an explanation of the ancient Roman method of alternating over and under tiles (Imbrex and Tegula), which developed into the profiled single lap tiles that we still refer to as 'Roman', and also into 'Spanish' tiling. There is then a clear explanation of the setting out of the gauge and lap of a plain tiled roof, including the difference between rafter pitch and effective pitch, followed by a description of details such as verges, ridges, abutments and valleys. The final section covers single-lap interlocking tiles and different ways to detail hips and valleys.

The next three chapters discuss roofing with asbestos-cement based materials, asphalt shingles, and asbestos felt. Although most of these materials are not used today, some, like diamond slating and fibre cement slating, are being reused or repaired in conservation areas. We still need to learn about these products, as it is not only important to understand how to repair and possibly re-lay them, but also to be aware of the risk of asbestos and consequent health issues.

Chapter X describes the use of wood shingles, which was increasing in popularity at the time. This section is rather basic, but is a useful introduction. Unfortunately it doesn't differentiate between the durability of cedar and oak, or between sawn and split shingles. We now understand that oak shingles, particularly if they have been split (to follow the grain), will last considerably longer than cedar.

Emergency repairs to roofs after an air raid are described in Chapter XI. It offers useful advice on how to keep a building watertight until financial resources or materials can be found to re-cover the roof properly (a concern these days when trying to save a redundant building from further decay). This includes guidance on laying felt or corrugated iron over a roof, and the best ways to finish edges. There is also a suggestion about how to lay slates in 'extended order' (i.e. with vertical gaps) if there is a shortage of materials. This is advocated as a temporary measure, but there are examples of roofs laid this way, to be found today, that are still serviceable. Slightly worryingly, the text also makes reference to 'slurrying' to avoid damaging undisturbed areas of a roof. Presumably this refers to the application of a cement slurry or bitumen (the latter known as 'turnerising'), both of which cause damage to slates and tiles in the long term.

The final chapter is titled 'Roofing Tables'. This gives information on the sizes of timbers required for different rafter lengths on pitched roofs, in tabular form.

This book, with its simple but comprehensive description of roofing methods, is likely to have saved many damaged buildings from further decay during the war. As well as the chapter on emergency repairs, the other chapters give enough information for a practical person to lay a slate or tile roof properly. Tim Ratcliffe has photos of his grandfather, a vicar in Dagenham during the war, on the roof of the church, refixing slates after a bombing raid. He seems to be doing a reasonable job and it would be nice to think that he, and the curate with him, had a copy of *Roof Construction and Repair* to refer to!

We should be clear, however, that this is not just a beginner's guide to roofing. Mr Molloy's knowledge means that the level of information and detail goes far beyond this. This is a book that deserves to be more widely known and will prove useful to anyone concerned with the skills and craft of roofing.

Richard Jordan & Tim Ratcliffe
August 2009

Richard Jordan (Roofer)
Richard Jordan is a slater who followed in his father's footsteps, and learnt his trade working with him on site. In 1999 he was awarded a 'William Morris' travelling fellowship by the Society for the Protection of Ancient Buildings (SPAB). He has worked on the repair and replacement of roofs on historic buildings for a variety of clients, including the National Trust. He now also provides specialist consultancy advice on roofs and roofing projects, and is involved with encouraging training in traditional craft skills for building owners, architects, contractors and other construction professionals.

Tim Ratcliffe (Architect)
Tim Ratcliffe was awarded a 'Lethaby' travelling scholarship by the SPAB in 1987 and has also worked as a labourer for a number of specialist conservation contractors. He worked for two architectural firms specialising in historic building work (Rodney Melville & Partners and Donald Insall Associates) before setting up in practice with his wife, Jan, in 2000. Based in Oswestry, they work and give advice on churches, houses, castles and old industrial buildings in the Midlands and North Wales.

ROOF CONSTRUCTION AND REPAIR

ROOF CONSTRUCTION AND REPAIR

DEALING WITH SLATE, TILE, ASBESTOS-CEMENT, FELT, AND CONCRETE ROOFS, WITH A SPECIAL CHAPTER ON EMERGENCY REPAIRS

Prepared by a Staff of Technical Experts under the direction of

E. MOLLOY

WITH ONE HUNDRED AND EIGHTY-ONE ILLUSTRATIONS

GEORGE NEWNES LIMITED
TOWER HOUSE, SOUTHAMPTON STREET, STRAND
LONDON, W.C.2

FIRST PUBLISHED . . . 1942
SECOND EDITION . . . 1945

PRINTED IN GREAT BRITAIN BY HAZELL, WATSON & VINEY, LTD., LONDON AND AYLESBURY

PREFACE

ROOF construction may be divided broadly into two sections:

(*a*) carpentry work, which is concerned with the construction of roof framework, and

(*b*) roof covering, which involves the application of slates, tiles, asbestos cement, and similar materials, to the roof structure. The present book deals with both aspects of the subject.

In the first chapter will be found a clear explanation of the various components which together form the roof structure. All the main types, including the collar-and-tie roof, the valley roof, the purlin roof, and the Mansard roof are described and illustrated.

The second chapter is devoted to the construction of trussed roofs, which are used in most cases where the span exceeds about 20 ft.

Flat roofs constructed of either timber or reinforced concrete form the subject of Chapter III, and in this section will be found, in addition to the structural details, useful information concerning the chief types of coverings which are employed for flat roofs, namely, asphalte, copper, and zinc. An item of particular interest which is also dealt with in this chapter is the subject of roof lights employing "Glass-crete," i.e. a series of glass prisms embedded in concrete. Another important feature which is closely allied to the subject of flat roofs is that of heat insulation. This also receives adequate treatment in the section under review.

The various calculations involved in determining the sizes and spacing of the various roof members form the subject of the next chapter.

In spite of the growing popularity of natural tiles and also composition tiles, the slate roof still holds pride of place. All the practical details which are necessary in connection with roof slating are given in Chapter V, a particularly valuable feature being the trade descriptions of the various sizes and types of roofing slates, which range from Princesses, size 24 in. by 14 in., down to Small Doubles, size 12 in. by 6 in. In this chapter also will be found some most useful information enabling the quantities of slates required for a given job to be accurately estimated.

After these preliminary details, practical instructions are given for the actual operation of slating. Similar information is also given concerning all the important forms of tiles, both interlocking and plain.

Asbestos-cement tiles, under which classification are included a number of well-known proprietary makes, are dealt with in Chapter VII. Although some of these are similar in appearance and dimensions to the natural clay or slate product, the methods of fixing vary considerably. All these variations have been carefully explained from the point of view of the practical roofer and tiler.

The method of applying asbestos-felt, and the use of wood shingles as a roof covering, form the subjects of the succeeding chapters. Emergency repairs to roofs have been dealt with in considerable detail in the final chapter. Preliminary inspection, emergency slating repairs, covering roofs with bitumen roofing felt, the use of corrugated iron and ruberoid roofing materials are all carefully explained in detail with a wealth of illustration.

We should like to take this opportunity of thanking the suppliers of roofing materials for the valuable assistance which they have rendered us in the preparation of this work. In particular we would express our indebtedness to the Westmorland Green Slate Quarries Ltd., Messrs. Langley London Ltd., The Marley Tile Co., Messrs. Turners Asbestos Co. Ltd., The Universal Asbestos Manufacturing Co. Ltd., The Atlas Stone Co. Ltd., W H. Colt Ltd., Messrs. D. Anderson & Sons Ltd., and Messrs. Frazzi Ltd. for supplying technical data and trade information concerning their respective products.

It is hoped that the collection of this information into one volume, convenient for reference, will prove of maximum utility for all concerned in the design and construction and repair of roofs.

E. M.

PREFACE TO SECOND EDITION

In revising this book the opportunity has been taken of adding a new chapter on Covering Roofs with Asphalte Shingles. New material has also been included relating to materials for covering flat roofs, together with many useful diagrams.

E. M.

CONTENTS

ROOF CONSTRUCTION AND REPAIR

Chapter I

ROOF CONSTRUCTION FOR SMALL BUILDINGS

ROOF construction is an interesting subject at any time to all engaged in the work of house building and repair. At the present time, however, the subject is one of vital importance owing to the enormous amount of damage which has occurred to roofs as a result of enemy air activity. When such damage occurs, the subject of speedy repair is of the utmost importance if the building is to be rendered habitable.

Before roof work can be undertaken, it is essential to understand the various forms of roof construction that are to be met with. This aspect receives attention in the first four chapters of the present work. Special attention is given to the methods employed for domestic dwellings in which timber construction is largely employed. The remaining chapters deal with the materials used for coverings, and how these coverings are placed on the roof members. This section includes a chapter on the emergency repair of roofs.

Types of Roofs

There are several types of roofs, which are designated by various names according to outline or form of construction. Many considerations are taken into account when determining the type of roof to be adopted, such as span, material used for the covering, and climatic conditions.

Span

The *effective* span of a roof is the horizontal distance between the centres of the bearings on the supports, and the *clear* span the horizontal distance between the walls.

Pitch of Roof for Various Coverings

The term *pitch* is applied to the amount of slope given to the side of a roof, and may be stated in terms of the number of degrees in the angle which the slope makes with the horizontal, or the ratio of the rise to the span which is usually designated by a fraction. Thus, suppose the rise to be 12 ft. and the span 48 ft., then the pitch is :

$$\frac{\text{rise}}{\text{span}} = \frac{12}{48} = \frac{1}{4}$$

The minimum pitch or inclination it is desirable to use for the various materials used for coverings is given in the table on the next page.

PITCH OF ROOF FOR VARIOUS MATERIALS

Materials	*Pitch*	
	Minimum Angle with Horizon	*Ratio of Rise to Span*
Slates (small)	33°	$\frac{1}{3}$
,, (ordinary)	26°	$\frac{1}{4}$
,, (large)	21°	$\frac{1}{5}$
Tiles (single-lap)	35°	$\frac{7}{20}$
Plain tiles	45°	$\frac{1}{2}$
Corrugated sheets	20°	$\frac{9}{50}$
Copper and zinc	1°	$\frac{1}{80}$
Lead and asphalte	0°	$\frac{1}{120}$
Ruberoid	20°	$\frac{9}{50}$

In exposed positions these pitches should be increased over the amounts given above.

Parts of a Roof

The lowest part or edge of a sloping roof is called the *eaves,* and may or may not project beyond the wall face. Where the roof finishes over a gable end, the edge is termed the *verge. Valley* is the line of intersection of two roof planes containing an external angle less than 180°, and a *hip* the line of intersection of two roof surfaces which contain an angle greater than 180° A *hipped end,* the triangular surface formed by the slope being continued round the end. These terms are illustrated in Fig. 1. *Rafters* (common) are inclined members running from ridge to eaves. Where they finish against hip or valley rafters they are termed *jack rafters.*

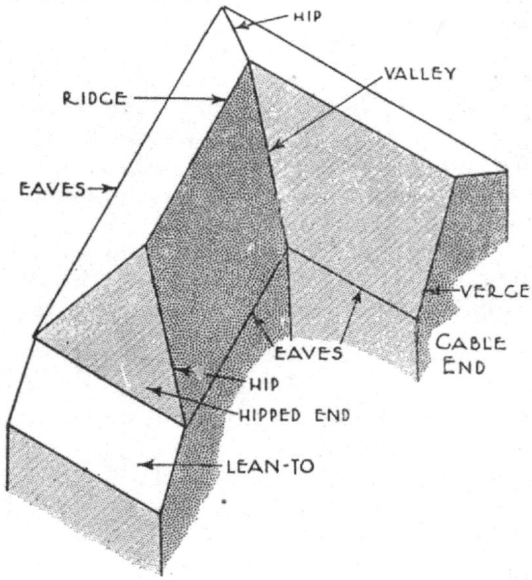

Fig. 1.—SKETCH OF ROOF, ILLUSTRATING THE TERMS EMPLOYED TO DESCRIBE PARTS

A series of rafters 12 in. to 16 in. apart is usually placed over the entire surface. If they exceed about 8 ft. in length, intermediate supports termed *purlins* must be provided for them. Generally, they run from the roof ridge or apex down to

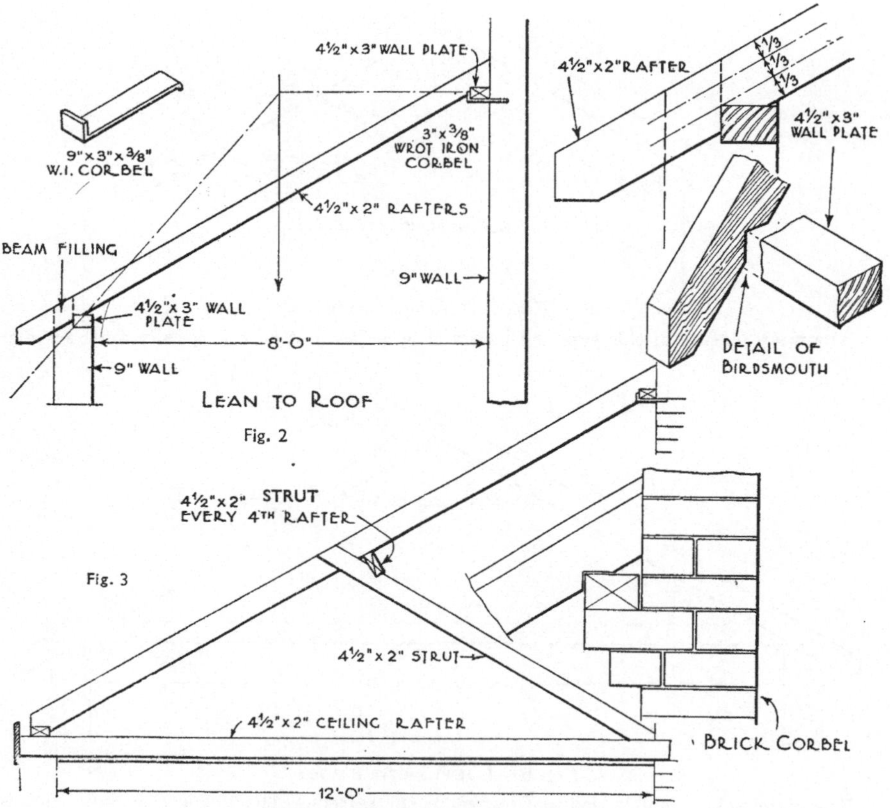

Figs. 2 *and* 3.—LEAN-TO ROOFS

The span suitable for the type shown in Fig. 2 is 8 ft., but it can be increased if suitably tied and braced by the use of purlins and struts at intervals if necessary, as in Fig. 3. Fig. 3 also shows the construction of a brick corbel.

the eaves, but occasionally are placed in a horizontal position. *Wall plates,* to which the lower ends of the rafters are usually fitted with a bird's-mouth joint and nailed, should be bedded on the wall, preferably placed along the inside. For convenience of fixing the roof covering, it is necessary either to nail battens transversely at intervals or to board the rafters entirely over.

Roofs may be classified as single, trussed, composite (wood and steel), and steel.

Single Roofs

Single roofs are those which consist of a framework of common rafters alone, with a wall plate and a ridge piece, and with or without purlins. These include the following types : lean-to, couple, couple-close, collar-tie,

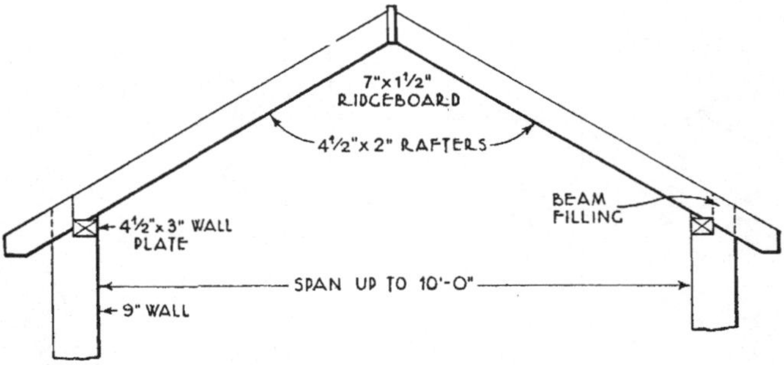

Fig. 4.—Couple roof

The weak feature of this type is that its weight does not bear vertically on the walls.

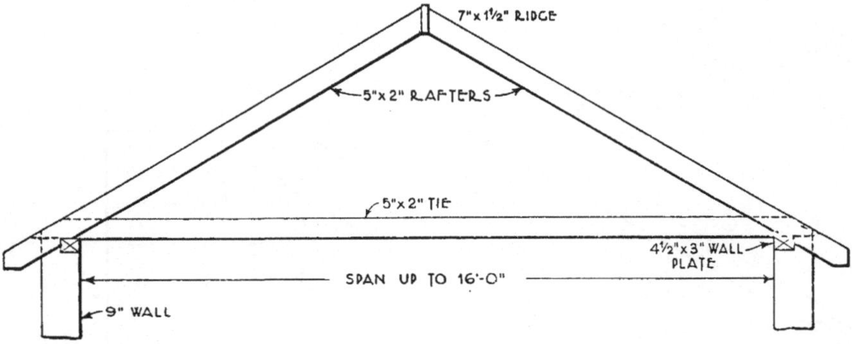

Fig. 5.—Couple-close roof

The couple-close roof is tied at the feet of the rafters. The ties act as ceiling joists where a ceiling is required.

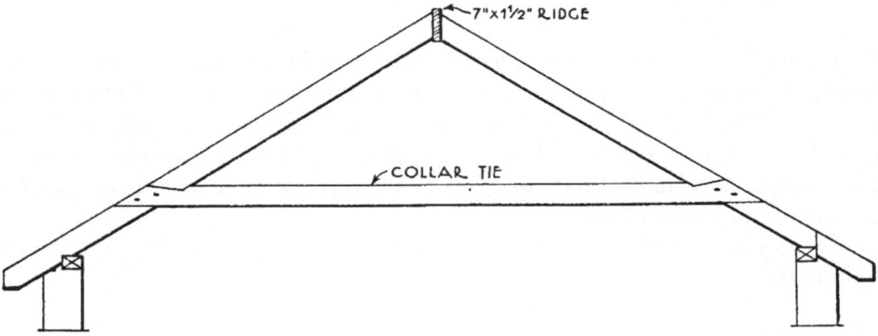

Fig. 6.—Collar-tie roof

The tie is placed some distance above the wall plate, and is called a tie-rod if of steel and a tie-beam if of wood. It is usual to place the tie at one-third the vertical height from wall to ridge.

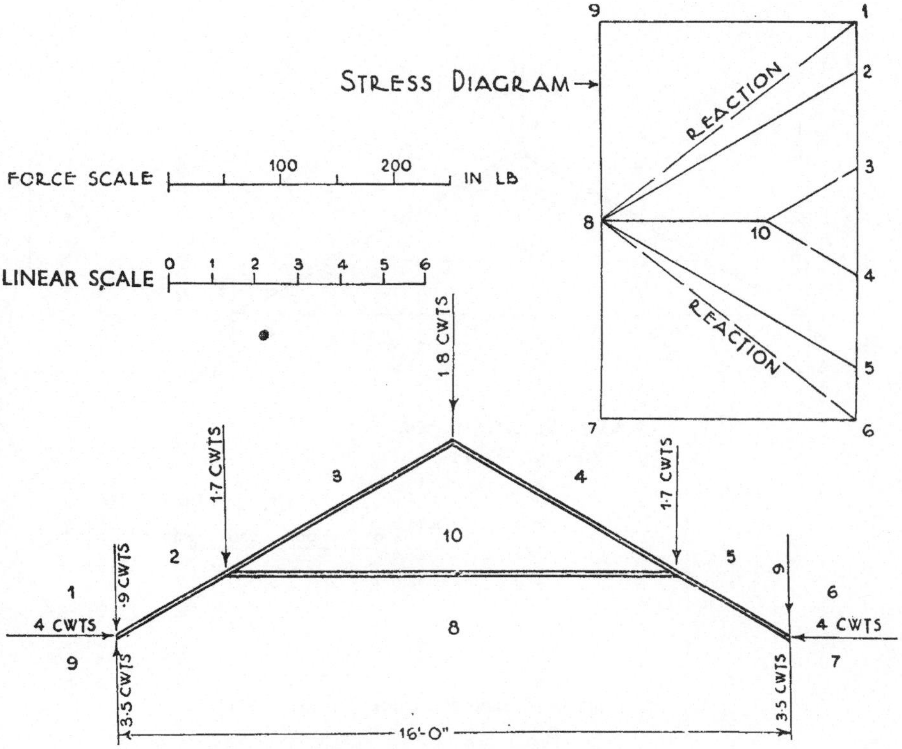

Fig. 7.—FRAME DIAGRAM FOR RIGID WALLS

V-roof, and flat roof. When purlins are used they are sometimes called double or purlin roofs.

Lean-to

This is formed with only one slope, and is used for sheds and buildings attached to the main buildings (see Fig. 2). The span suitable for this type is 8 ft., but it can be increased if suitably tied and braced by the use of purlins and struts at intervals if necessary (see Fig. 3). If the distance from ridge to eaves is less than 5 ft., it is not necessary to use rafters at all, but simply to board the surface over, the boards running with the slope, and a suitable support provided for them at top and bottom.

The upper ends of the rafters are fixed to a wall plate which is either built into or attached to the back wall at the desired height. When the wall plate is not built into the wall, or rests on an offset, it may be supported on a projecting course of bricks, or corbels of brick or wrought iron, at about 3-ft. intervals, built in or fixed for the purpose (see Figs. 2 and 3), The lower ends of the rafters are fitted to the wall plate in the usual way

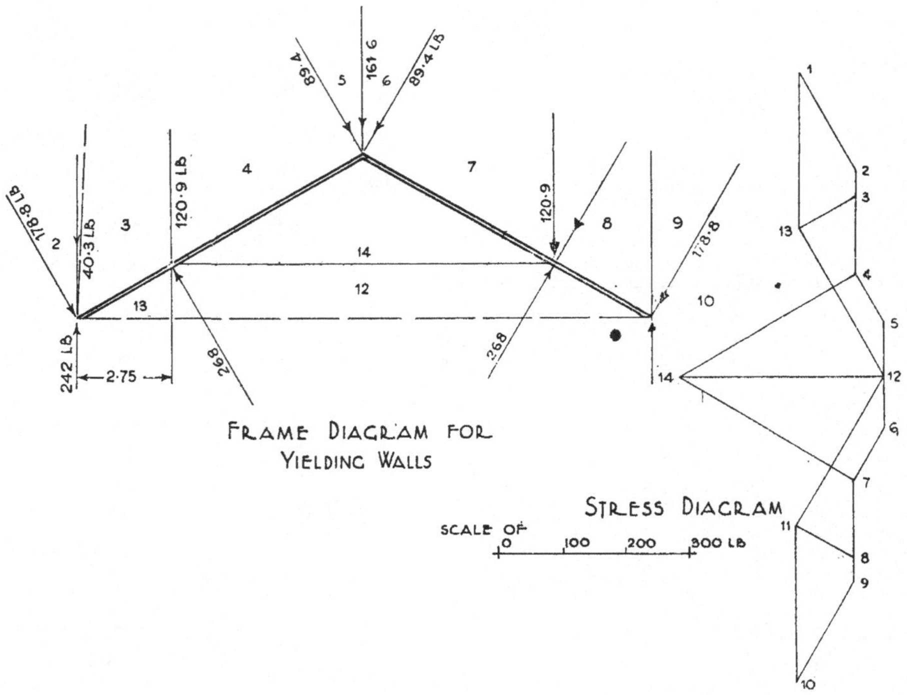

Fig. 8.—STRESSES IN COLLAR-TIE ROOF

Couple Roofs

As their name implies, couple roofs are roofs consisting of pairs of rafters fixed at their feet to a wall plate (see Fig. 4), and pitching against the ridge. The weak feature of these roofs is that their weight does not bear vertically on the walls, but tends to thrust them apart unless the walls are sufficiently strong to resist the thrust, but it is quite easy to modify its form so that all the outward thrust, or most of it, can be prevented. They are only suitable for spans up to about 10 ft.

Couple-close Roof

When the couple roof is tied at the feet of the rafters it is termed a *couple-close* roof (see Fig. 5). The weight of the roof, etc., tends to depress the ridge, and therefore the feet of the rafters will tend to spread and push the wall outwards. The tie prevents the feet from spreading, and consequently the danger of the walls overturning is avoided.

These ties also act as ceiling joists where a ceiling is required. Although the tie beam is in tension it requires to be of good depth to prevent sagging.

Where a ceiling is to be fixed a good rule is to make the depth of the joist ½ in. for every foot of span.

Collar-tie Roof

When the tie is placed some distance above the wall plate, it is called a *collar-tie* roof (see Fig. 6). This tie is called a tie-rod if of steel, and a tie-beam if of wood. If it is placed at half the vertical height from the wall plate to the ridge, the bending in the rafter would be prevented, but in this position the tie would not be very efficient to prevent the overturning thrust on the walls. It is therefore usual to compromise, and place it at one-third the vertical height from the wall to the ridge. The collars have a dual function, according to changing circumstances. If the walls are rigid and the rafters are sufficiently stiff to stand without deflection, the collar tie will be in compression (see Fig. 7), as also will be the case under wind pressure. However, the slightest degree of settlement or the spreading of the supports and they at once become ties (see Fig. 8). In view of this alternating change in function it is well that every fourth or fifth collar should be halved to the rafters in order to form a shoulder, but it is not wise to weaken the rafter at this point by cutting into it to form the joint. These rafters should be proportionately increased in width, so as to maintain the same sectional area, as the weak point of the roof is the amount of deflection that may occur in the rafter between the ends of the collars and the wall plate.

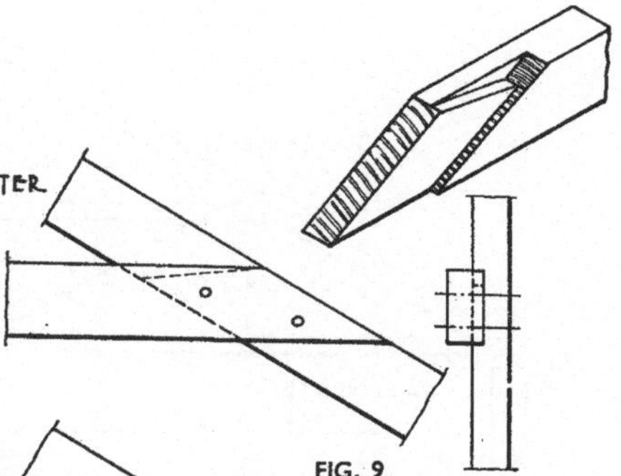

FIG. 9
DOVETAIL HALVING JOINT

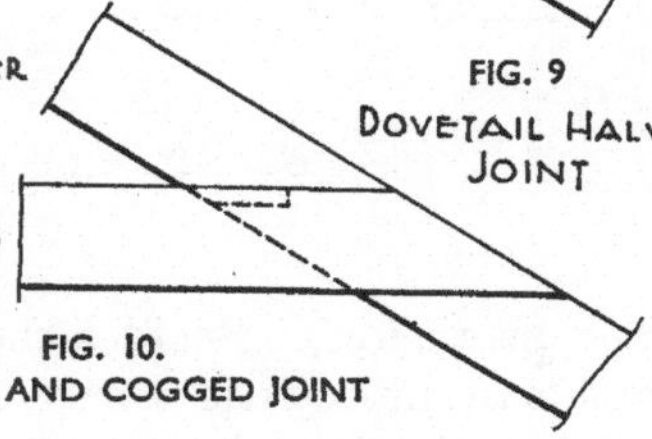

FIG. 10.
HALVED AND COGGED JOINT

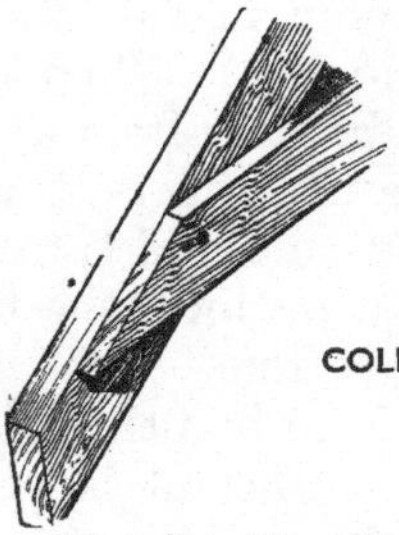
FIG. 11.
COLLAR HALVED

Figs. 9 *to* 11.—Details of joints

The joint connecting the collar beam to the roof may be a dovetail-halved joint, as shown in Fig. 9, or a halved and cogged joint (Fig. 10), or the collar alone may be halved (Fig. 11).

Collar-and-tie Roof

Though the generality of textbooks deal almost entirely with roofs constructed with trusses, the greater number of small buildings are

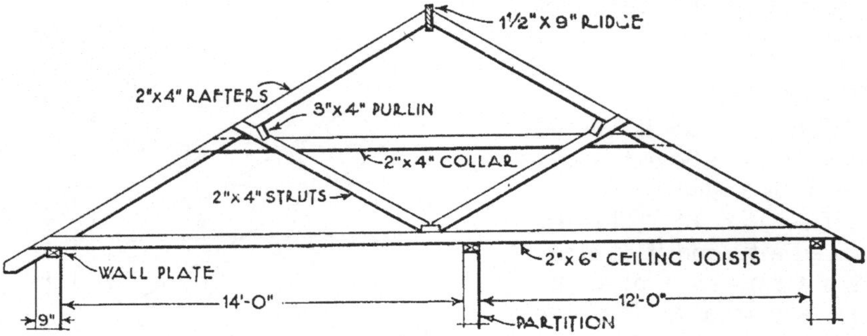

Fig. 12.—Collar-and-tie roof

without such provision. Besides the various forms of single roofs shown, larger spans can be satisfactorily constructed by the use of struts and ties. When constructed in this way they are known as *collar-and-tie* roofs (see Figs. 12 and 13). When this last type of roof is further strengthened by placing pairs of rafters at about 5 or 6 ft. apart, and securing with collars, struts, and hangers, they are termed *purlin* or *double-rafter* roofs. An alternative method is to carry the roof on a Howe or N girder, which forms a trussed purlin ; the top boom carries the rafters, and the lower one the ceiling rafters.

If the roof space is to be utilised as a room, then the collars will have to be raised to allow sufficient head room. The purlins can be used as ashlaring along the sides of the room and covered with a plaster board or fibre board, or the purlin filled in with studs to receive the laths for plastering.

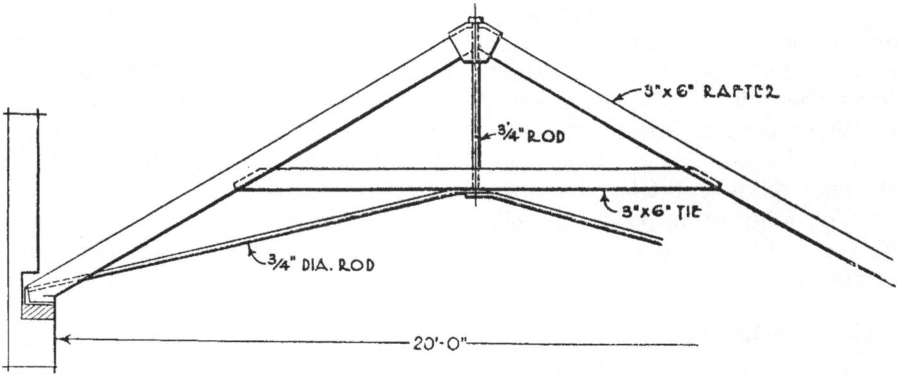

Fig. 13.—Collar-and-tie roof

Valley or Double Lean-to Roof

Another form of roof is the valley or double lean-to (see Fig. 14). The roof is inclined from the party or main walls, towards a gutter in the centre usually over a partition wall or some other support. The rafters rise from a pole plate, or sometimes from a pair of parallel plates which form the sides of the gutter, and which are supported by a partition. The upper ends of the rafters are carried on plates resting on wrought-iron or brick corbels from the party walls. The front of the building is usually finished with a wall and parapet, and the back of the building with gable ends, the roof finishing with a verge.

Purlins

Purlins are horizontal members introduced to provide an intermediate support to the common rafters, and in turn are supported by gable walls, roof trusses, or by the use of struts supported on partition walls where the rafters are hipped on each end. Care should be taken that the struts, when used, have a good bearing at their feet. Stud partitions, rising from a timber floor below, are not altogether satisfactory.

Spacing of Purlins

The spacing of the purlins is governed to a large extent by the roof covering, and to some extent by the type of roof design. In order that the common rafters may have economical dimensions, the purlins that carry them require to be within a spacing of not more than 10 ft. The purlins should be placed in position before the rafters are fixed, although they are sometimes added afterwards.

Trussed Purlins

Where, owing to the length of the roof, the purlins would become inconveniently large (see Fig. 15), a useful construction that may be used, and might be more often adopted, is the trussed purlin. It will also be found suitable where there is not the necessary room for a principal, and the space inside the roof is to be utilised.

The purlins should extend from wall to wall, and rest on stone templates built into the wall. They should be kept clear of the floor joists, otherwise, when wind pressures come suddenly on one side of the roof,

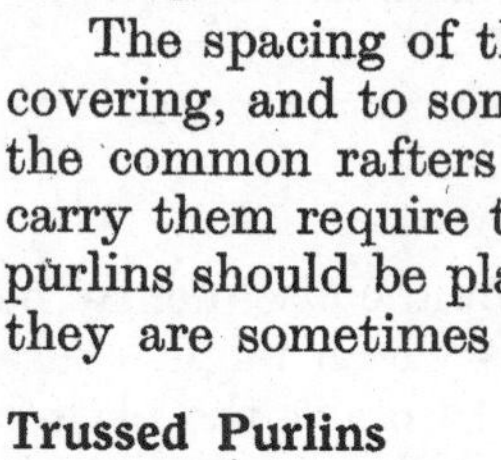

Fig. 13A (*left*).—JOINT BETWEEN RAFTERS, PURLIN, AND STRUT WHERE LATTER IS AT ABOUT RIGHT ANGLES TO RAFTERS

Fig. 13B (*right*).—JOINT WHERE STRUT IS NOT SET AT ABOUT RIGHT ANGLES TO RAFTERS

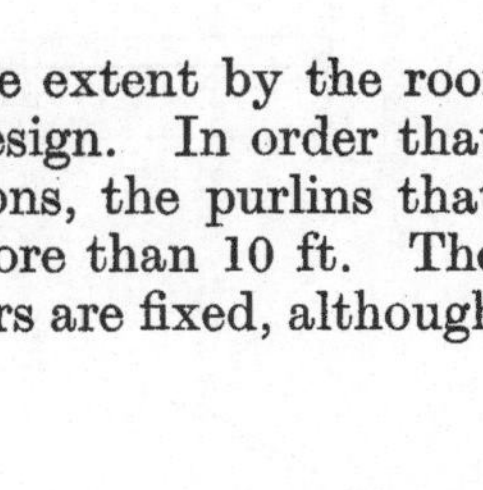

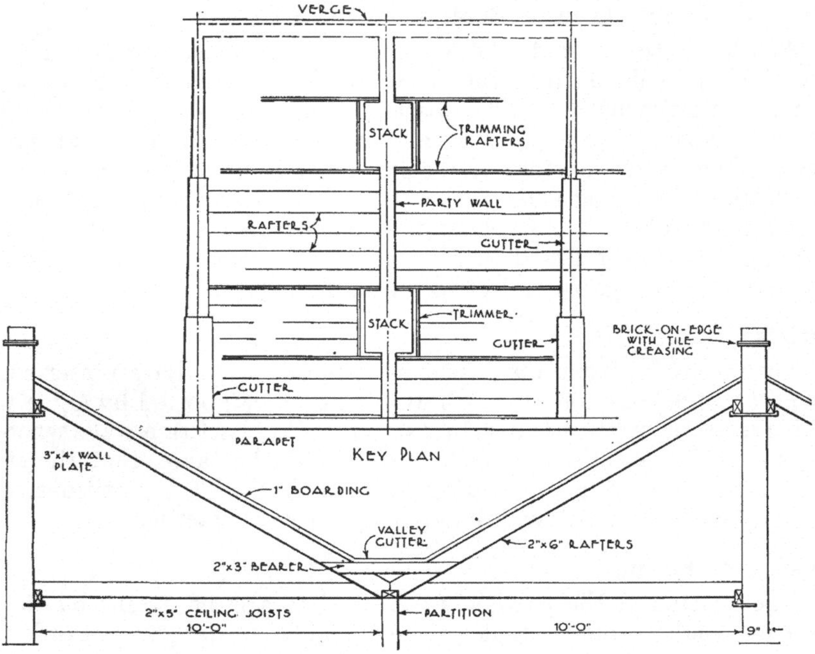

Fig. 14.—Valley roof

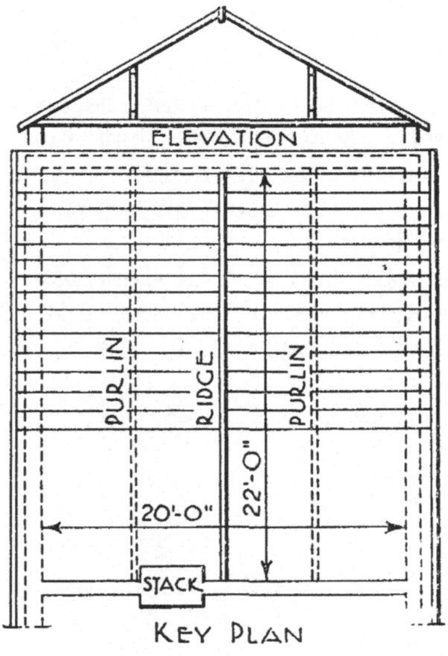

Fig. 15.—Purlin roof

the trussed purlin would consequently be subjected to stresses which might cause sufficient deflection to crack the plaster ceiling below. The bottom member is usually made 4 in. by 4 in., and the struts 3 in. by 4 in., with $\frac{1}{2}$-in., $\frac{5}{8}$-in., or $\frac{3}{4}$-in. bolts, but, if desired, the stresses could be calculated to obtain the exact sizes required (see Fig. 16). The truss usually forms the ashlaring along the sides of the room, and may be filled in with studding to receive the plaster or to be covered with a fibre board.

Roofs Constructed of Short Timbers

Other simple types suitable for comparatively large spans can be built up by placing pieces of various lengths side by side with the use of a truss. In these types it is usual to place the two rafters a few inches apart, to allow for

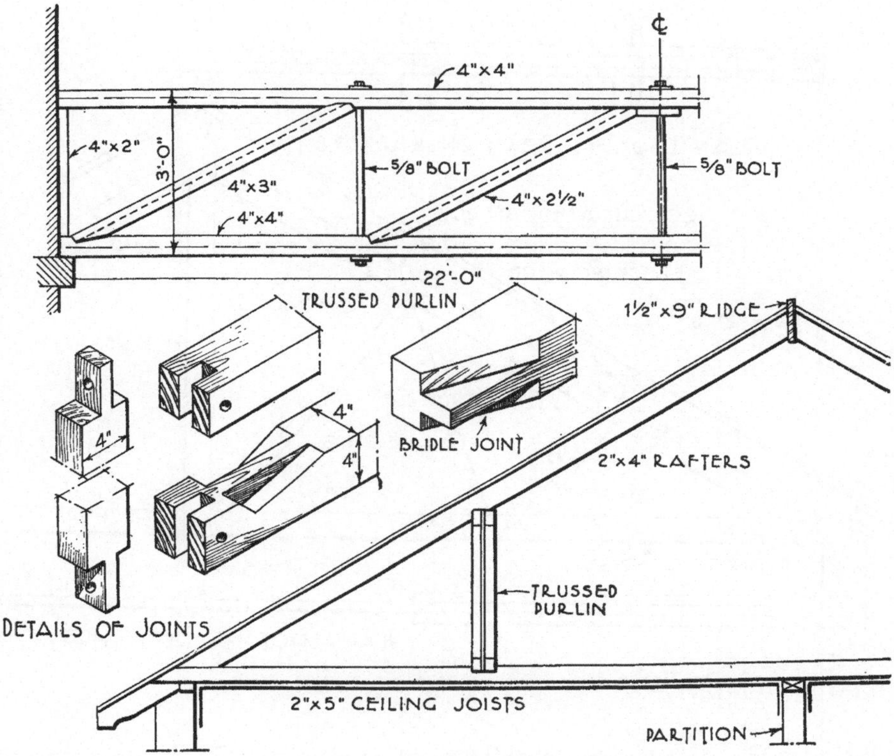

Fig. 16.—PURLIN ROOF

the internal members being fitted securely between the built-up rafters and main tie. The members A, in Fig. 17, are formed at their ends with shoulders which bear on the double rafters and the members, and part formed to extend between the rafter and tie as a tenon. Member B is similar, excepting that at the lower end it notches over the ties and finds a bearing on them. The rafter back near the apex of the truss is formed with two 2-in. by 5-in. pieces placed together, one acting as a joint-plate in lieu of a fish-plate.

When properly fastened together by nailing and bolting, the short pieces are equally as strong as single pieces, and are cheaper and easier to obtain.

Single Mansard Roof

This type is being much used in domestic work. For small spans, it provides an economical means of containing and roofing upper floors and bedrooms. When properly built, it is constructionally sound, and

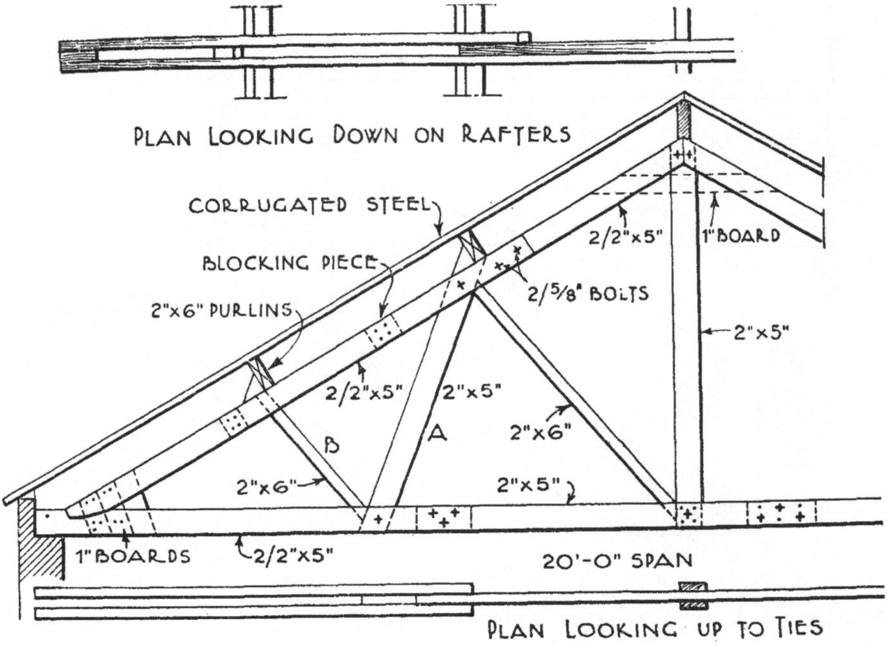

Fig. 17.—Roof construction of pieces of timbers

also capable of pleasing architectural treatment. It is unnecessary to use trusses to support this type of roof over small spans up to 20 ft.

There are many variations in the outline, usually obtained by using one or other of the original French methods of setting out adopted by Mansard, the inventor. Fig. 18 shows the methods used. A semicircle is drawn equal in diameter to the effective span. This is divided into four or five equal parts, giving slightly different outlines. In some cases the lower pitch is inclined at 60° until sufficient headroom is obtained, and then the upper slope inclined at 30°. In modern work the lower slope is usually made 75°, which is the maximum allowable under the Building Acts. For small buildings the lower slope is inclined at 75°, and the upper at from 26° to 45°, according to the covering used.

To obtain the maximum amount of room it is usual to finish with gable-end construction, at least to the height of the lower pitch or kerb. Fig. 19 shows a type commonly adopted, as it gives more floor space. The type shown in Fig. 20 is of stronger construction, but a certain amount of floor space has to be sacrificed. Additional strength can be obtained by nailing cross-pieces between the ashlaring or upright pieces and the

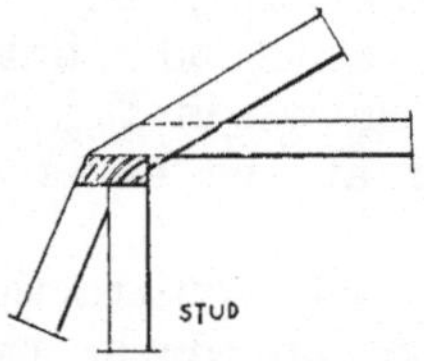

Fig. 20.—ANOTHER TYPE OF MANSARD ROOF CONSTRUCTION

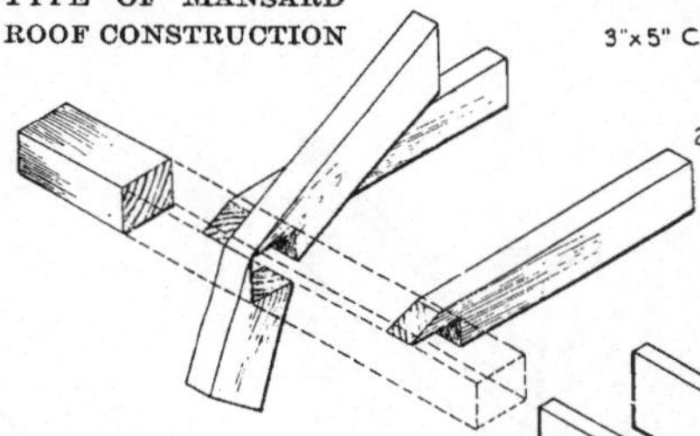

Fig. 21.—ALTERNATIVE METHODS OF FINISHING AT CURBS

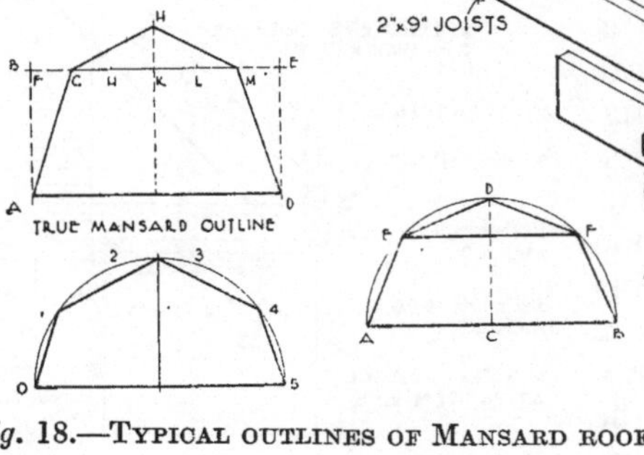

Fig. 18.—TYPICAL OUTLINES OF MANSARD ROOF

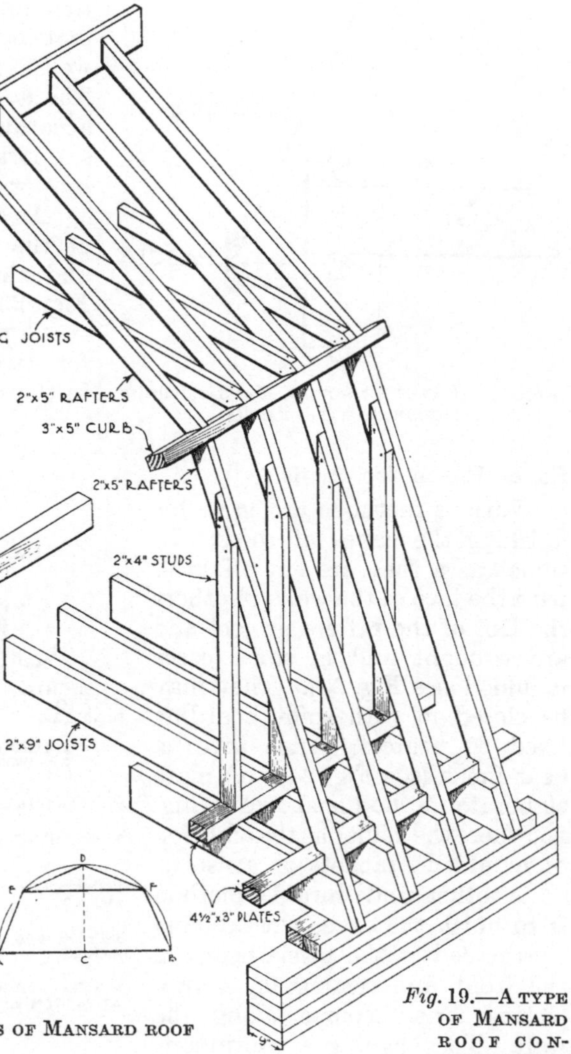

Fig. 19.—A TYPE OF MANSARD ROOF CONSTRUCTION COMMONLY ADOPTED

Figs. 18 *to* 21.—SINGLE MANSARD ROOF DETAILS

rafters, usually about every fourth member. This bracing will considerably stiffen the frame and lessen its liability to rack. The rafters should be bird's-mouthed to the wall plate, and also fixed to the side of joists. This will help to stiffen the roof. Every fourth or fifth stud should be tenoned into the cill and curb. Where wind bracing is employed, the

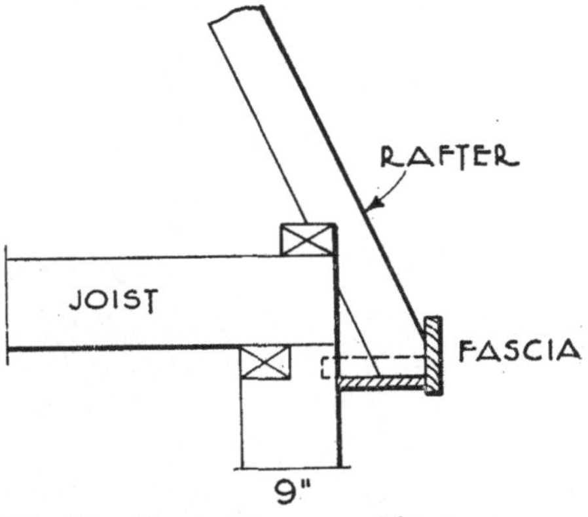

Fig. 22.—Eaves of single Mansard roof finished with fascia

tenoning of the studs may be omitted provided the joints are well made and securely fixed. The floor joists will vary in depth according to span. They are often supported at intermediate points by party walls or partitions.

An alternative method of finish at the curb is shown in Fig. 21, and the finish at the eaves in Fig. 22.

Types of roof construction for larger spans are dealt with in the next chapter.

Eaves Finish for Roofs

Various methods are used for finishing the eaves of roofs. In some cases they are cut off flush with the face of the wall; in others the feet of the rafters project and are wrought and in some cases moulded (see Fig. 23). They may be closed in with soffit boarding fixed to bearers, which gives a neat finish (see Fig. 24). A more elaborate method is shown in Fig. 25, where the soffit has the addition of moulded brackets or consoles.

Another and durable method is to finish the eaves with roofing tiles nailed to the fascia board in the front and resting on a projecting brick course along the wall. Tiles having a continuous nib along the top look best, and therefore make a more suitable finish than the un-nibbed variety. Fig. 26 illustrates this treatment.

Tilt at the Eaves

Tiled roofs do not require any exaggerated tilt at the eaves such as is given by the use of sprocket

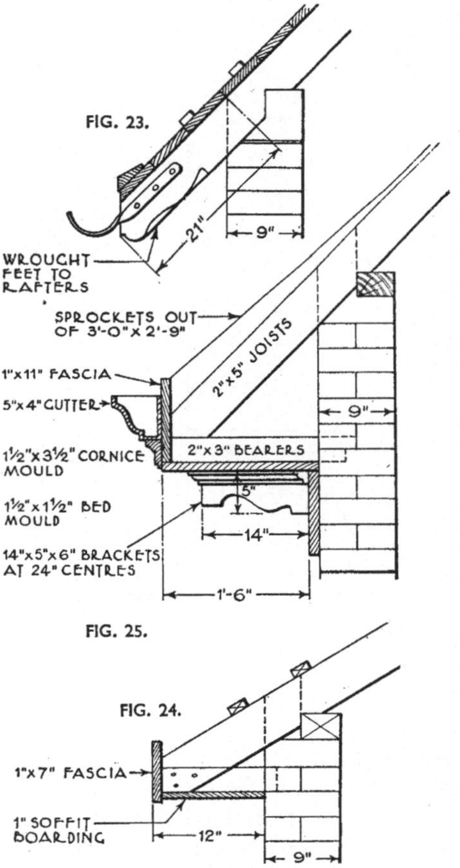

Figs. 23 *to* 25.—Eaves details

pieces (see Fig. 25), but where such are employed care should be taken that the difference in pitch between the sprocket and the roof proper is not too great, nor that the pitch adopted for the covering at this point is too flat where a large volume of water has to be dealt with.

Sprockets may be fixed to the top of the rafters or nailed to their sides.

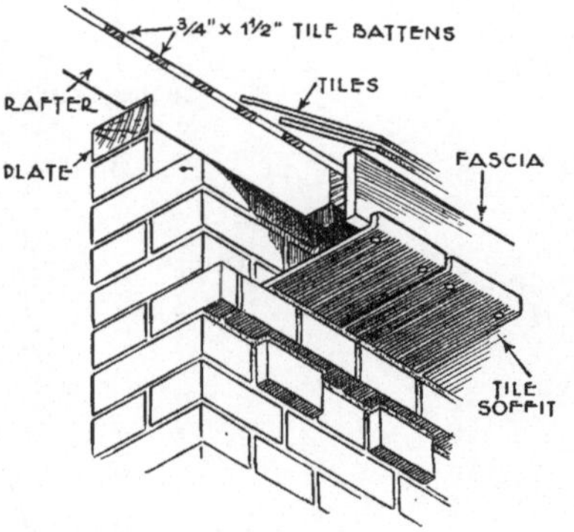

Fig. 26.—Eaves formed with fascia board and tile soffit

Precast Concrete Roofing Units

A recent development in the construction of roofs of comparatively small span is the introduction of precast concrete units suitable for supporting lightweight roof coverings. This type of construction is likely to develop rapidly to meet the urgent need for speed in erection and saving in timber occasioned by the post-war construction programme.

TRIMMING

Chimneys, etc.

Where chimneys, dormer windows, skylights, or other openings occur in a roof, it is generally necessary to trim the rafters in order to leave sufficient open space. The trimmers are tenoned into the trimming rafters, and these are generally made ½ in. thicker than the ordinary rafters. The trimmed rafters are notched to the trimmers. A frame is thus provided in the roof surface without any rafters crossing it (see Fig. 27).

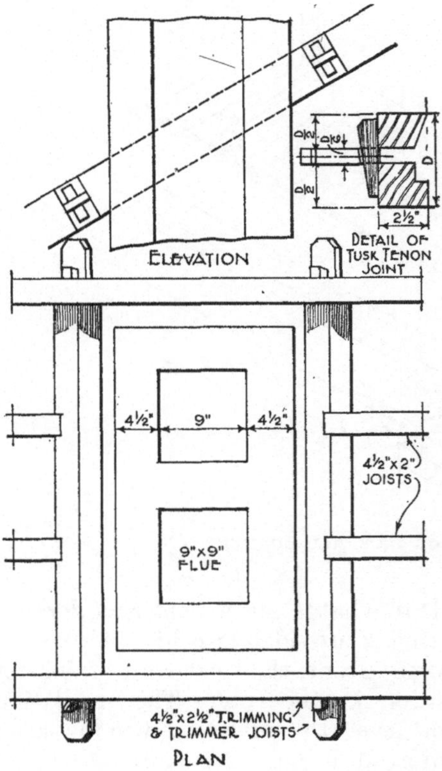

Fig. 27.—Trimming to chimney stack

Dormer Windows

The trimming for a dormer window is shown in Fig. 29.

Owing to building laws the projection of dormers is in some

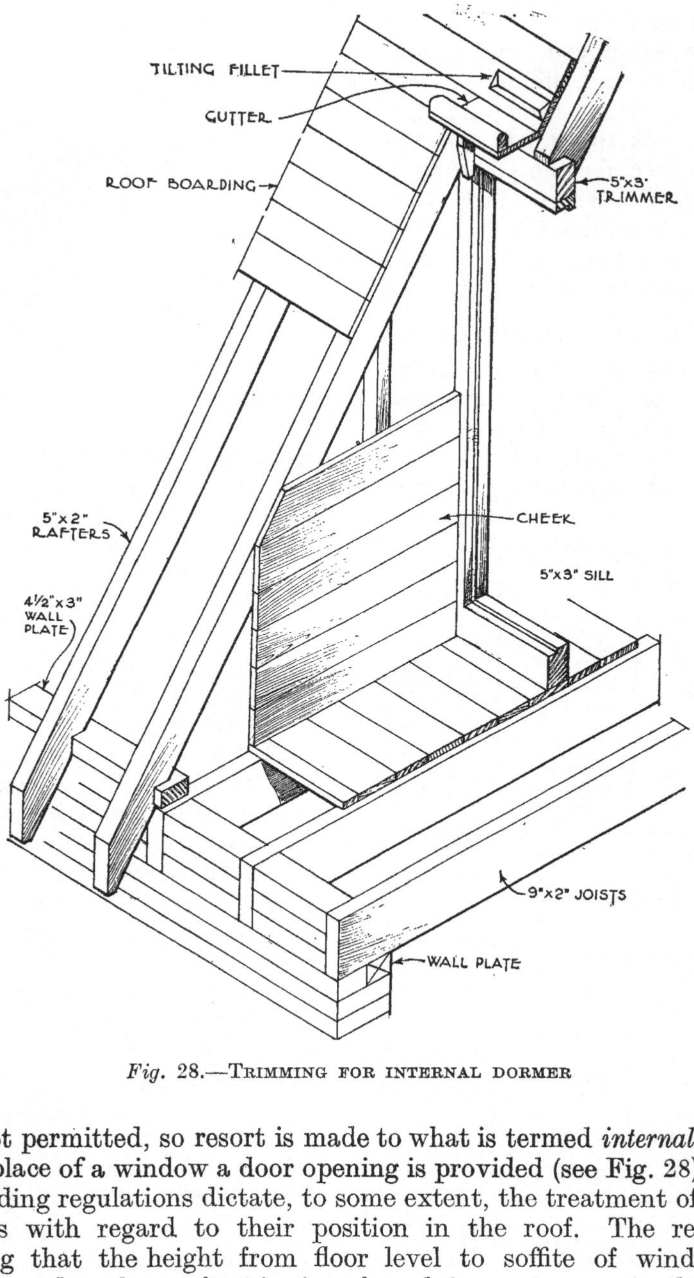

Fig. 28.—Trimming for internal dormer

cases not permitted, so resort is made to what is termed *internal dormer*, and in place of a window a door opening is provided (see Fig. 28).

Building regulations dictate, to some extent, the treatment of dormer windows with regard to their position in the roof. The regulation requiring that the height from floor level to soffite of window-head shall be not less than 6 ft. 6 in. is enforced, in most areas, in the case of dormer windows, as is also the regulation that the ashlaring in rooms

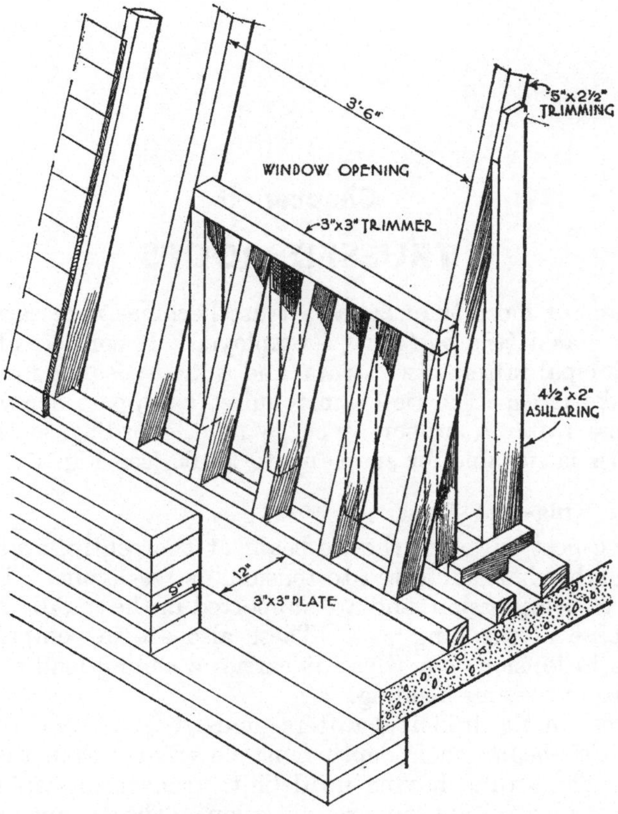

Fig. 29.—Trimming for dormer window

occupying part of the roof space shall have a minimum vertical height of 4 ft. 6 in.

The combination of these two requirements results in a reasonably attractive appearance both externally and internally.

From the æsthetic standpoint dormer windows look best if they project above the roof slope either one-third or two-thirds their own height. They do not look so well if the projection approximates to half their own height.

Chapter II

TRUSSED ROOFS

FOR spans of more than 20 ft. a truss becomes necessary, and what is known as a *king-post truss* is employed. It consists of a tie-beam, two principal rafters, two struts, and a king-post. As a rough guide we may take it that the tie-beam requires a support every 15 ft., and the principal rafter a support every 8 ft. According to this rule this type of truss is suitable for spans up to 30 ft. (see Fig. 1).

Principle of King-post Truss

The king-post supports the tie-beam at the centre, and although a vertical member it is subjected to tensional stress alone. The principal rafters are in compression, and are supported in the middle by the struts from the base of the king-post. These also are in compression. The tie-beam is in tension, but where it carries a ceiling load it will also be subjected to transverse bending.

The stress in the principal rafters tends to bend, and consequently, as with the tie-beam, their depth must be greater than their width or thickness. The struts, having no definite transverse strain, should be made as nearly as possible square in section. The purlins are supported by the truss, and in turn support the roofing, i.e. common rafters, boarding, battens, slates, or tiles.

The dimensions given in the Table below are minimum sizes, and may be increased if desired. This has been done on the diagrams, Fig. 1.

DIMENSIONS OF TIMBERS FOR KING-POST ROOF TRUSSES
10 FT. APART, PITCH 30°, SLATED

Span	*Thickness of All Truss Members*	*Minimum Breadth on Elevation*			
		Tie-beam	*Principal Rafter*	*King-post*	*Struts*
ft.	*in.*	*in.*	*in.*	*in.*	*in.*
20	4	8	4	3	2
22	4½	9	4	3½	2¼
24	5	10	4¼	3½	2½
26	5½	10	4¼	4	2¾
28	6	11	4½	4	3
30	6½	12	4½	4½	3¼

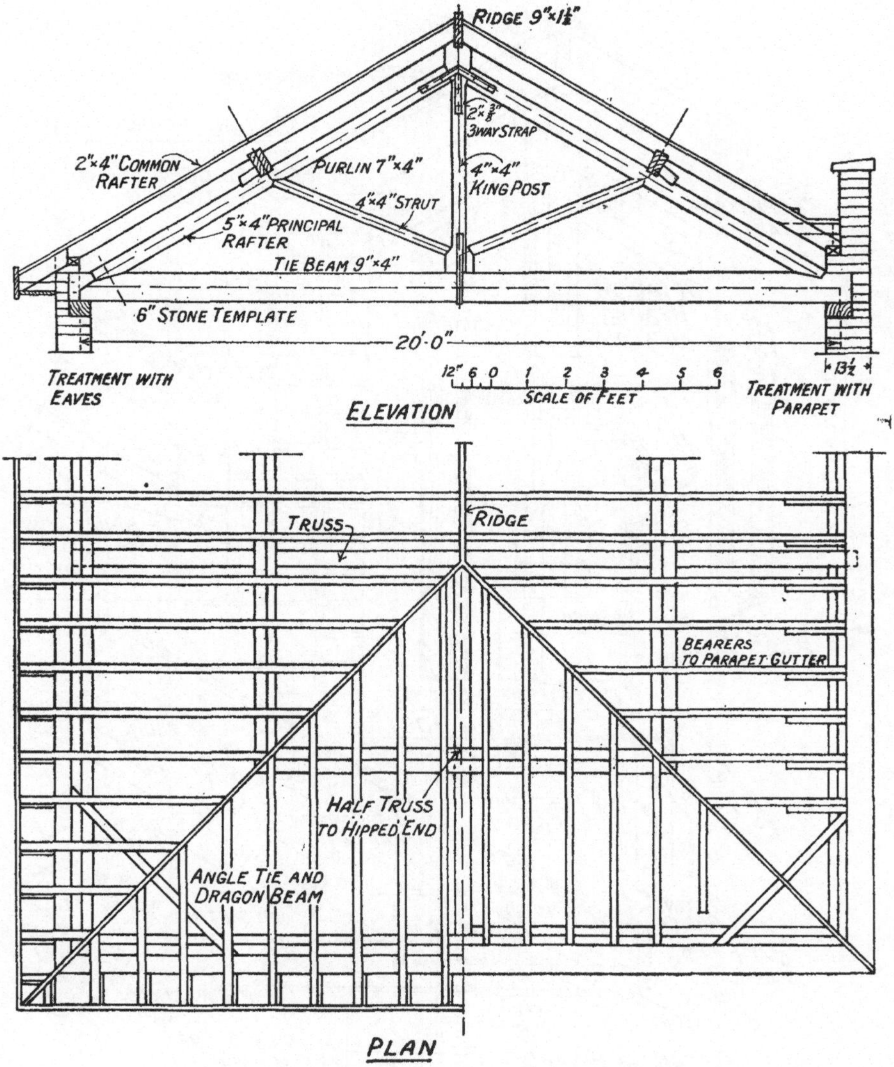

Fig. 1.—KING-POST ROOF TRUSS WITH HIPPED END

All the members of a king-post roof truss are made the same thickness with the exception sometimes of the struts. This allows the iron straps to be bolted to the surface to hold the joints together.

The Purlins

The purlins are generally placed over the top of the struts, and as there are only two struts in a king-post truss the purlins are consequently

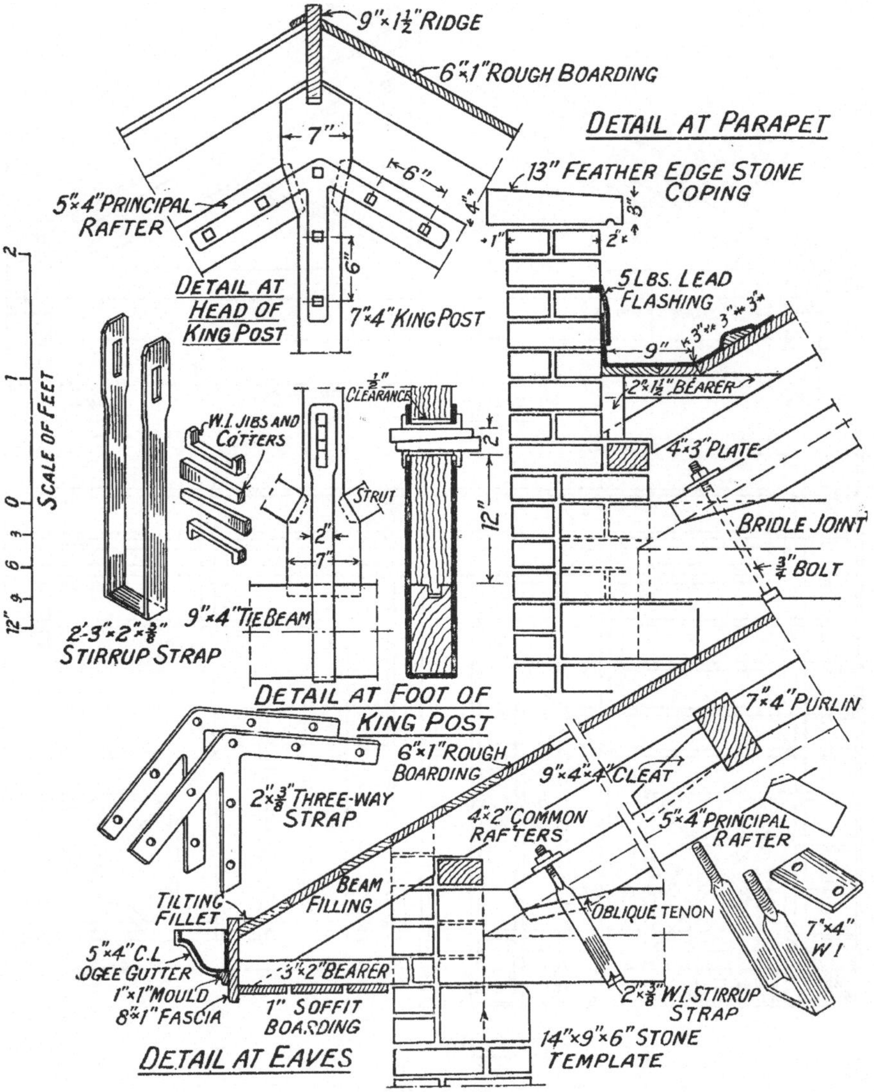

Fig. 2.—King-post details

Showing details at head and foot of king-post, eaves, and parapet.

two in number. The purlins are cogged or recessed about ½ in. or so, to fit over the principal rafters, and are fixed by nailing. They are further secured and supported by cleats to prevent them from turning over or slipping down. Details of joints are shown in Fig. 2.

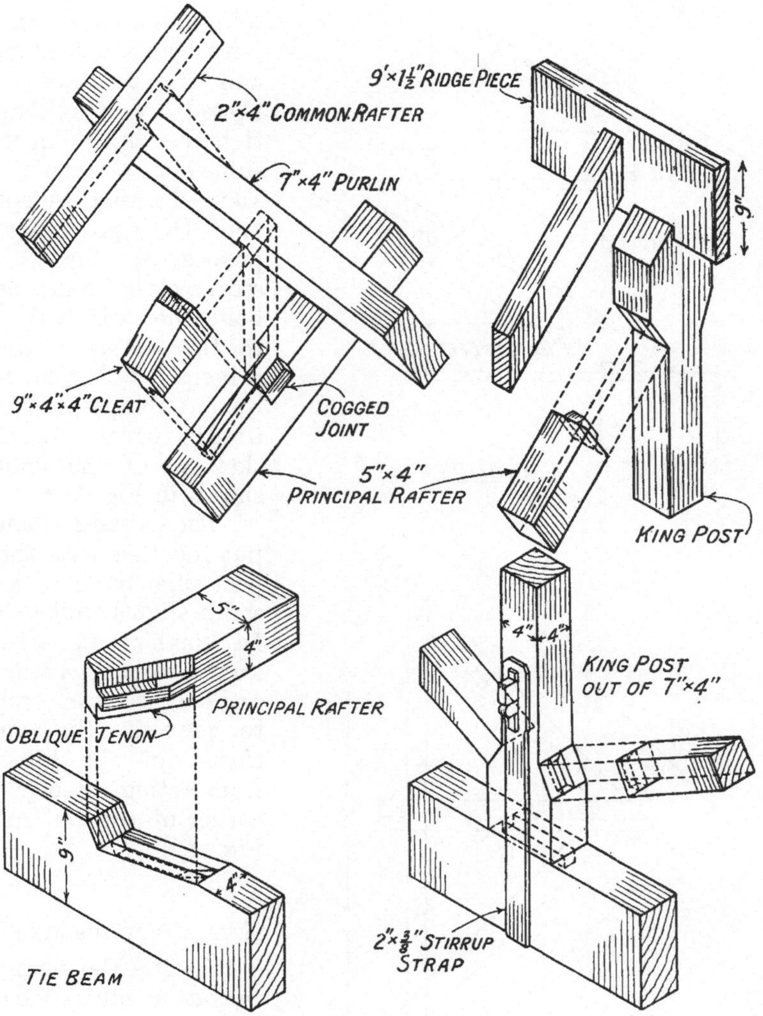

Fig. 3.—King-post truss joints

To form an abutment as nearly as possible at right angles to the inclination of the member, the king-post is reduced in size to about half its width in the middle, and to secure the joints further, iron straps are used (see Fig. 2).

Joints

The joint between the top of the principal rafter and the king-post is strengthened and made more secure with two three-way straps and

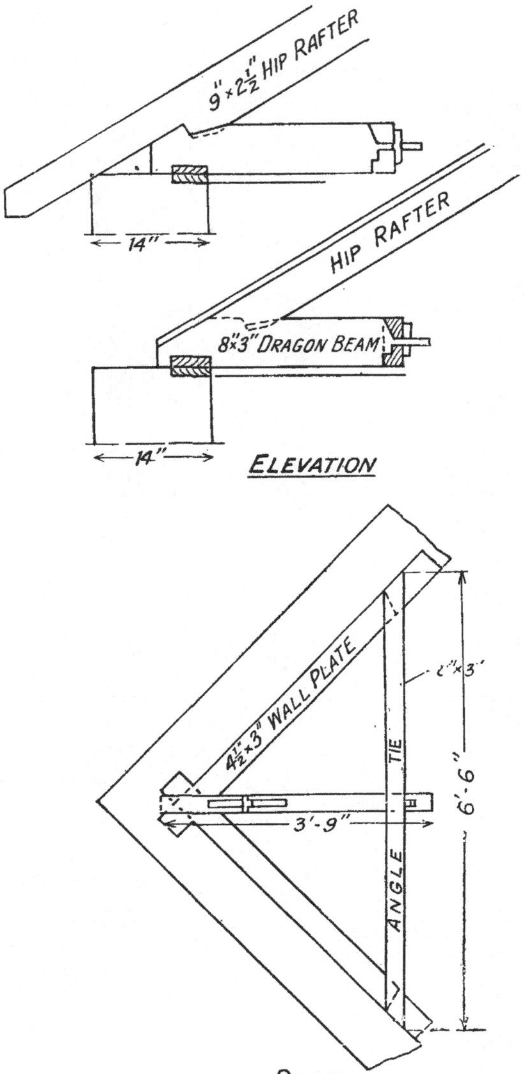

Fig. 4.—ANGLE TIE AND DRAGON BEAM

½-in. bolts, as shown. The joint between the king-post and the tie-beam is connected by a stirrup and tightened by folding wedges, sufficient clearance being allowed in both the stirrup and the post for this purpose (see Fig. 2). Heel-straps or bolts are used to hold the principal rafters to the tie-beam, and the principal rafter is formed by an oblique tenon or a bridle joint. Isometric sketches of the joints are shown in Fig. 3.

The trusses should be put together with the king-post slightly short, and the struts slightly full, to length. In small roofs what are known as *dragon beams* and angle ties are employed to prevent the outward thrust of the hip rafter from acting directly on the corner of the building (see Fig. 4).

Sizes of Various Members

To find the sizes of the various members the following rules may be employed. For the thickness of all members, take ¼ span in feet — 1, = thickness in inches. The breadth of the members on the elevation will be : tie-beam, ½ span in feet — 2 ; centre of king-post, ⅙ span in feet. Make king-post ends twice width of centre less ½ in. ; struts 2 in. for 20 ft., increasing ¼ in. in width for every 2 ft. Reduce thickness of truss by ½ in. and depth of tie-beam by 1 in. if there is no ceiling.

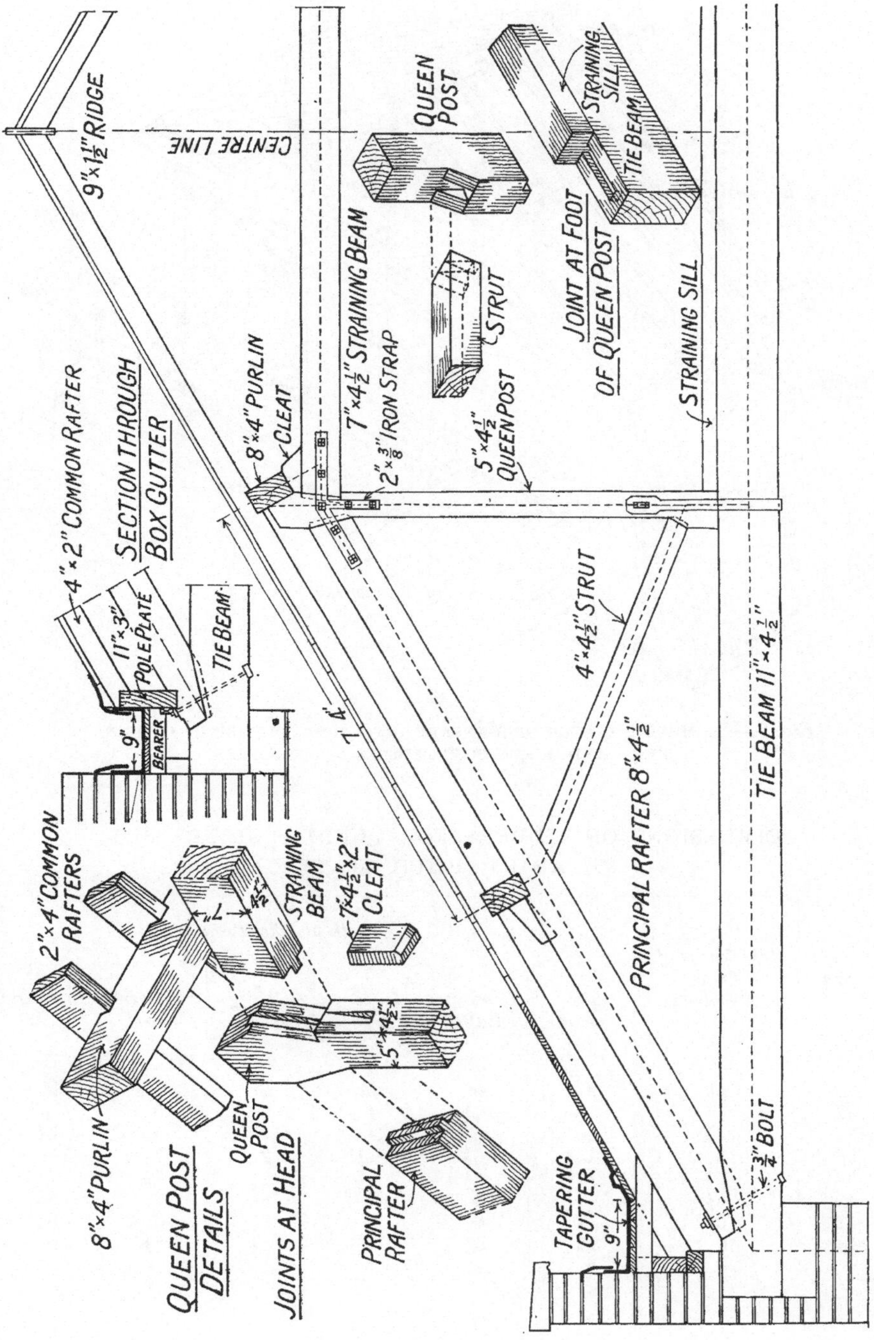

Fig. 5.—QUEEN-POST ROOF TRUSS

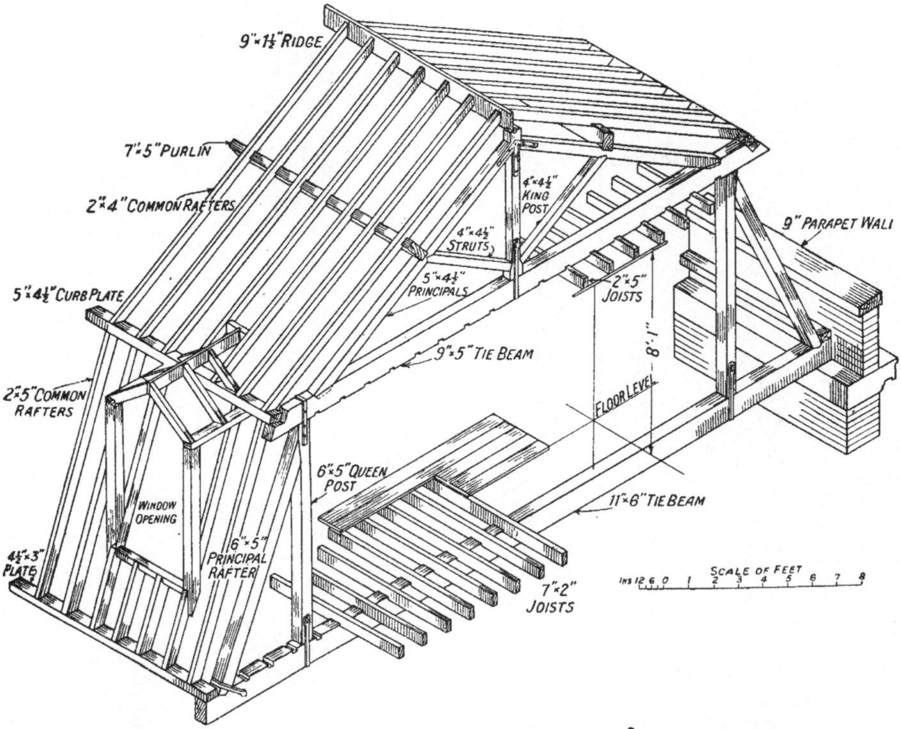

Fig. 6.—ISOMETRIC SKETCH OF MANSARD ROOF, SHOWING USE OF COMBINED KING- AND QUEEN-POST TRUSSES AS SUPPORTS

DIMENSIONS OF TIMBERS, FOR QUEEN-POST TRUSSES 10 FT. APART, PITCH 30°, SLATED

Span	*Thickness of Truss Members*	*Breadth on Elevation*					
		Tie-beam	*Principal Rafter*	*Queen-post*	*Struts*	*Straining Beam*	*Straining Cill*
ft.	*in.*	*in.*	*in.*	*in.*	*in.*	*in.*	*in.*
32	4	9	4½	4	2	6	3
34	4½	10	5	4	2	6½	3½
36	5	10½	5½	4½	2	7	4
38	5½	11	5½	4½	2¼	7½	4
40	5½	11½	6	5	2½	8	4½
42	6	12	6	5	2½	8	5
44	6	12	6½	5½	2½	8½	5

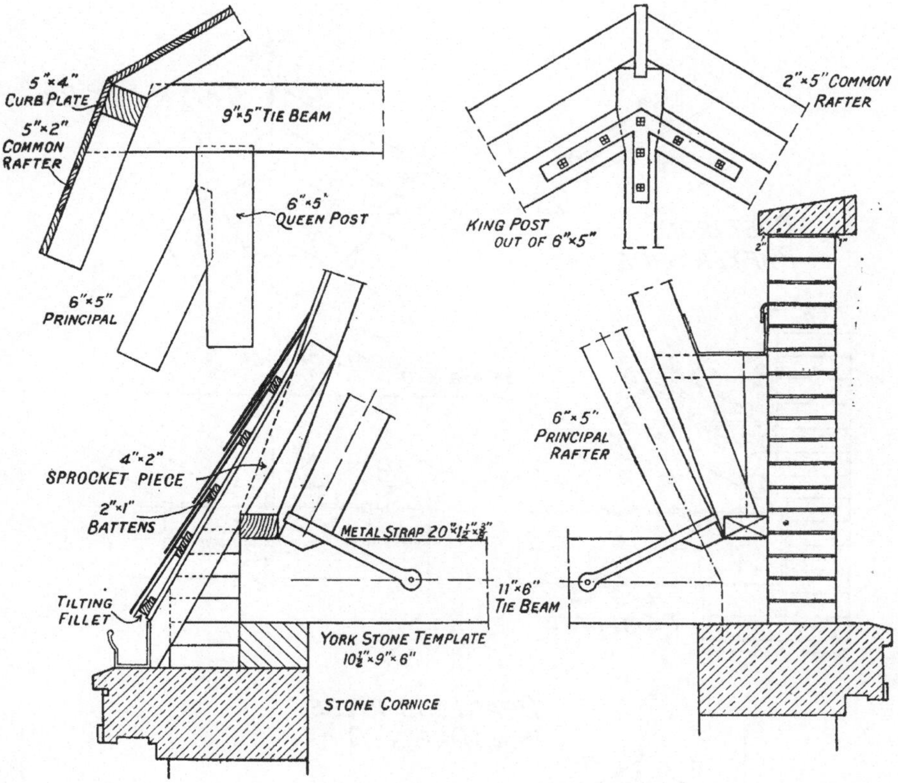

Fig. 7.—MANSARD ROOF DETAILS

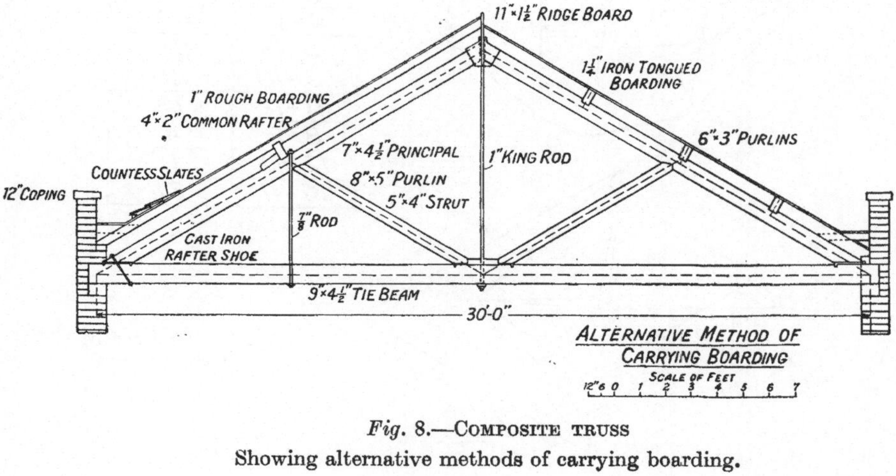

Fig. 8.—COMPOSITE TRUSS

Showing alternative methods of carrying boarding.

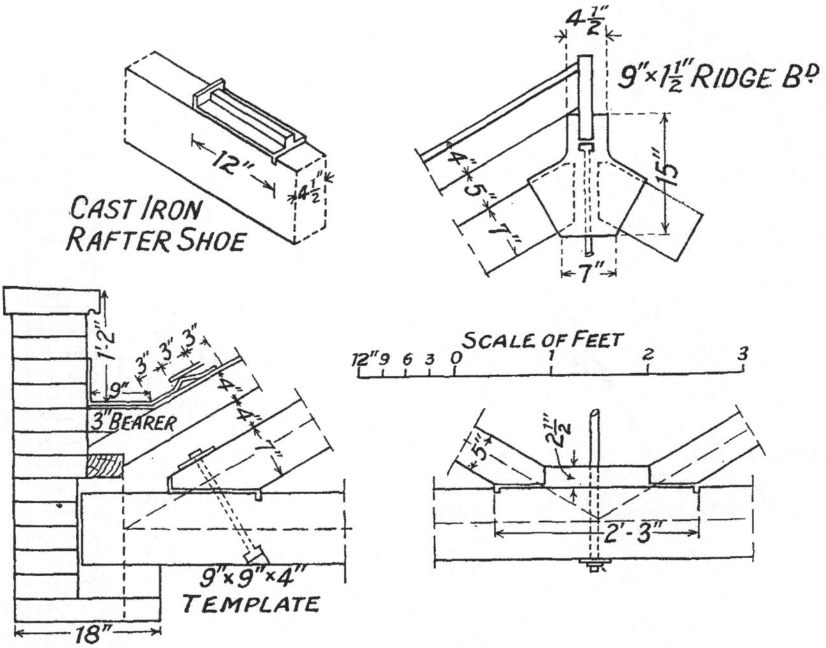

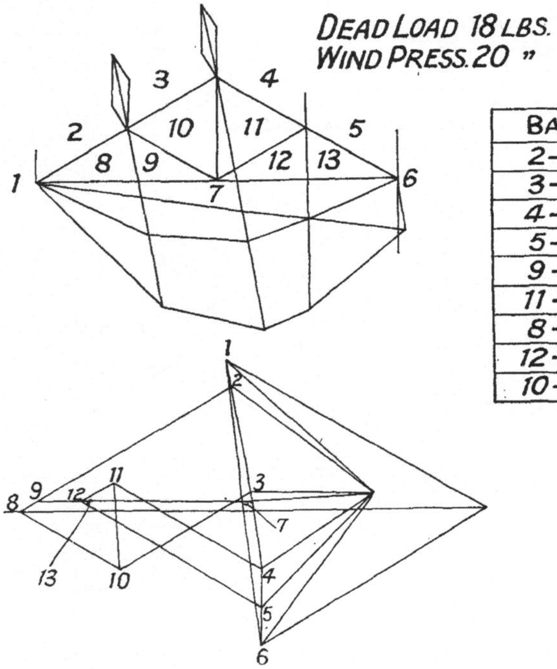

BAR.	STRESS IN CWTS
2-8	60
3-10	38
4-11	43
5-13	55
9-10	29
11-12	13
8-9	4
12-13	0
10-11	21

Fig. 9.—DETAILS OF COMPOSITE TRUSS

Queen-post Trusses

These are used for spans of from 30 ft. to 45 ft., the tie-beam and rafters being supported at two intermediate points in their length, instead of only at one. The two queen-posts are connected at their tops by a horizontal member called a *straining beam,* and the junction of these affords a support at one point for the rafters (see Fig. 5). The principal rafter ends at this point, and is not carried to the ridge as in the king-post roof truss. A support for the middle of the principal rafter is obtained by the strut which springs from the base of the queen-post. The purlin over this point occurs at about a third of the distance along the common rafter, the second purlin at the top of the queen-post being another third, which provides the necessary support to the common rafters.

The thrusts from the struts are resisted by a tenon on the foot of each post, and a member called a *straining sill.* Many of the details of this truss are the same as those of the king-post truss previously described and illustrated (see Fig. 5).

Queen-post roof trusses are not much in use at the present time, owing to the increased use of steel for large-span roofs, but they can be used with advantage where a lantern light has to be fixed in the centre. The Table on page 24 gives the scantlings for queen-post roof trusses.

Mansard or Curb Roof

The Mansard or curb roof is essentially one with two pitches, and is usually employed as a means of economising space. In roofs of ordinary pitch a great amount of the space is lost, due to the sharp pitch of the sides, but in the Mansard roof this is overcome by making the sides of the lower pitch nearly vertical. The upper slope is then made relatively flat to avoid an acute ridge. Fig. 6 is an isometric view of this roof, and Fig. 7 shows the details of the joints.

Composite Roof Trusses

Roofs formed or built up of a combination of timber and steel members are known as composite trusses, the compression members being of timber and the tension members of steel, which from its great tensile strength is more suitable, but these roofs are not very frequently used (see Fig. 8). Alternative methods of construction are illustrated.

Chapter III

FLAT ROOFS

In practice, flat roofs are formed with timber, concrete and steel, reinforced concrete, or hollow tiles as a base, and covered with asphalte lead, copper, or zinc, or concrete slabs over asphalte, or asbestos-cement tiles on asphalte. The construction is similar to floor construction, but a slight fall is necessary to drain off the water.

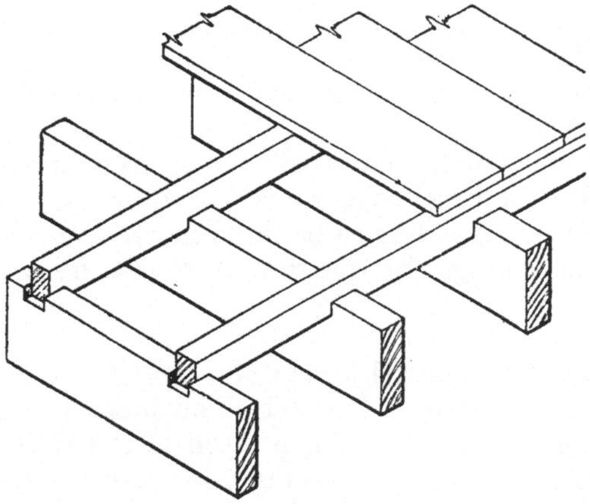

Fig. 1.—Flat roof—joists parallel to flow

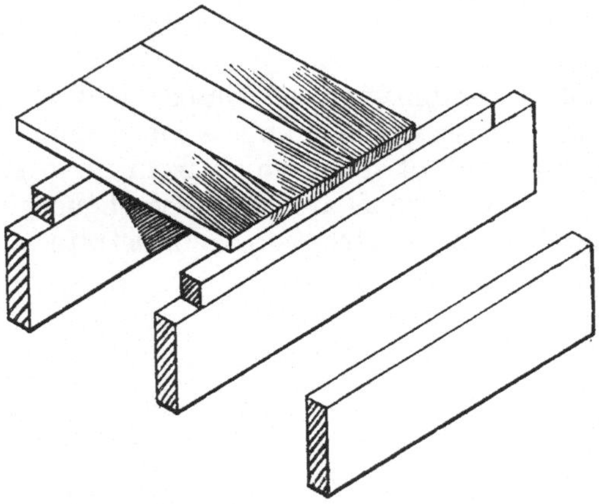

Fig. 2.—Flat roof—joists at right angles to flow

Timber Construction

When timber is employed the joists are furred to falls (Fig. 1). Where the span of the joists exceeds about 16 ft., rolled-steel joist binders are introduced to form an intermediate support for the joists. For lead-covered flats, the roof is given a fall of $1\frac{1}{2}$ in. in 10 ft., or 4°. The boards should run in the direction of the flow, because if placed at right angles to it, and the boards should warp slightly, hollows would form in which the water may lie (Figs. 1 and 2). For good-class work the boarding should be in narrow widths, and $1\frac{1}{4}$-in. nominal thickness, and the roof covered with felt to give a smooth surface for the lead or other covering.

Lead Flats—Drips

The joint along the end of the lead sheet is formed by

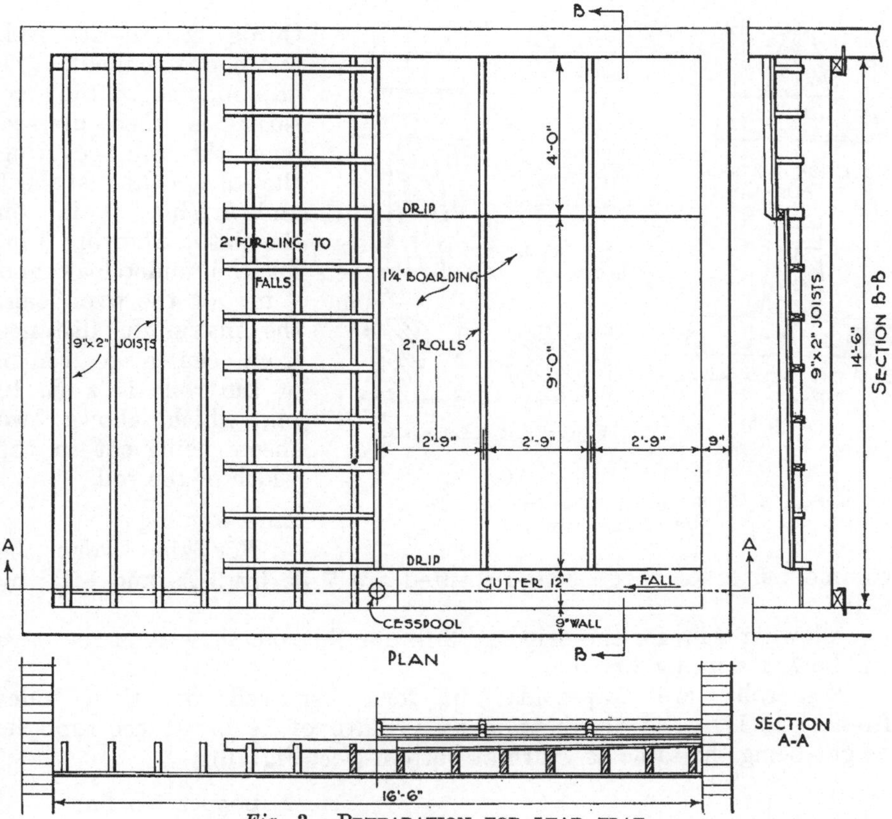

Fig. 3.—PREPARATION FOR LEAD FLAT

means of a *drip*—an abrupt change in the level of the roof, usually 2½ in. deep. The face of the drip may be vertical (see Fig. 4), or an angle fillet may be introduced.

The end of the boarding at the top is rebated to a depth equal to the thickness of the sheet, and a width of 1 in. or 1½ in. The upper end of the lower sheet is dressed over the drip and turned down into the rebate, and fixed with copper nails. The upper sheet is next dressed down over the drip, and is either finished about ½ in. short of the lower flat or carried down and dressed about 1 in. on the flat below. The amount of lead required to form a 2½-in. drip is 7 in., and this amount, deducted from the maximum length of sheet it is desirable to use, i.e. 10 ft., gives the distances between the drips or length of bay at 9 ft. 5 in.

Rolls for Lead

The joint along the edge of the sheet and parallel to the fall is formed by means of a roll, over which the lead sheets are dressed (see Fig. 5). The edge of one sheet, or *undercloak* as it is called, is dressed about two-

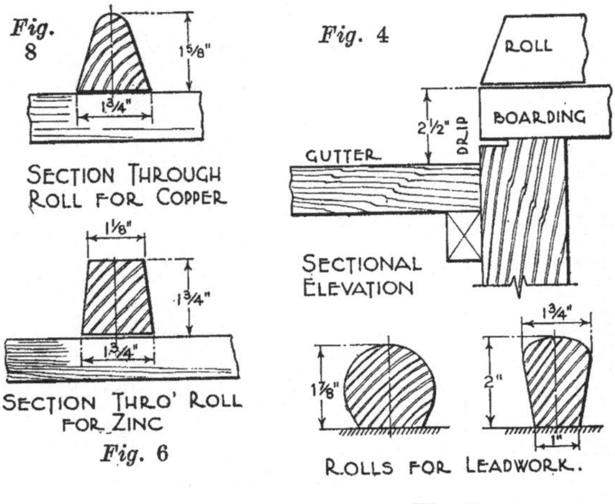

Figs. 4, 5, 6, *and* 8.—DETAILS OF ROLLS FOR SHEET METAL

thirds round the roll, and copper nailed. The adjoining sheet, the *overcloak,* is then dressed over the roll, covering the edge of the first sheet and finishing 1 in. on the flat. Allowing 3 in. for the undercloak and 7 in. for the overcloak, the maximum distance from centre to centre of the rolls is 2 ft. 10 in., which allows two sheets being cut in the width of the roll.

Zinc Roofing

For zinc work the common sizes of sheets manufactured are 7 ft. by 3 ft. and 8 ft. by 3 ft.

Allowing 6 in. for the drip and 3 in. for the roll, the size of the bays will be 7 ft. 6 in. by 2 ft. 9 in.

The rolls are trapezoidal in form, splayed on their sides from $1\frac{5}{8}$ to $1\frac{3}{4}$ in. at the bottom to a width of $1\frac{1}{8}$ in. at the top, the height being the same as width at bottom (see Fig. 6).

Copper Roofing

For copper roofing the sheets employed measure 5 ft. 3 in. by 2 ft. 8 in., and 4 ft. by 3 ft. 6 in., both having the same area. After making allowances for roll and drip, the bays will measure 4 ft. $10\frac{1}{2}$ in. by 2 ft. $4\frac{1}{2}$ in. when using a 5-ft. 3-in. by 2-ft. 8-in. sheet (Fig. 7). The rolls are made conical shape in section, measuring $1\frac{3}{4}$ in. at the bottom and $1\frac{5}{8}$ in. or $1\frac{3}{4}$ in. in height (see Fig. 8).

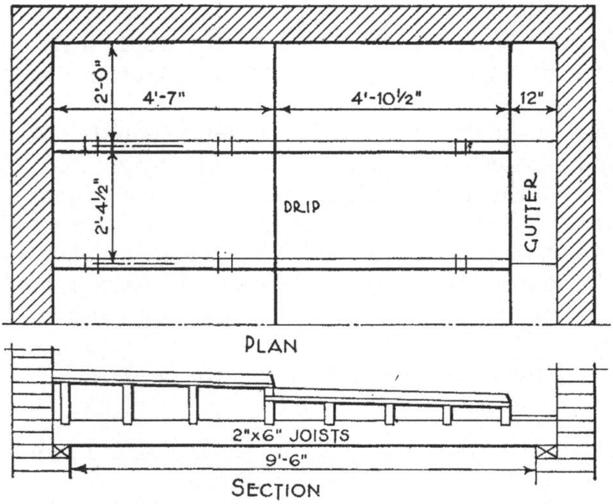

Fig. 7.—PREPARATION OF ROOF FOR COPPER COVERING

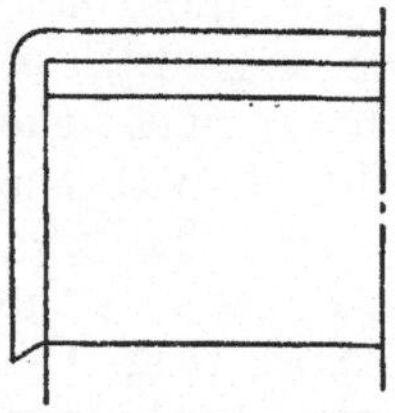

Fig. 9.—Asphalte apron with undercut drip

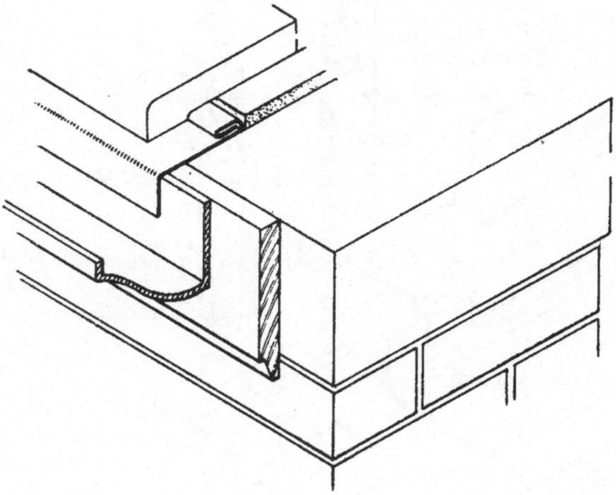

Fig. 10.—Asphalte dressing to welted lead or copper apron on rebated edge

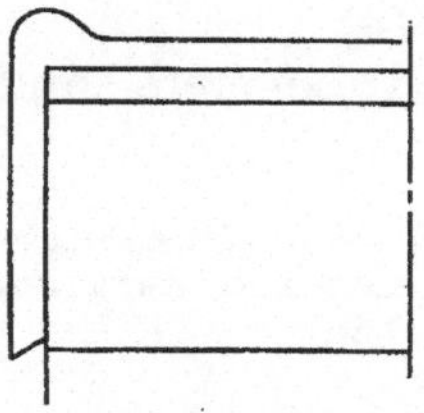

Fig. 11.—Asphalte finish at verge

Asphalte Roofing

This material can be laid on concrete or boarding ; when laid on boarding an underlay of felt must be employed, but the use of wire or expanded metal lathing in addition is not considered essential. For flat roofs the surface should be finished to a fall of 1 in 10. On sloping roofs the surface should be formed with grooves to provide a key, as the material is apt to run if exposed to the sun. The grooves are formed by fixing $1\frac{1}{2}$-in. by $\frac{3}{8}$-in. battens horizontally along the roof at 18-in. centres, and then rendering the surface level with the top of the battens in cement and sand (1 to 2). The battens are removed after the cement has set, leaving grooves in the surface. Where a flat roof finishes with an eaves gutter the asphalte is dressed over on to the face of the wall to form an apron (see Fig. 9), the lower edge being splayed back to form a drip. An alternative method is to dress the asphalte to a welted lead or copper flashing on a rebated edge of the flat, the asphalte being set back $\frac{3}{4}$ in. from the edge (see Fig. 10). Where verges occur on a concrete pitched roof, the edge is slightly tilted to divert the water from the edge (see Fig. 11).

Junction of Roof with Lantern Lights

Where a flat roof abuts against a lantern light, a curb is formed in concrete or wood, the asphalte carried up the face of the curb and finished

Fig. 12

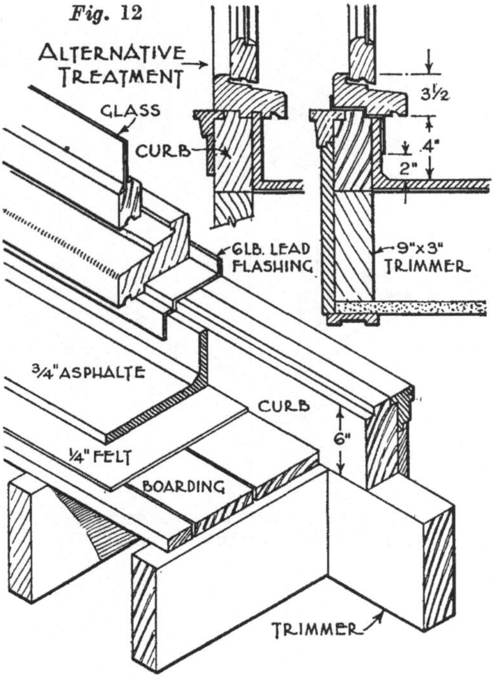

Fig. 13.—TREATMENT OF TIMBER ROOF ABUTTING LANTERN LIGHT

in a groove in the under side of the cill (see Fig. 12), or it may finish against the under side of the cill with the addition of a lead flashing, a groove being formed in the cill for the purpose (Fig. 13). For a concrete curb the asphalte is taken up the face of the curb under the cill, and finished against the water bar (see Fig. 14).

Steel and concrete and glass are now largely used in the construction of lantern lights.

Fig. 14 (*below*).—TREATMENT FOR CONCRETE ROOF ABUTTING LANTERN LIGHT

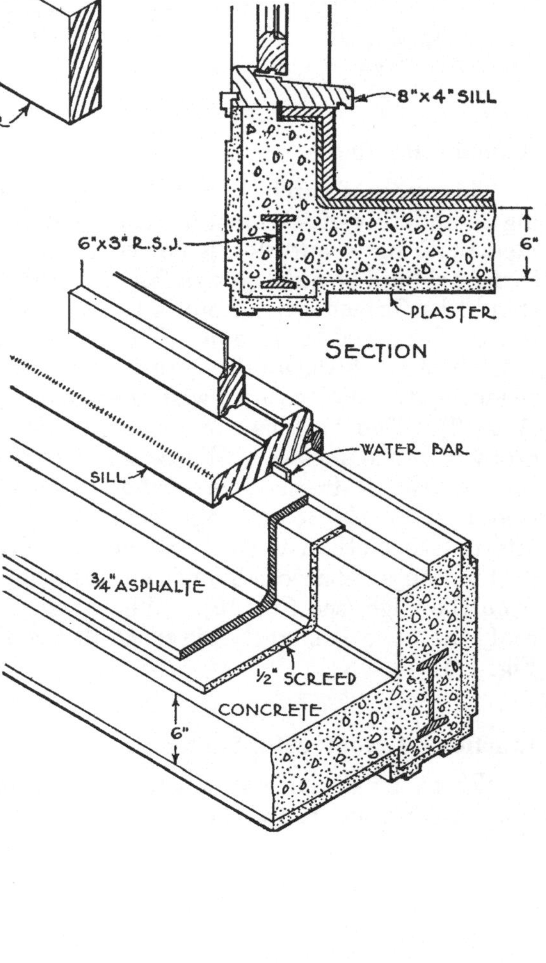

Steel Construction

Fig. 15 shows a lantern light in all-steel construction. The angle shafts are $2\frac{1}{4}$ in. square, and the metal $\frac{3}{16}$ in. thick; the cill is also of the same section. The cill is fixed to the concrete curb by means of a lug, as shown, or by the use of a coachscrew, where the curb is formed with timber.

" Glass-crete "

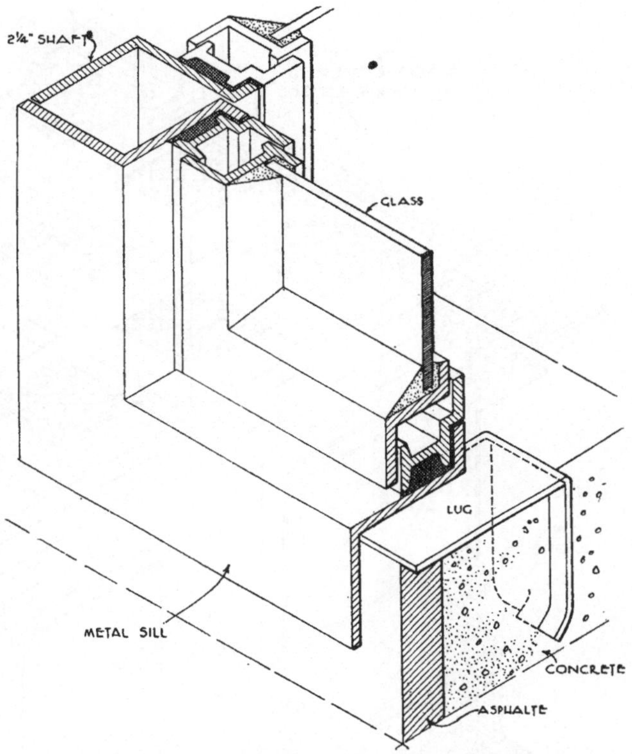

Fig. 15.—LANTERN LIGHT IN ALL-STEEL CONSTRUCTION

The use of glass prisms embedded in concrete gives a strong construction which allows considerable carrying power over large spans. The glass units are produced in dimensions to conform to structural requirements as to thickness and weight, depending on the type of structure. The use of concrete permits of greater possibilities, and the older methods of glazing, which would not meet the higher standard of modern practice, have been superseded.

All the disadvantages which arose from the use of wrought iron are removed by the use of reinforced concrete. In addition, there are no surfaces to rust,

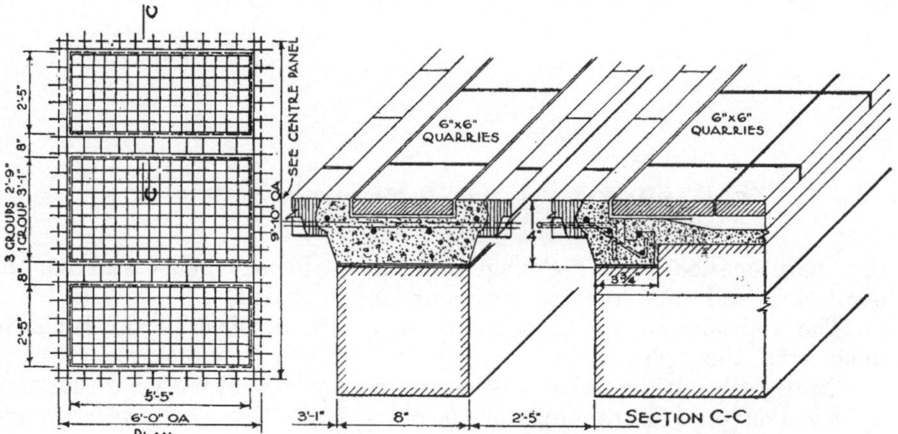

Fig. 16.—DETAIL OF ROOF LIGHT ON FLAT REBATED CURB

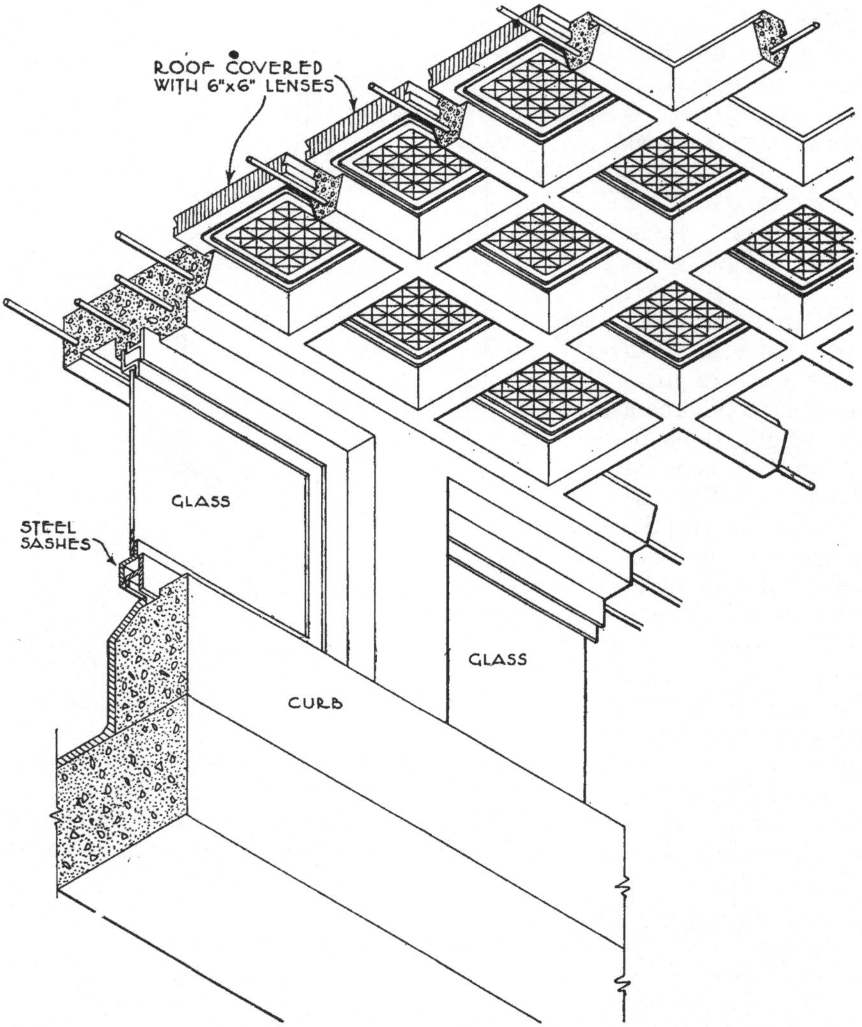

Fig. 17.—Lantern light in "Glass-crete" on raised curb

the maintenance costs are negligible, and efficient heat- and sound-insulation and resistance to corrosion are provided.

The top surface of the concrete may be finished with asphalte flush with the lights.

Quarry tiles, stone slabs, or other finish may be adopted where the roof light is fixed on a flat rebated curb (see Fig. 16). Fig. 17 shows a lantern light on a raised curb in the same materials. The sides of the lantern are

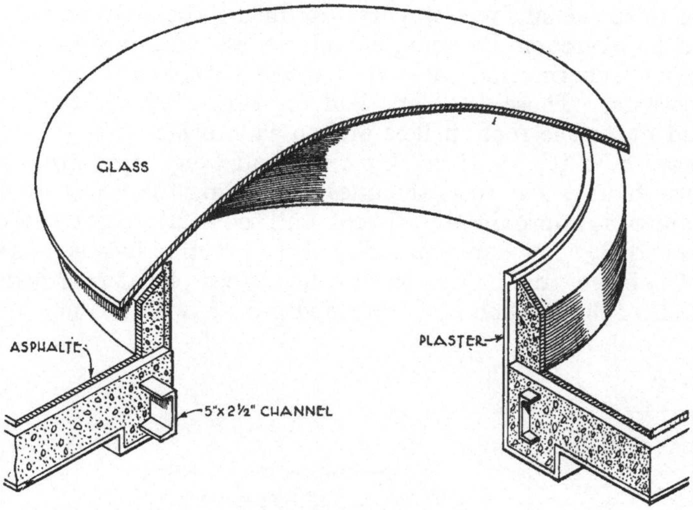

Fig. 18.—Isometric sketch of glass dome light

fitted with steel sashes, and the roof is constructed with 6-in. by 6-in. lenses. Fig. 18 shows a glass dome formed in one piece, and suitable for spans up to 6-ft. diameter. The dome is fixed to the curb by means of special fittings.

Roof Insulation

Flat roofs generally require some form of insulation. Where the roof is of timber construction a certain amount of insulation in some cases is adequate by fixing a wall board to the ceiling. A more even distribution of temperature would be obtained if the insulating board were placed directly under the roof boarding or bitumen sheeting, and using a lath-and-plaster ceiling. When the insulating board is placed directly under the bitumen sheeting or asphalte, it

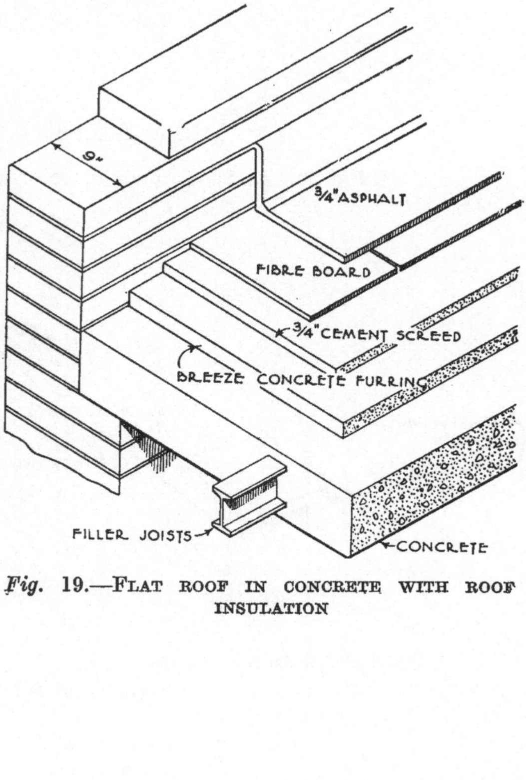

Fig. 19.—Flat roof in concrete with roof insulation

tends to raise the surface temperature during the summer (see Fig. 19). This can be overcome by using asbestos tiles. An excellent tile for this purpose is "Thermotile," which is made with a mixture of asbestos-cement waste. These tiles are laid on three layers of bitumen felt, cemented on to the roof surface and to each other with bitumen. The tiles measure 12 in. by 12 in. by 1 in., and weigh approximately 8 lbs. per square foot. The total thickness, including the waterproof sheeting and bitumen, is approximately 1½ in., and the total weight approximately 10 lbs. per sq. ft. The damp-proofing of the junction between parapet wall and roof is important in this as in other types of flat-roof construction, and details of the method recommended are shown in Fig. 20. Details

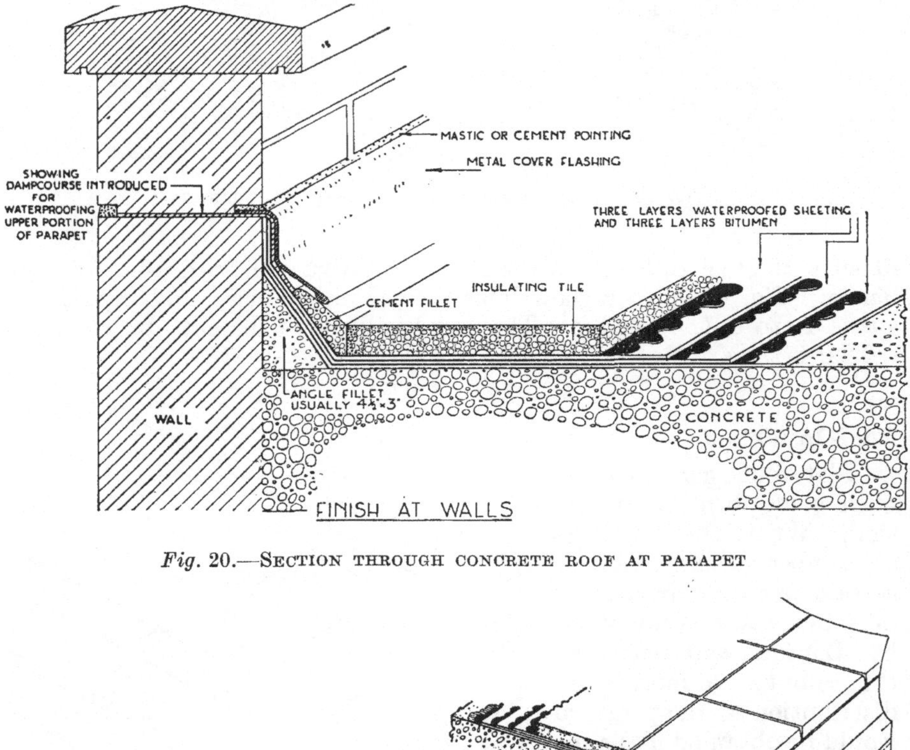

Fig. 20.—Section through concrete roof at parapet

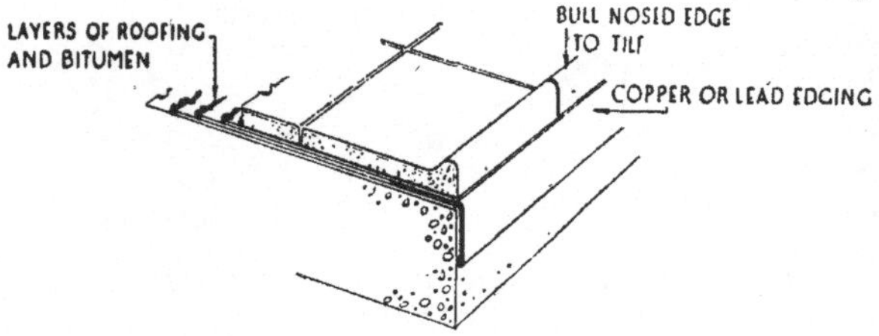

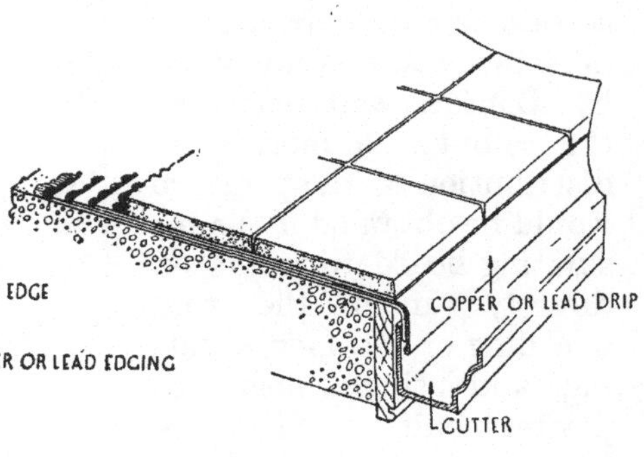

Fig. 21.—Section at verge *Fig.* 22.—Section at eaves

(*D. Anderson & Son Ltd.*)

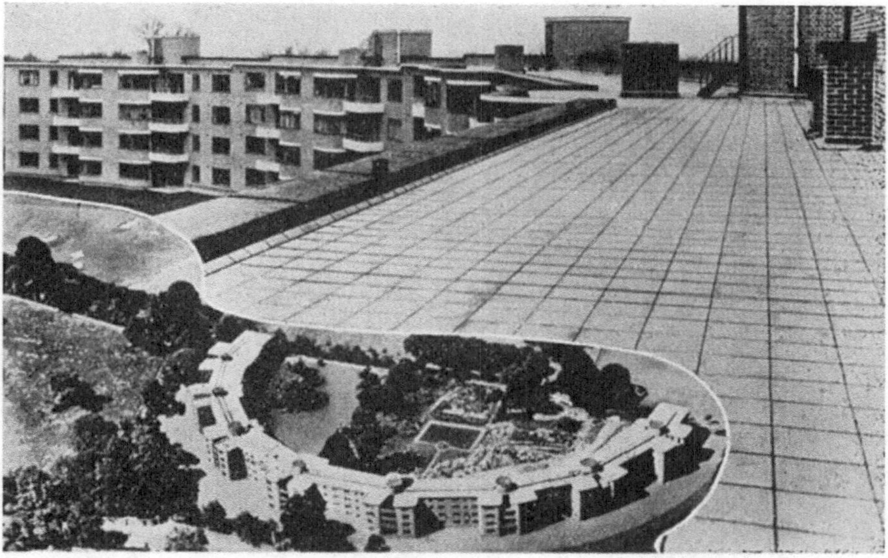

Fig. 23.—Roofs covered with Thermotile at Fairacres, Roehampton Lane, London, S.W. (*D. Anderson & Son Ltd.*)

Architects: Minoprio and Spenceley, A.A.R.I.B.A.
Consulting Architect: B. de Helsby, Esq., A.I.A.A.
General Contractors: C. F. Kearley, Ltd.

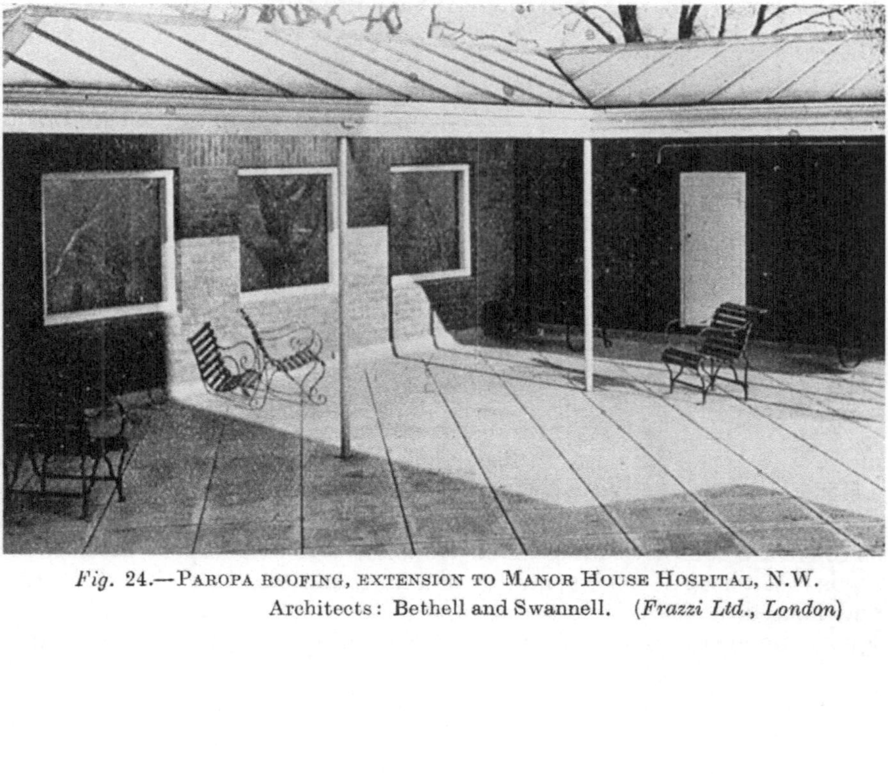

Fig. 24.—Paropa roofing, extension to Manor House Hospital, N.W.
Architects: Bethell and Swannell. (*Frazzi Ltd., London*)

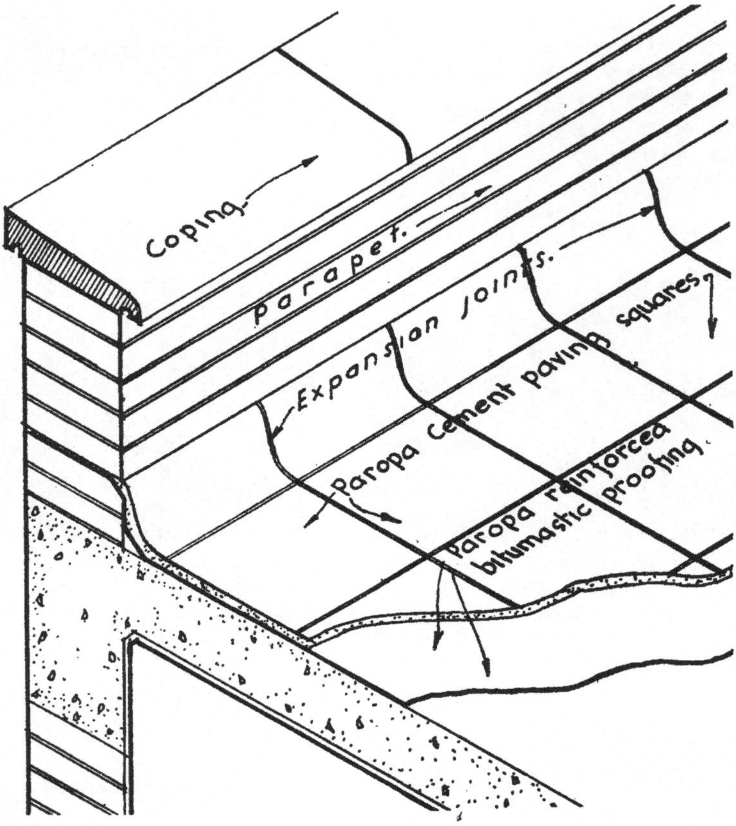

Fig. 25.—Paropa roofing on concrete, showing treatment against a brick parapet. (*Frazzi Ltd.*)

of the treatment at verge and eaves are given in Figs. 21 and 22. The metal cover flashings to walls and eaves are particularly important, and the makers of "Thermotile" roofing, Messrs. D. Anderson & Son Ltd., prefer to execute this work themselves to ensure that it is carried out to exact requirements.

Another excellent type of insulated flat-roof covering is "Paropa," made by Messrs. Frazzi Ltd., which consists of a well-primed surface having a slope of 1 per cent., on which a bituminous mat is built up with layers of pure bitumen, wood felt, and hessian. This waterproof mat is so composed as to ensure complete adhesion to the base. On this impermeable covering is laid a coat of cement mortar of 1 in. thickness, which is well tamped and floated, and while soft is divided into panels, approximately 24 in. square, by means of special tools. The dividing joints framing the panels

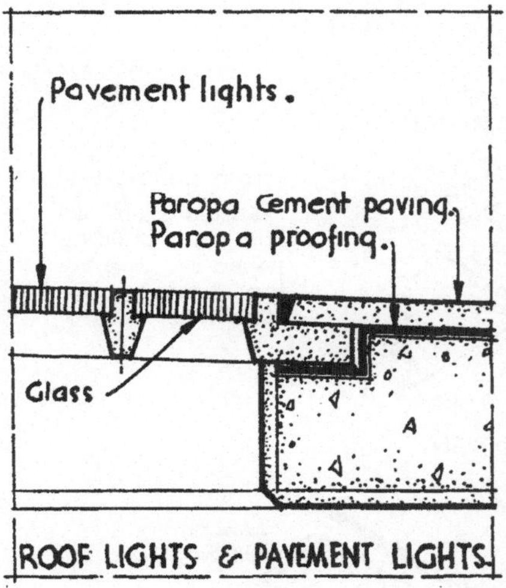

(a)

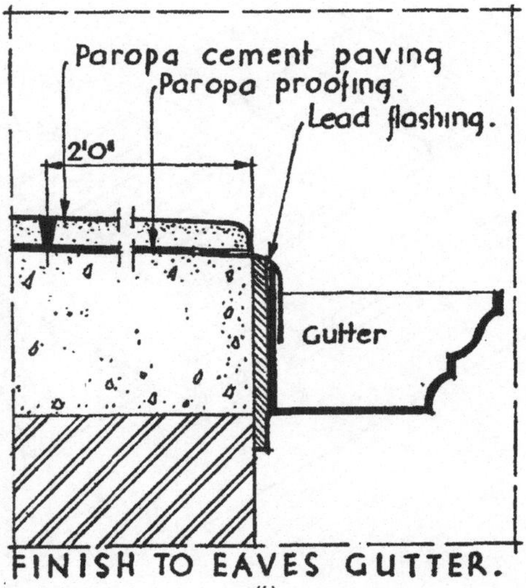

(b)

Figs. 26A *and* B.—Paropa roofing on concrete

a—Junction between Paropa and roof-light. *b*—Showing finish to eaves gutter.

(*Frazzi Ltd.*)

are cut to the bitumen below, thus forming most efficient expansion joints. After hardening of the cement topping the expansion joints are primed and filled with an elastic bitumen.

"Paropa" can be finished in various designs and colours, and forms a good non-slip surface. The weight is 12 lbs. per sq. foot. The junction between roof and parapet, and the treatment at gutters and outlets, together with the treatment of roof lights, are shown in Figs. 25, 26A, B, and C.

Both Thermotile and Paropa can be applied to wood as well as to concrete surfaces, the bitumen layers being applied, preferably, to a layer of insulating board laid on top of the normal roof boarding.

Where a high degree of insulation is required, the use of 2-in. insulating blocks such as "Fosalsil" is a proved method, these being laid on

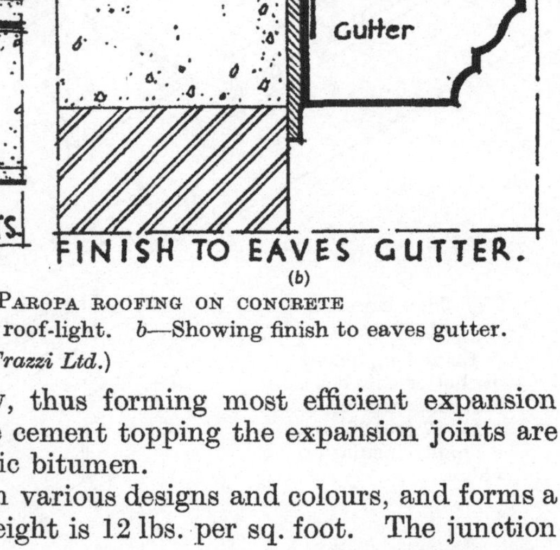

Fig. 26C.—Showing treatment of rain-water outlet in Paropa roofing on concrete

(*Frazzi Ltd.*)

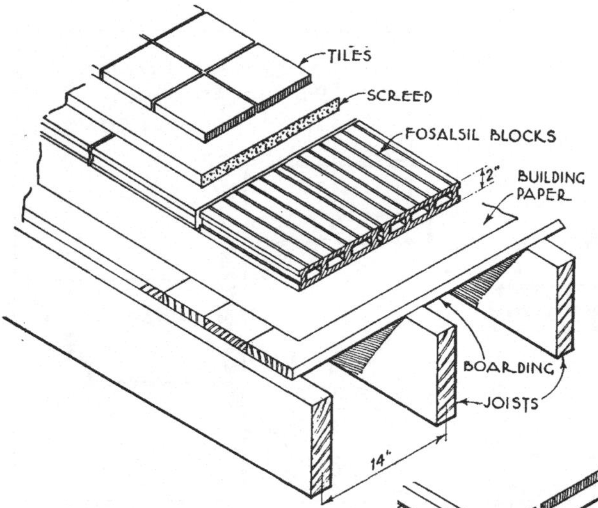

Fig. 27 (*left*).—ROOF INSULATION

Insulating blocks laid on building paper, the base being timber construction.

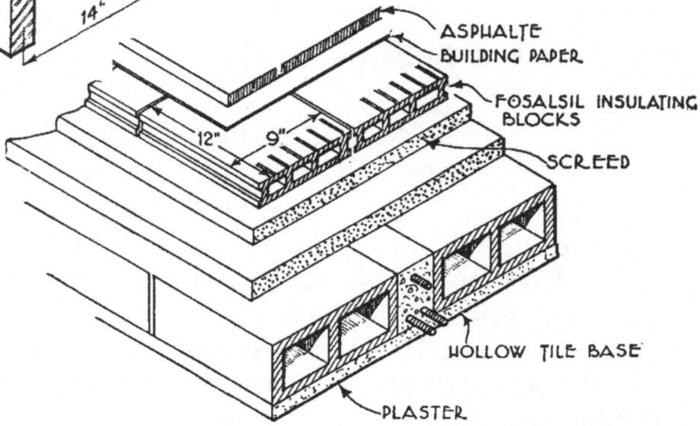

Fig. 28.—ROOF INSULATION

Insulating blocks on hollow-tile base. Methods shown in Figs. 27 and 28 give a high insulation value.

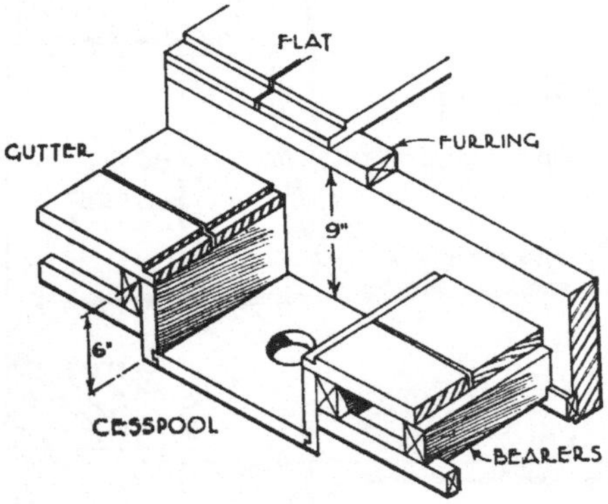

Fig. 29.—PARALLEL GUTTER TO FLAT ROOF

Showing detail of cesspool with joists parallel to gutter.

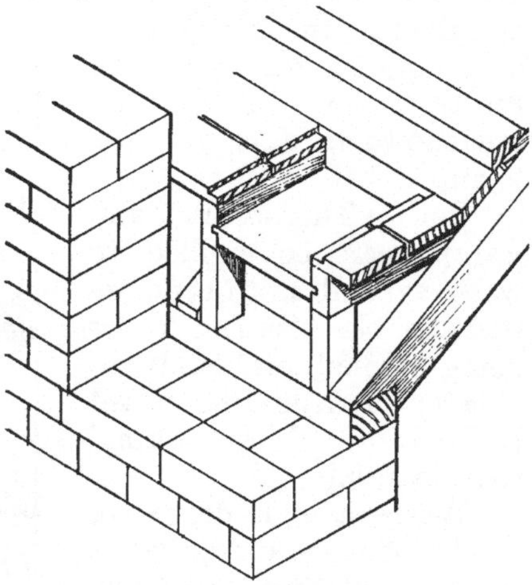

Fig. 30.—TAPERING GUTTER

Isometric sketch of chute to parapet gutter. Note bearers are nailed to side of rafters.

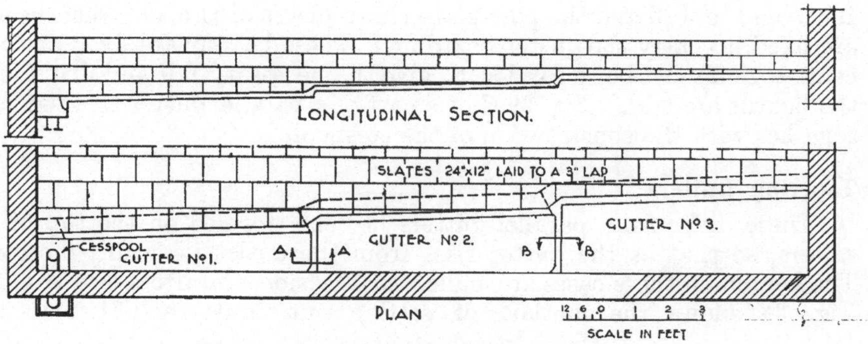

Fig. 31.—Lead gutter to parapet wall

top of boarding or screed for wood or concrete roofs respectively, followed by normal asphalte or paving tile construction. Figs. 27 and 28 illustrate the method for both types of roof.

Preparation for Gutters

Gutters may be either parallel or tapering on plan.

Parallel Gutters

These are formed by fixing a pole-plate at a distance of from 9 in. to 12 in. from the wall. This pole-plate carries the lower ends of the rafters.

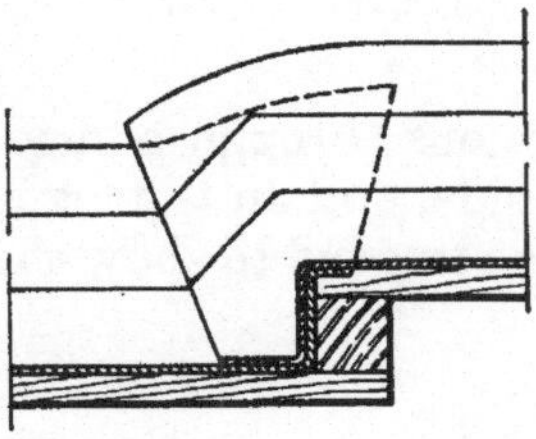

Section through drip A–A from wall side.

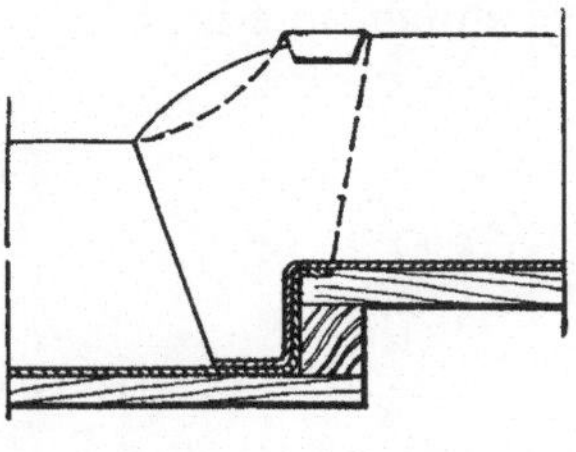

Section through drip showing finish of lead against wall.

Fig. 32

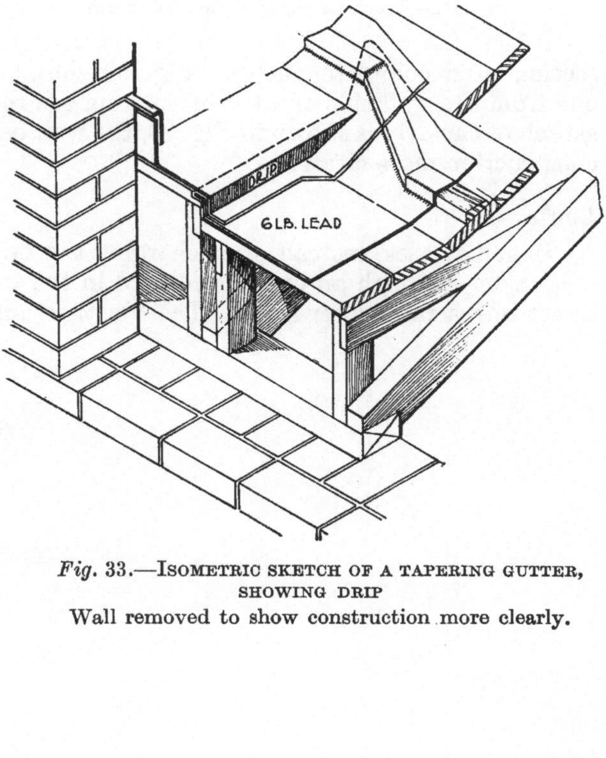

Fig. 33.—Isometric sketch of a tapering gutter, showing drip

Wall removed to show construction more clearly.

Between the wall and the pole-plate short pieces of timber called bearers are fixed, to carry the gutter boarding. These bearers are fixed at 15-in. centres, and must be so fixed as to give the necessary fall and drips when the boards are laid. Fig. 29 shows part of a parallel gutter to a flat roof, together with the construction of the cesspool.

Tapering Gutters

These differ from parallel gutters in being formed on the top of the rafters, so that as the gutter rises from the outlet its width increases. The bearers in these cases are nailed to the side of rafters (see Fig. 30). Fig. 34 shows the method of setting out, and Fig. 31 plan and

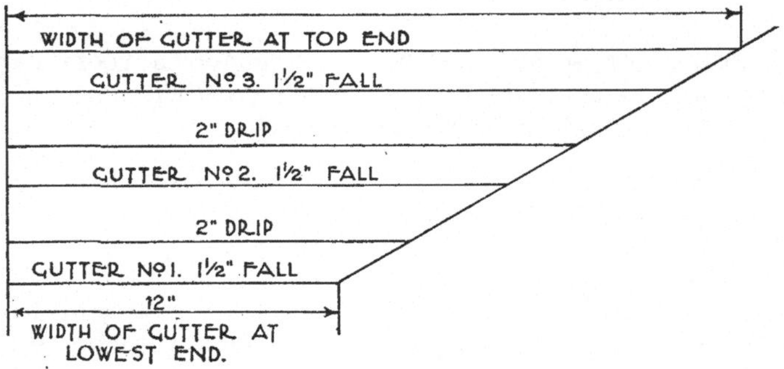

Fig. 34.—DIAGRAM SHOWING WIDTH AT TOP AND BOTTOM OF EACH GUTTER

section of a complete gutter. Fig. 32 shows sections through a drip, one from the wall side and the other from the roof side, and an isometric sketch of the drip is shown in Fig. 33, the wall being removed to show the construction more clearly.

Chute

In some cases, instead of discharging the rain-water into a cesspool, it is taken, through an opening formed in the wall by means of a chute, direct into a rain-water head. The construction is shown in Fig. 31

Chapter IV

SIZES AND SPACING OF ROOF MEMBERS

ALTHOUGH suitable sizes for roof members are given in the tables and illustrations in this and other chapters, everyone interested in building work should be able to calculate the most economical spacing of the rafters, and also the safe load on the beams.

Under the Code of Practice, 1932 (sec. 35), sloping roofs of over 20° pitch may be designed for a combined superimposed and wind load of 15 lbs. per square foot, assumed acting normal to the surface inwards on the windward side, and 10 lbs. per square foot of surface similarly acting outwards on the leeward side, provided this requirement applies only in the design of the roof structure. Snow may be taken at 3 lbs. per sq. ft.

The weight of the truss is given by Fowler's formula: ·04 span + ·4 for light roofs, and ·06 span + ·6 for heavy roofs; or by Ricker's formula: $W = \frac{\text{span}}{25} + \frac{\text{span}^2}{6{,}000}$.

Working Stresses for Rafters

A list of sizes for purlins is given on page 44.

In calculating the safe load on timber beams, rafters, or joists, various methods are used. The following assumes good-quality timber.

One method is based on the results of numerous tests on small pieces of timber 1 in. by 1 in. in section, supported at both ends, over a span of 12 in., and loaded in the middle, the breaking weight being used as a constant. When the test piece is loaded in this way it is said to be under transverse stress, the fibres at the top being in compression and those at the bottom being in tension, while the intensity of each stress diminishes towards the centre of the beam, or the centre of gravity of the section, at which point they both vanish. Where this occurs it is called the *neutral layer* on the elevation of the beam, and the *neutral axis* in the cross-section. In beams of symmetrical section it is found at the geometrical centre of the section. The unit of transverse stress is called the *modulus of rupture*. It is sometimes supposed to be the same as the maximum fibre stress, but it is found to be greater than this.

The strength varies as $\frac{bd^2}{L}$, where b = breadth in inches, d = depth in inches, and L = span in feet. This formula does not make provision for any variation in the class of material used. This provision is expressed by the constant c, or unit load to break unit beam. It varies with the variety of wood used. For spruce or fir it is found to be 3·5 cwts., for red deal 4 cwts., for oak 4·5 cwts., and for pitch pine 5 cwts.

In the ordinary way the beam is required to carry a load safely, and to do this it is necessary to reduce the load to a fraction of the breaking weight, say $\frac{1}{5}$ or $\frac{1}{6}$, and the factor of safety F is then said to be 5 or 6, as the case may be.

The formula now becomes $\frac{cbd^2}{FL}$.

WEIGHTS OF ROOFING MATERIALS

Material	*Average Weight per Ft. Super in Lbs.*
Slates—North Wales: Firsts	5·5
Seconds	6·5
Thirds	7·5
Cornish: Firsts	6·72
Seconds	7·84
Thirds	11·20
Westmorland: Firsts	8·4
Seconds	10·1
Thirds	12·32
Tiles—Machine-made	11·25
Hand-made	12·25
Pantiles	11·25
Asbestos tiles	3·0
Asbestos corrugated sheets	3·1
Steel corrugated sheets—18 B.W.G.	2·75
20 B.W.G.	2·25
Roof boarding—1 in.	2·5
$\frac{7}{8}$ in.	2·25
$\frac{3}{4}$ in.	1·87
Tiling battens (4-in. gauge)—2 in. by 1 in.	1·5
2 in. by $\frac{3}{4}$ in., or $1\frac{1}{2}$ in. by 1 in.	1·125
1 in. by 1 in.	0·75
Felt.	0·5
	Average Weight per Sq. Ft. in Lbs.
2-in. by 3-in. common rafters at 15-in. centres, 6-ft. span	1·2
2-in. by 4-in. ,, ,, ,, ,, ,, 7-ft. 6-in. span	1·6
2-in. by $4\frac{1}{2}$-in. ,, ,, ,, ,, ,, 9-ft. span	1·8
2-in. by 5-in. ,, ,, ,, ,, ,, 10-ft. ,,	2·0
2-in. by 6-in. ,, ,, ,, ,, ,, 12-ft. ,,	2·4

PURLINS FOR ALL ROOFS

Clear Span	*Distance Apart Not Exceeding*					
	6 ft.		*7 ft. 6 in.*		*9 ft.*	
	in. in.	*lb./sq. ft.*	*in. in.*	*lb./sq. ft.*	*in. in.*	*lb./sq. ft.*
6	3 × 5	·62	3 × $5\frac{1}{2}$	·55	3 × 6	·50
8	3 × 6	·75	3 × 7	·70	4 × 7	·70
10	4 × 7	1·2	4 × 8	1·1	5 × 8	1·1
12	4 × 9	1·5	$4\frac{1}{2}$ × 9	1·35	5 × 9	1·25
14	5 × 9	1·6	$4\frac{1}{2}$ × 10	1·50	$4\frac{1}{2}$ × 11	1·37

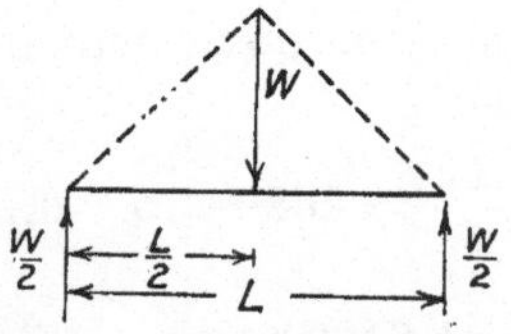

Fig. 1.—BENDING-MOMENT DIAGRAM FOR CONCENTRATED LOAD

Example.—Required the safe concentrated load in cwts. on a beam of red deal 5 in. deep, 2 in. wide, and 10-ft. span. F = 5.

$$W = \frac{cbd^2}{FL} = \frac{4 \times 2 \times 5^2}{5 \times 10} = 4 \text{ cwts.}$$

Resistance Moment

As a means of comparison we will now ascertain the load based on the moment of resistance of the beam. This is given by the following equations :—

$$BM = MR = Zf, \text{ in which—}$$

BM = bending moment.
MR = moment of resistance.
Z = section modulus of the beam.
f = permissible fibre stress in the material, usually referred to as the extreme fibre stress.

The bending produced by the load on a simply supported beam tends to shorten or compress the upper fibres, and to lengthen or put in tension the lower fibres. In the case of a simply supported beam, with a load at the centre, the maximum bending moment is $\frac{WL}{4}$, and is obtained by multiplying the reaction $\frac{W}{2}$ by the leverage $\frac{L}{2}$ (see Fig. 1). The modulus of section, $Z = \frac{bd^2}{6}$, is obtained as follows : on the section shown in Fig. 2 draw two diagonals, forming triangles, the two middle triangles showing the quantity and distribution of stress. Rectangular sections are assumed as if they were two triangles joined together at their apexes, and in consequence equally stressed in every fibre. The area ACE will be the equivalent area for compression, and EBD the equivalent area for tension. The area of each hypothetical triangle would be $\frac{b}{2} \times \frac{d}{2} = \frac{bd}{4}$.

Given that the centre of gravity of every triangle is at one-third the height from the base, and the height of the triangle is $\frac{d}{2}$, the leverage will be $\frac{d}{2} \times \frac{2}{3} = \frac{d}{3}$, and for the two triangles $\frac{2}{3}d$. The section modulus Z for any rectangular section will be the area of one triangle multiplied by the lever arm, $= \frac{bd}{4} \times \frac{2}{3}d = \frac{bd^2}{6}$.

For the specimen under consideration, the value of $Z = \frac{1 \times 1^2}{6} = 0{\cdot}166 \text{ in.}^3$. Since the specimen broke at 4 cwt., and the factor of safety

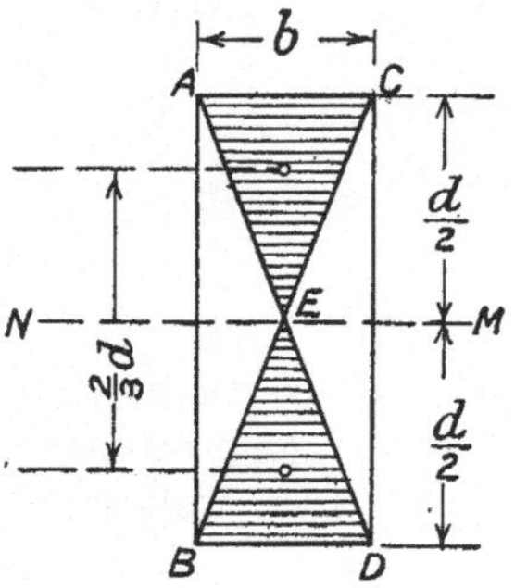

Fig. 2.—DIAGRAM SHOWING RESISTANCE AREA

is 5, the safe load will be 0·8 cwt., which gives a bending moment of—

$$\text{BM} = \frac{\text{WL}}{4} = \frac{0{\cdot}8 \times 112 \times 12}{4} = 268{\cdot}8 \text{ lb. in.,}$$

$$\text{therefore } f = \frac{\text{BM}}{\text{Z}} = \frac{268{\cdot}8}{0{\cdot}166} = 1{,}619 \text{ lb.}$$

Now to complete the problem :—

$$\text{If } \frac{\text{WL}}{4} = \text{Z}f, \text{ then W} = \frac{4\text{Z}f}{\text{L}}.$$

$$\text{W} = 4\,\frac{bd^2 \times f}{6 \times \text{L} \times 12} = \frac{4 \times 2 \times 5^2 \times 1619}{6 \times 10 \times 12}$$

$$= 448 \text{ lbs. or 4 cwts.}$$

The value of f_0 obtained by experiment is called the *modulus of rupture*, and will be found to be 18 times the weight that will break the beam across. This will be seen by substituting the values of l, b, and d for the experimental beam in the equation.

$$f_0 = \frac{\text{WL}}{4} \times \frac{6}{bd^2} = \frac{\text{W} \times 12 \times 6}{4 \times 1 \times 1^2} = 18\text{W}$$

The value of f obtained by the experiments above referred to is in most cases too high, because the specimens selected for tests are usually small pieces.

WORKING UNIT STRESSES FOR STRUCTURAL TIMBER IN POUNDS PER SQUARE INCH

Timber	*Extreme Fibre Stress*		*Modulus of Elasticity, Average*	*Shearing Stress*	
	Average Ultimate	*Safe Stress*		*Parallel to Grain*	*Bending*
Spruce	5,000	1,000	1,300,000	100	80
Redwood	5,600	1,100	1,200,000	150	100
Douglas fir	6,100	1,200	1,510,000	180	120
Pitch pine	6,500	1,400	1,600,000	180	120
Oak	6,500	1,400	1,200,000	200	120

Design of Boarding

In making up the load carried by the various members it will be found convenient to determine the resultant load carried by one square foot. From the Table previously given, slates (thirds) weigh 7·5 lbs., battens (2 in. by ¾ in.) 1·125 lbs., felt 0·5 lb., and boarding 2·5 lbs., per square foot respectively. The dead load will then be 11·625 lbs. per square foot of roof area. To this must be added half the proposed snow load (1·5 lbs.), as a maximum wind pressure (15 lbs.) and a snow load are not likely to occur at the same time. Adding these amounts together the total load including the boarding will be 28·125 lbs. per square foot.

Assuming that the rafters are spaced at 15-in. centres, the moment due to the load will be $\frac{1}{8}\ Wl^2 = \frac{28{\cdot}2 \times 1{\cdot}25^2 \times 12}{8} = 66$ in. lbs. approximately.

This moment is resisted by a $\frac{7}{8}$-in. by 12-in. section of boarding, for which the resulting fibre stress will be $f = \frac{\text{BM} \times 6}{bd^2} = \frac{66 \times 6}{12 \times \frac{7}{8}^2} = 43$ lbs. per square inch, which is very low, and indicates that for ordinary conditions the design for boarding need not be carried out.

Design of Rafters

For the rafters assume a 2-in. by 4-in. section, and 8-ft. span. At 2 lbs. per foot run the dead weight per foot of rafter is $\frac{2 \times 8}{8 \times 1{\cdot}25} = 1{\cdot}6$ lbs. Adding the weight of the rafter the total load to be carried by the rafter is a uniform load of 29·8 lbs. per square foot.

The moment is $\frac{Wl^2}{8} = \frac{29{\cdot}8 \times 8 \times 1{\cdot}25 \times 8 \times 12}{8} = 3{,}576$ lbs. in.

The section modulus of a 2-in. by 4-in. rectangle is $\frac{1}{6}bd^2 = \frac{1}{6} \times 2 \times 4^2$ $= 5{\cdot}33$ in.^{3}, and the fibre stress is $f = \frac{\text{BM} \times 6}{bd^2} = \frac{3576 \times 6}{2 \times 4^2} = 670{\cdot}5$ lbs. per square inch. As the allowable fibre stress is 1,000 lbs. per square inch, the assumed section is sufficient.

The maximum span for the rafters to carry the above loading of boarding, battens, and slates, and also a wind pressure of 15 lbs. per square foot, making a total of 29·8 lbs. per square foot, may be worked out as follows :—

Assuming a safe fibre stress of 1,000 lbs. per square inch, and a nominal breadth b of the rafters as 2 in., spaced at 15-in. centres :—

Then, $\quad \text{BM} = \frac{\text{WL}}{8}, \quad \text{W} = \text{L} \times \frac{15}{12} \times 29{\cdot}8 \text{ lbs.} = 37{\cdot}25\text{L}.$

Therefore $\text{BM} = \frac{37{\cdot}25\text{L} \times \text{L} \times 12}{8} = 55{\cdot}87\text{L}^2.$

The moment of resistance $\text{MR} = \frac{bd^2}{6} \times f = \frac{2 \times d^2 \times 1000}{6} = \frac{1000d^2}{3}.$

Equating the bending moment to the moment of resistance :—

$$\text{BM} = \text{MR}$$

$$55{\cdot}87\text{L}^2 = \frac{1{,}000d^2}{3}$$

$$\frac{55{\cdot}87\text{L}^2 \times 3}{1000} = d$$

$$d = \sqrt{{\cdot}1676\text{L}} = {\cdot}409\text{L}.$$

The depth of the rafters will therefore be, say, ·41 of the span in feet. For $f = 1{,}100$ lbs., $d = \cdot 39L$.

Where hand-made tiles are used in lieu of slates, the loading will be increased by the difference between the weight of the slates and the weight of the tiles, i.e. the difference between 7·5 and 12·3 lbs., or 4·8 lbs., making a total load of 34·6 lbs. Working this out in the same way as that used for slates, the depth will be found to be ·441L for $f = 1{,}000$ lbs., and ·42L for $f = 1{,}100$ lbs. These rules are shown plotted in the graph, Fig. 3.

When the rafters are required to carry a plaster ceiling, the deflection is usually limited to $\frac{1}{360}$ of the span to minimise cracks in the plaster. This condition will necessitate the rafters being designed for stiffness instead of strength. Taking the safe fibre stress at 1,000 lbs. per square inch, and E the modulus of elasticity at 1,510,000 :—

The deflection of a rectangular beam under a uniform load is given by the formula $\Delta = \frac{5}{384}\,\frac{WL^3}{EI}$, or for a maximum deflection of $\frac{1}{360}$:—

$$\frac{5}{384}\,\frac{WL^3}{EI} = \frac{L}{360}.$$

Dividing by L and substituting the given value of E, we get :—

$$\frac{5WL^2}{384 \times 1{,}510{,}000\, I} = \frac{1}{360}$$

$$\frac{WL^2}{322133} = I \qquad (1)$$

Again, for a beam of any symmetrical section, we know that :—

$$\frac{\text{Moment of inertia of section}}{\text{Modulus of section}} = \frac{\text{depth}}{2}.$$

Now Z = moment of resistance ÷ stress $= \frac{MR}{f}$. Hence, substituting for Z :—

$$I = \frac{MR}{f} \times \frac{D}{2}.$$

But for a beam with a distributed load, BM $= \frac{WL}{8}$,

$$I = \frac{WL}{8f} \times \frac{D}{2} = \frac{WLD}{16f} \qquad (2)$$

Combining results (1) and (2) we have :—

$$\frac{WL^2}{322{,}133} = \frac{WLD}{16f}$$

$$\frac{L}{D} = \frac{322{,}133}{16 \times 1000} = \frac{20}{1}.$$

Hence the depth of a uniform beam must not be less than $\frac{1}{20}$ of the span in feet, or $\frac{1 \times 12}{20} = \cdot 6$ of the span in inches if the deflection has not to exceed $\frac{1}{360}$ of the span (see graph, Fig. 3).

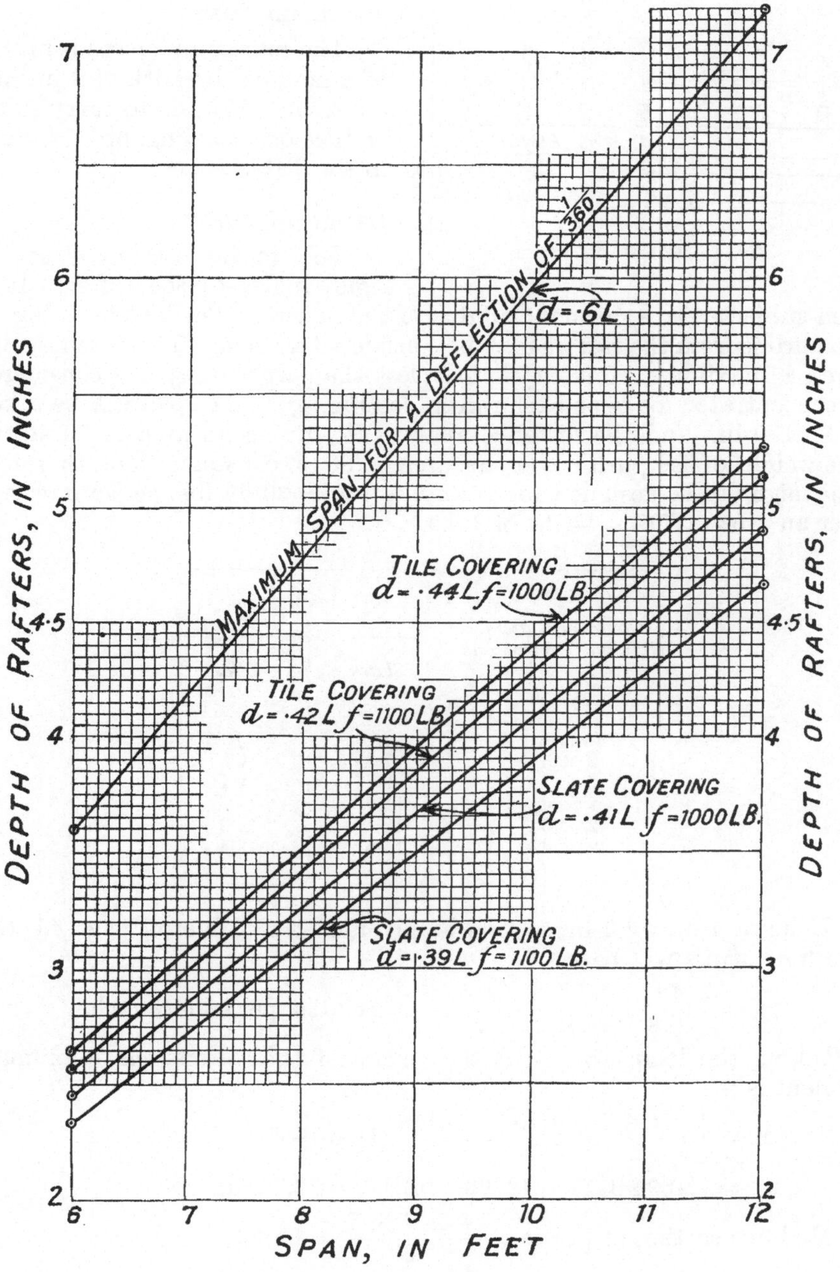

Fig. 3.—GRAPH TO DETERMINE DEPTH OF 2-IN. RAFTERS, AT 15-IN. CENTRES, FOR SLATES AND TILES

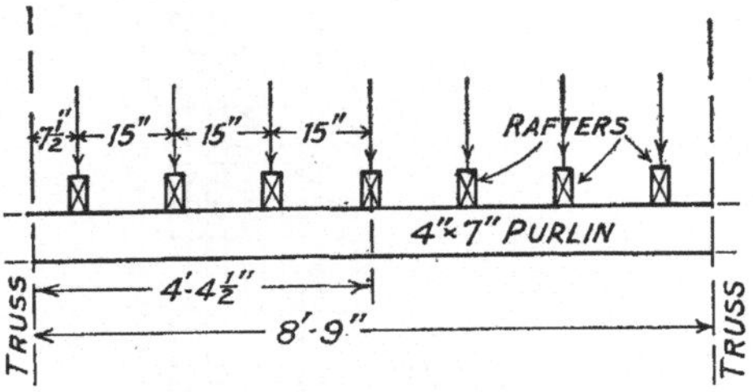

Fig. 4.—LOADS ON PURLIN

Maximum Span

The maximum span for rafters of a nominal breadth of 2 in. and a spacing of 15 in., to carry slates or tiles on boarding, etc., is given in the Table below.

Design of Purlins

The purlin section is set at right angles to the rafter. It is then subjected to a normal load due to the rafters. The loads coming on the purlins from the rafters may be considered as being distributed, which gives a maximum moment slightly less than when they are considered as concentrated loads on each rafter (see Fig. 4). The span will be taken as 8 ft. 9 in., and the distance apart 8 ft., giving an area of 70 sq. ft. The weight of the purlin over this area is ·86 lb. per square foot, therefore the weight to be designed for is 29·8 + ·86 = 30·66 lbs. per square foot over an area of 70 ft., = 2,146·2 lbs.

Common Rafters Nominal Dimensions	*Maximum Span*	
	Slates	*Tiles*
in. in.	*ft.*	*ft.*
2 × 3	7·3	6·8
2 × 4	9·75	9·1
2 × 4½	11·0	10·2
2 × 5	12·1	11·3
2 × 6	14·6	13·4

Using a 4-in. by 7-in. section as given in the Table on page 44, the safe fibre stress will be :—

$$f = \frac{2146 \times 8{\cdot}75 \times 12 \times 6}{8 \times 4 \times 7 \times 7} = 860 \text{ lbs. per square inch.}$$

Taking the loads to act at the centre of the rafters, the maximum moment is :—

$$M = \left[\left(\frac{2146}{2} \times \frac{8{\cdot}75}{2}\right) - \frac{2146}{7}(1{\cdot}25 + 2{\cdot}5 + 3{\cdot}75)\right]12$$

$$= [(4694{\cdot}375) - (2299{\cdot}125)]12 = 28{,}743 \text{ in. lbs.}$$

$$\text{Modulus section of purlin} = \frac{4 \times 7 \times 7}{6} = 32{\cdot}66.$$

$$\text{Maximum stress in the timber} = \frac{28743}{32{\cdot}66} = 880 \text{ lbs.}$$

Stress Diagrams for Roof Trusses

The method by which the stress in each member of a roof truss is found graphically is explained in the following example of a king-post roof truss. Suppose the span to be 24 ft., trusses placed at 10-ft. centres, the roof slope 30°, and the covering, slates on battens and boarding (see Fig. 5).

Assume weight or dead load as previously worked out is 15·66 lbs. per square foot, but to this must be added the weight of the truss. Using Jacoby's formula for wooden roofs, $W = \cdot075 \text{ span} + \cdot5 = 24 \times \cdot075 + \cdot5 = 2\cdot3$ lbs. per square foot, making a total load of 17·96 lbs. per square foot. The wind pressure of 15 lbs. per square foot of surface is assumed to be acting normal to the surface inwards on windward side, and 10 lbs. per square foot of surface similarly acting outwards on the leeward side, and a ceiling load of 10 lbs. per square foot.

The slope length is $\dfrac{\text{half-span}}{\cos\ 30°} = \dfrac{12}{0\cdot866} = 13\cdot85$ ft.

Then *dead load* $= 13\cdot85 \times 10 \times 17\cdot96 = 2{,}487\cdot4$ lbs.

Load on central points $= \dfrac{2487\cdot4}{2 \times 112} = 11\cdot1$ cwts.

Load on end points $= \dfrac{2487\cdot4}{4 \times 112} = 5\cdot5$ cwts.

Wind load $= 13\cdot85 \times 10 \times 15 = 2{,}077\cdot5$ lbs.

Load on central point $= \dfrac{2077\cdot5}{2 \times 112} = 9\cdot27$ cwts.

Load on end points $= \dfrac{2077\cdot5}{4 \times 112} = 4\cdot63$ cwts.

Suction $= 13\cdot85 \times 10 \times 10 = 1{,}385$ lbs.

Load on central point $= \dfrac{1385}{2 \times 112} = 6\cdot2$ cwts.

Load on end points $= \dfrac{1385}{4 \times 112} = 3\cdot1$ cwts.

Ceiling load $= 24 \times 10 \times 10 = 2{,}400$ lbs.

Load on central point $= \dfrac{2400}{2 \times 112} = 10\cdot7$ cwts.

Load on end points $= \dfrac{2400}{4 \times 112} = 5\cdot35$ cwts.

The latter are taken directly by the walls, and need not be considered.

To a scale of $\frac{1}{4}$ in. to a foot, draw the frame diagram, and indicate on the figure the forces combining the wind and dead loads. The dead load and wind pressure acting on the same point can be represented in magnitude and direction by two adjacent sides of a parallelogram, and their resultant is represented by the diagonal of the parallelogram

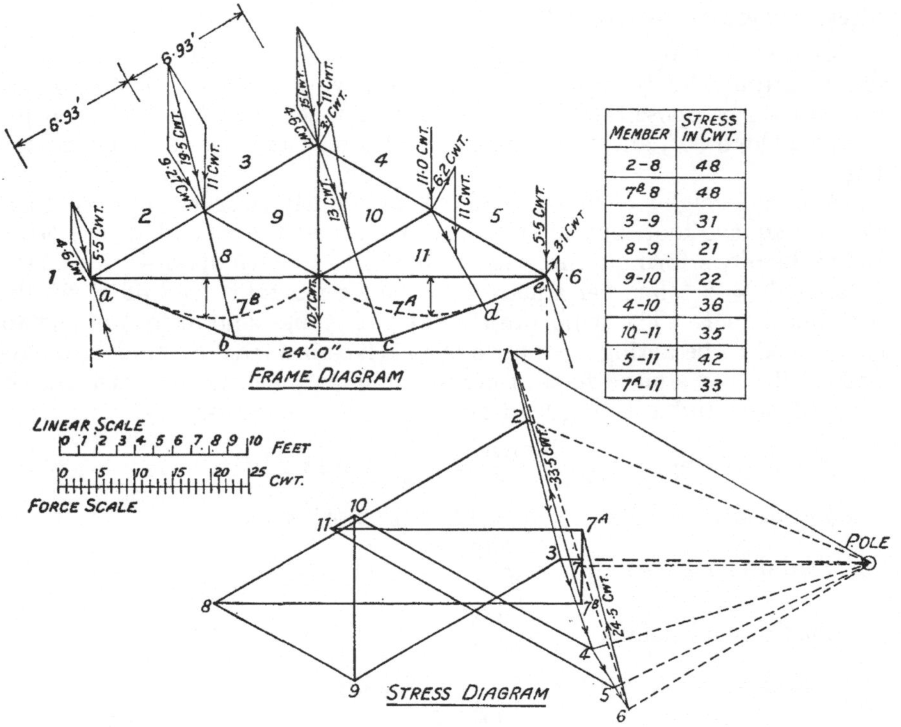

MEMBER	STRESS IN CWT.
2–8	48
7^B8	48
3–9	31
8–9	21
9–10	22
4–10	36
10–11	35
5–11	42
7^A–11	33

Fig. 5.—FRAME DIAGRAM OF KING-POST WITH STRUCTURAL LOAD, WIND PRESSURE, AND SUCTION

drawn from the point of application. The spaces must next be numbered or lettered between the forces acting on the frame.

Draw the load line 1, 2, 3, 4, 5, 6, and take any pole O. Draw the radial lines O1, O2, etc., and across the corresponding spaces 2, 3, 4, etc., on the frame diagram, draw parallel lines forming the funicular polygon *abcde*. Draw the closing line *ae*, and from the pole O draw a parallel line cutting the load at point 7. If there had been no ceiling load the lines drawn from this intersection to the points 1 and 6 would have given the magnitude and direction of the reactions 1–7 and 6–7. The addition of the ceiling load will obviously increase the reactions, and also cause the reactions to assume a more vertical direction. From the point 7 on the temporary reaction line, set up on each side half the magnitude of the central ceiling load, giving points 7^A and 7^B. Join point 1 to 7^B, and 6 to 7^A This gives the magnitude and direction of the two reactions (see Fig. 5). Next draw the stress lines parallel to the members of the truss : 2–8, 7–8 ; 3–9, 8–9 ; 9–10, 4–10 ; 10–11, 7–11 ; and 5–11. The forces in the frame can now be scaled off, and the magnitude of the stress in each member of the truss tabulated as below :—

Member	2–8	7^B–8	3–9	8–9	9–10	4–10	10–11	7^A–11	5–11
Magnitude of stress, in cwts.	48	48	31	21	22	36	3·5	42	38

The usual formula for roof members in compression is the Rankine-Gordon formula, and is :—

$$P = \frac{fA}{1 + \frac{1}{ac}\frac{l^2}{r^2}}$$

Where P = ultimate load in pounds

$f = \frac{2}{3}$ of the ultimate compressive strength of the material in pounds per square inch, say 4,000 lbs. for fir.

a = constant = 1 for column with round ends ; 2 for column with one end rounded.

c = constant = 750 for timber.

l = length of column in inches.

r = least radius of gyration of cross-section $= \sqrt{\frac{I}{A}}$ or $r^2 = \frac{I}{A}$

where I = moment of inertia $= \frac{bd^3}{12}$ for a rectangular section, and A = area of cross-section.

For the principal rafter the maximum stress is 5,376 lbs. and the unsupported length 6·94 ft.

Assume a scantling of 5 in. by 4 in., then :—

$$P = \frac{4000 \times 20}{1 + \frac{1}{2 \times 750}\frac{(6{\cdot}94 \times 12)^2}{1{\cdot}33}} = 17{,}937 \text{ lbs.}$$

Adopting a factor of safety of 4, the safe load will be $\frac{17937}{4} = 4{,}480$ lbs. or 40 cwts. The section 5 in. by 4 in. is too small. Try a 5-in. by 5-in. section and work out as before.

For the struts with a maximum compression of 21 cwts., and an unsupported length of 6·94 ft., try a section 5 in. by $2\frac{1}{2}$ in., then :—

$$P = \frac{fA}{1 + \frac{1}{ac}\frac{l^2}{r^2}} = \frac{4000 \times 12{\cdot}5}{1 + \frac{1}{2 \times 750}\frac{(6{\cdot}94 \times 12)^2}{1{\cdot}33}}$$

$$P = 11{,}185 \text{ lbs.}$$

and $\frac{11185}{4} = 2{,}796$ lbs. or 24 cwts. safe load.

The king-post has a tensional stress of 22 cwts.,and allowing 2·5 cwts. per square inch on the net area in tension, the king-post will require an area of $\frac{24}{2 \cdot 5} = 9 \cdot 6$ sq. in., say, 4 in. by 3 in.

The tie-beam has a maximum tension of 48 cwts., and a maximum bending moment $\frac{WL}{8} = \frac{10 \cdot 7 \times 12}{8} = 16$ cwts. ft. or 192 cwts. in.

Try a 10-in. by 5-in. section, then :—

$$-\frac{W}{A} \pm \frac{M}{Z} = -\frac{48}{50} \pm \frac{192}{\frac{1}{6}(5 \times 10^2)}$$

$= - \cdot 96 \pm 2 \cdot 3 = 3 \cdot 26$ cwts. per square inch in tension, and $1 \cdot 34$ cwts. per square inch in compression, which is satisfactory.

OBTAINING ROOF BEVELS

To obtain the roof bevels for a span roof first draw a plan of the roof, as shown in Fig. 1. The bevels for the members may then be obtained as follows :—

Common Rafter

The bevels and lengths may be obtained direct from the section FLH, FH being the rise or height of the roof (Fig. 6).

Hip Rafter

At right angles to the plan of the hip, as AE or ED, set out height of ridge E_1 E_1, that is, the top point of the rafter. Join E_1A or E_1D : then the bevels are obtained as shown. For backing the hip, draw the line 1—2 at right angles to the plan of the hip, and at the point of intersection of these two lines draw the line 3—4 at right angles to AE_1. Rotate 3—4 down to 3—5, and join 1—5, 5—2, and the backing is obtained. A similar construction gives the length, bevels, and backing for the adjacent hip, which is, of course, different owing to the irregular shape of the hipped end.

Jack Rafter

From the true length of the common rafter LH, turn over line to position LF_1. Next produce line of jack rafter as shown at GG_{11}, then top bevel is at G_{11}. The side bevel will be as for the common rafter.

Roof Boarding

Find development of side and end slopes by turning F_1 to F_{11} and drawing $F_{11}E_{11}$ parallel to CD. A complete roof plan is shown in Fig. 7.

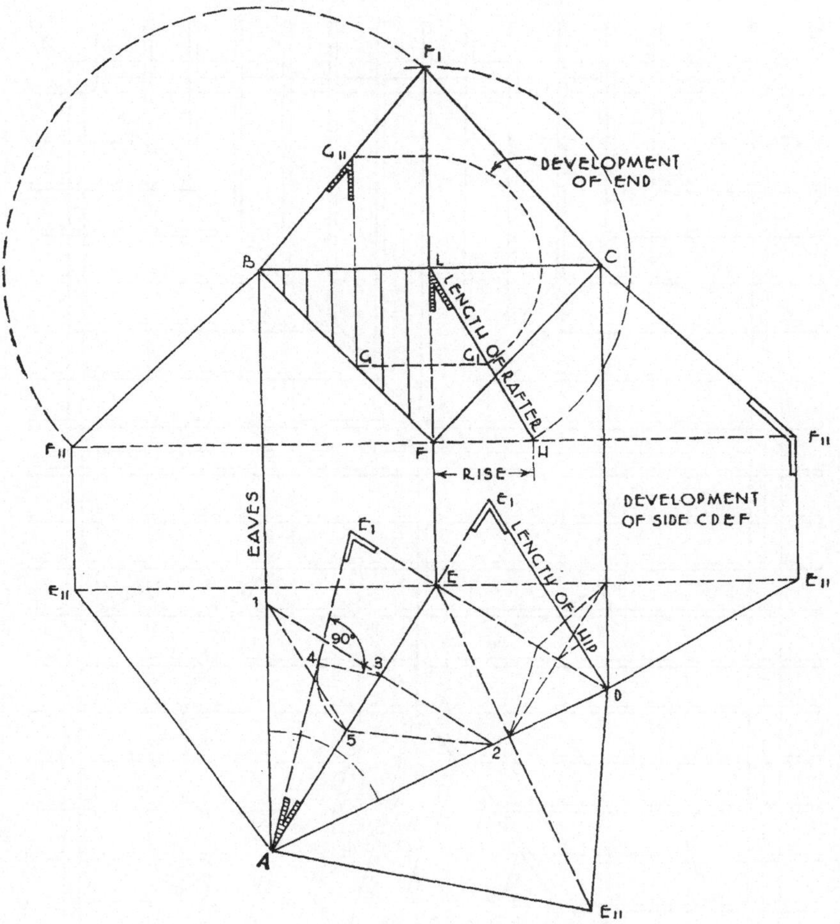

Fig. 6.—THIS ILLUSTRATES THE METHOD OF OBTAINING ROOF BEVELS

A plan of the roof is first drawn. The bevels of the members may then be obtained as described in the text.

Purlins

The bevels for the purlins are shown in Fig. 8. Set up the pitch of the roof, in this case 30°, and draw the plan of the hip at 45°. Place the purlin in position, and letter the points ABC. With B as centre, and radius BA, turn A into a horizontal position A^1. Next drop verticals from A, A^1 on to the plan of the hip as shown, and join A^1A^{11} horizontally. The line drawn through B^1A^{11} gives the top cut for the purlin. The side is obtained in a similar manner.

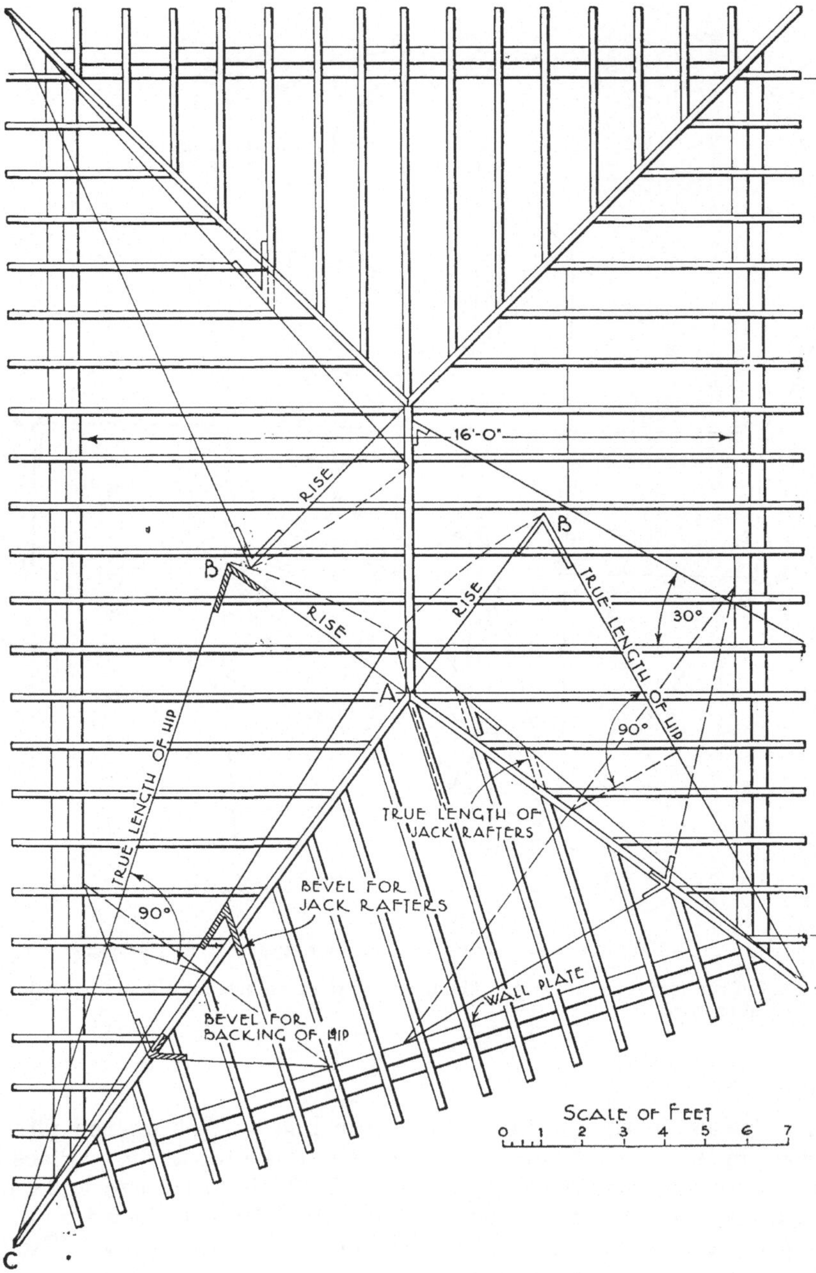

Fig. 7.—PLAN OF ROOF WITH IRREGULAR HIP END

Where Wall Plates Are at Obtuse or Acute Angles

Where the wall plates are at obtuse or acute angles, and the hips do not bisect the angle between them, the finding of the bevels will be slightly different, though based on the same geometrical principles (see Fig. 9). Draw lines ABC to represent the lines of the wall plates, and BD the centre line of the hip. Fix upon any point in it and draw IE, IC parallel to BC, AB respectively. At any convenient point E draw E2 at right angles to BC, and (2) draw 2–3 at right angles to E2. From E set up the pitch of the roof, and 2—4 at right angles to 2C.

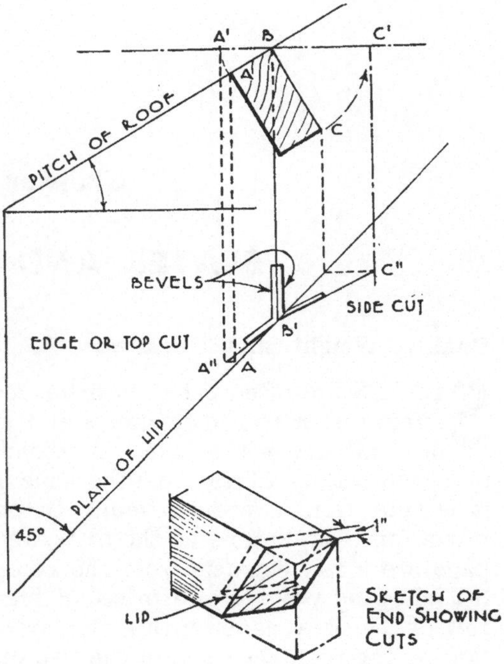

Fig. 8.—BEVELS FOR PURLINS

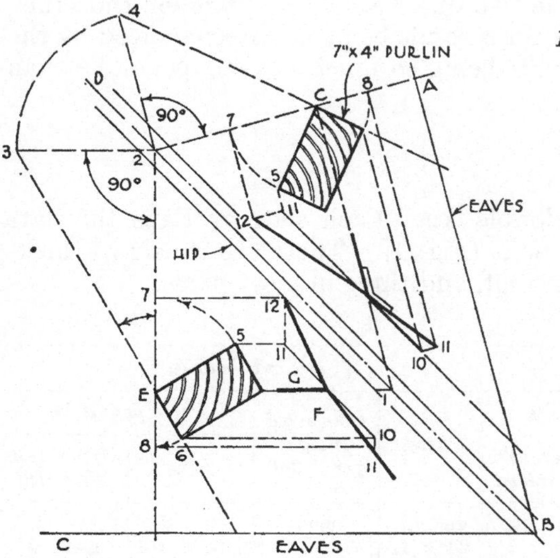

Fig. 9.—BEVELS FOR PURLINS WHERE HIP DOES NOT BISECT ANGLE, AND WALL PLATES ARE NOT AT RIGHT ANGLES TO EACH OTHER

Make 2—4 equal to 2—3; joining C4 should give the pitch of that side of the roof; continue the lines 4C and 3E, and set out the sections and plans as shown in Fig. 4. Then with E as centre and 5 and 6 as radii, obtain the points 7 and 8; projecting down from these points, parallel to CB, points 10 and 11 are obtained, and thus the bevels FG. The bevels for the other side are obtained in a similar manner.

Chapter V

SLATES AND SLATING

Quality, Weight, and Thickness

SLATES are often listed as firsts, seconds, and thirds. This grading refers rather to the thickness and weight than to the actual quality or durability of the slate. A seconds Welsh slate is generally thicker and coarser than a firsts from the same quarry, and hence heavier because it is split from a coarser vein. In practice, the seconds will usually prove quite as durable as the firsts, and perhaps more robust. On this page are a few extracts from the comprehensive Penrhyn slate quarry list, showing weights and prices of first- and second-quality slates of a few of the sizes made by this, the largest of the Welsh quarries. When laid on the roof, the costs of the two qualities work out much the same, the amount saved in initial cost for seconds being counterbalanced by the extra cost of carriage, the seconds being so much heavier per mille than the firsts.

Calculations for Quantities

All slates are laid with a double lap. Each slate overlaps the slate in the next course but one below it (Fig. 4). There are thus two thicknesses of slate in all parts of the roof, and three in most parts.

First Quality				*Second Quality*			
Size	*Computed Weight per 1,200*	*Price per Mille*		*Size*	*Computed Weight per 1,200*	*Price per Mille*	
		Blue	*Green and Wrinkled*			*Blue*	*Green and Wrinkled*
in. in.	*cwt.*	*s. d.*	*s. d.*	*in. in.*	*cwt.*	*s. d.*	*s. d.*
24 × 12	56	700 0	668 0	24 × 12	76	685 0	644 0
20 × 10	36	445 0	420 0	20 × 10	50	462 0	418 0
18 × 9	29	314 0	303 0	18 × 9	40	304 0	298 0
16 × 8	23	247 0	237 0	16 × 8	32	240 0	218 0

Prices are quoted for the purpose of comparison only; they are subject to revision for current rates.

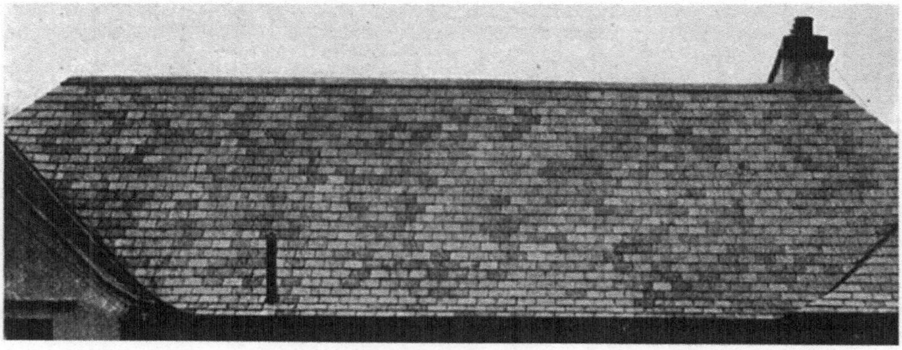

Fig. 1.—OLD DELABOLE SLATING—SLATES OF REGULAR SIZES

Sized Slates

The sizes of slates in common use range from 12 in. by 6 in. up to 24 in. by 12 in. and even 24 in. by 14 in. The practice of specifying any kind of roofing material by its gauge alone is bad, but it is particularly so in slating: it is always better to specify the lap. The standard minimum lap for plain tiling is $2\frac{1}{2}$ in. For slating, roof pitches are on the average lower, and the standard minimum lap has come to be recognised as 3 in. In any specification for slating, the size of slate and the lap should be stated.

The length of a slate on the roof may be considered as made up of twice the gauge plus the lap. In Fig. 4 we have an 18-in. by 9-in. slate laid to a 3-in. lap, and the gauge is therefore (18 in. — 3 in.) ÷ 2, or $7\frac{1}{2}$ in. To find the number of slates per square we divide the exposed area of each slate (in this case 9 in. by $7\frac{1}{2}$ in.) into one square of 100 ft. super. It is usually convenient in these calculations to work in inches, and our calculation of the number of 18-in. by 9-in. slates laid to a 3-in. lap required to cover a square becomes :—

$$\frac{14{,}400}{7\frac{1}{2} \times 9}, \text{ or } 213.$$

By a similar process it will be found that the number of 16-in. by 12-in. slates laid to a $3\frac{1}{2}$-in. lap required to cover one square is $\frac{14{,}400}{6\frac{1}{4} \times 12}$ or 192.

Calculating the Number of Slates Required

The following Table gives the number of slates of each of the ordinary sizes required to cover one square for $2\frac{1}{2}$-in., 3-in., and $3\frac{1}{2}$-in. laps. It

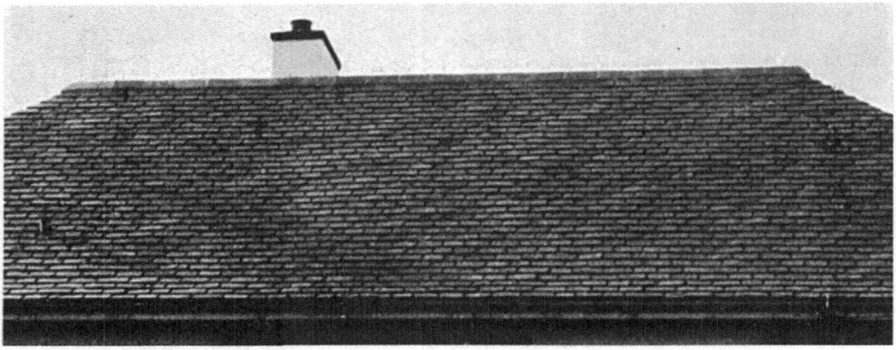

Fig. 2.—OLD DELABOLE SLATING—RANDOM-WIDTH SLATES OF A STANDARD LENGTH LAID TO A REGULAR GAUGE

also gives the old names for some of the sizes. (These names are rapidly dying out, and nobody really regrets their passing : it is undignified to speak of a Wide Countess or a Narrow Lady. Nowadays no countesses are wide, and all ladies are narrow.) But it is useful to know the names, as they do still appear in some specifications.

Size in Inches	*Name*	*Number per Square When Laid to a*		
		2½-in. Lap	*3-in. Lap*	*3½-in. Lap*
24 × 14	Princesses	96	98	100
24 × 12	Duchesses	112	114	117
22 × 12	Small Duchesses	123	126	130
22 × 11	Marchionesses	134	138	142
20 × 12	Wide Countesses	137	141	145
20 × 10	Countesses	165	169	175
18 × 12		155	160	166
18 × 10	Wide Viscountesses	186	192	199
18 × 9	Viscountesses	206	213	221
16 × 12		178	185	192
16 × 10	Wide Ladies	213	222	230
16 × 9	Broad Ladies	237	246	256
16 × 8	Ladies	267	277	288
14 × 10	Headers	250	262	274
14 × 8	Small Ladies	313	327	343
14 × 7	Narrow Ladies	358	374	392
12 × 6	Small Doubles	505	533	565

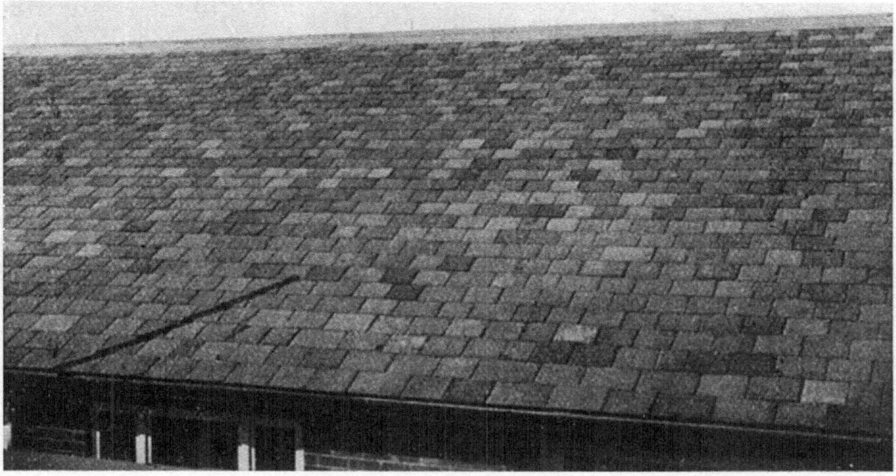

Fig. 3.—OLD DELABOLE SLATING—RANDOM SLATES LAID IN DIMINISHING COURSES

How Slates Are Sold—the Cover per 1,000

It is here necessary to digress for a moment to explain the methods by which slates are sold. Sized slates are sold at the quarry by the mille of 1,200. An order to a quarry for 3,500 slates would be interpreted as meaning three and a half times 1,200, or 4,200 actual slates. They are now usually retailed by slate merchants to builders by actual count; that is to say, 1,000 slates are sold as 1,000 actual count. In this article, "mille" means 1,200 and "thousand" or "1,000" means 1,000.

The cover per 1,000 is found by multiplying the exposed area of each slate by 1,000. The cover per 1,000 for a 16-in. by 10-in. slate laid to a 3-in. lap would therefore be :—

$$10 \text{ in.} \times 6\tfrac{1}{2} \text{ in.} \times 1{,}000 = 4{\cdot}52 \text{ squares.}$$

The cover per mille would be :—

$$10 \text{ in.} \times 6\tfrac{1}{2} \text{ in.} \times 1{,}200 = 5{\cdot}42 \text{ squares.}$$

There is a very simple method, not very well known, of finding the cover per mille. Suppose that a 16-in. by 12-in. slate is to be laid to a 3-in. lap. Then the gauge is $6\frac{1}{2}$ in., and the cover per mille is $6\frac{1}{2}$ squares. The cover per mille in squares for a slate 12 in. wide is always the same as the gauge in inches. The reason is easy to see. The cover per mille for a 16-in. by 12-in. slate laid to a 3-in. lap is $12 \times 6\frac{1}{2} \times 1{,}200$ sq. in. =

$$\frac{12 \times 6\frac{1}{2} \times 1{,}200}{14{,}400} \text{ squares.}$$

Cancellation of this fraction leaves only the $6\frac{1}{2}$.

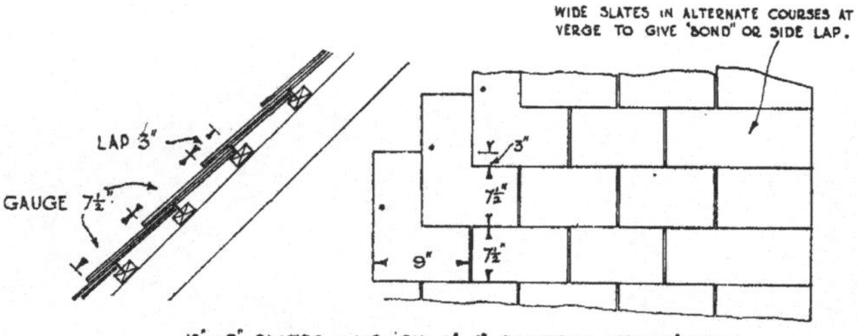

18" × 9" SLATES LAID ON 2" × 1" BATTENS TO 3" LAP.

Fig. 4.—GAUGE AND LAP IN SLATING

Then, for a 10-in. slate the cover will be five-sixths of that given by a 12-in. slate of the same length. Hence the cover for a 16-in. by 10-in. slate laid to a 3-in. lap would be five-sixths of 6·5 squares, or 5·42 squares.

One more example will make the point quite clear. What would be the cover in squares per mille of an 18-in. by 9-in. slate laid to a 3½-in. lap ? Gauge = (18 in. — 3½ in.) ÷ 2 = 7¼ in.

Then cover per mille for 18-in. by 12-in. slate = 7·25 squares,

∴ cover for 18-in. by 9-in. slate = ¾ of 7·25, or 5·44 squares.

Random Slates

Random-sized slates are of unequal length and width : generally, the longer a slate the wider it is, so on a roof covered with " randoms " the largest slates, which are always fixed in the lowest courses, may measure 26 in. by 14 in., and the smallest, in the top courses, 12 in. by 6 in. or even smaller. The intermediate courses grade downwards gradually between these extremes.

Slates of random widths have been mentioned above, and the distinction between the two kinds of randoms should be kept clear in the reader's mind, and the points about battening noted. For random-width slating the whole roof can be battened at once : where random-sized slates are to be used the carpenter cannot batten until the slater has given him the spacing for each course, and the slater cannot do this until he has sorted the slates into sizes on the job.

Peggies are small randoms of lengths from 8 in. up to 12 in. or 14 in., and of irregular widths.

Random slates of all kinds are sold by the ton. The covering capacities cannot be worked out by the purchaser, but all quarry owners who make such slates issue lists showing covering capacities per ton. Considerations of space forbid the reproduction of full lists here, but following are short extracts from two such quarry lists. It should be noted that the computed covers per ton are averages, and cannot be guaranteed accurate for any particular consignment.

Examples of Covering Capacity of Westmorland Random Slates

Random sizes, Buttermere Light Green.

Bests : 24 in. to 12 in., in proportionate widths, computed cover 27–28 sq. yds. per ton.

Seconds : 24 in. to 12 in., in proportionate widths, computed cover 21–22 sq. yds. per ton.

Thirds : 20 to 10 in. in proportionate widths, computed cover 15–16 sq. yds. per ton.

The computed *weights* for bests, seconds, and thirds of these slates work out at about 8, 10¼, and 14½ cwts. per square. Note that these slates follow the general rule in slates : the lower the quality, the thicker the slate, so in practice, although the bests given above cost more per ton than the seconds, we get better cover per ton, and the seconds, when laid on the roof, cost about as much as the bests.

The Buttermere Light Green is one of fourteen kinds listed by the Westmorland Green Slate Quarries Ltd., Keswick, Cumberland.

Delabole Randoms

Randoms for laying in graduated courses, Rustic Reds (25 per cent.) and Weathering Grey-Greens (varied mixed shades), 3-in. lap.

No. 1 *Grading :* 24-in. to 12-in. lengths, cover per ton 2·50 squares.

No. 2 *Grading :* 22-in. to 12-in. lengths, cover per ton 2·25 squares.

No. 2*a Grading :* 16-in. to 12-in. lengths, cover per ton 2·25 squares.

Random widths, ordinary grey-green, No. 1 grading :—

Length (× *Random Widths*)	*Cover in Squares per Ton*
20 in.	2·38
18 in.	2·37
16 in.	2·37
14 in.	2·44

Here is a point for careful note. As a general rule, the larger the slate the thicker it is : it is possible to cut a slate of small area to a lesser thickness than one of larger area. This explains why, say, the No. 1 grading in Delabole randoms, ranging from 24 in. to 12 in., gives much the same cover per ton as the No. 2*a* grading, which ranges from 16 in. to 12 in. If all the slates, large and small, were of the same thickness, the No. 1 grading would give by far the better cover, because with large slates less of the roof is covered with three thicknesses of slate than with small slates. The lesser thickness of the small slates just about compensates for the extra area covered with three thicknesses, and as a result the cover per ton given by large and small slates is about equal.

Calculations for Battening

For sized slating and for tiling, the calculations for battening are simple. If battens are fixed on a roof at 12-in. intervals, centre to centre, then on one square of roof there will be 100 ft. run of battens. If the spacing or gauge is 6 in., there will be 200 ft. run to the square. The rule is : Divide 1,200 by the gauge in inches. The following table gives the number of feet run per square for various gauges, and will be found useful for both slating and tiling :—

Gauge in Inches	*Feet run of Battens per Square*	*Gauge in Inches*	*Feet run of Battens per Square*
3½	343	7½	160
3¾	320	8¼	146
4	300	8½	141
4¼	283	9¼	130
4½	267	9½	127
5	240	10¼	117
6	200	10½	114
6¼	192	12	100
6½	185	13	92
7¼	166	13½	89

The battening for random-sized slates cannot be accurately calculated. For 24-in. to 12-in. random slating an average is 190 ft. to 200 ft. per square, but the actual figure depends upon the proportions of large and small slates in a consignment.

Preparation for Slating

The usual methods of preparation for slating are as follows :—

(1) Open battening or rafters. (2) Plain boarding. (3) Plain boarding and battens. (4) Plain boards, felt, and battens. (5) Plain boards, felt, counter-battens, and battens. (6) Untearable felt and battens.

Open battening is more satisfactory as a preparation for slating than for plain tiling. The slates " lie closer " on the roof, and there is little penetration of draught and dirt through a slated roof.

Plain boarding is rather better than open battening, and the appearance from the inside of the roof is improved : this is important where the roof space is used. Plain boarding is hardly ever used in plain tiling, since the nibs of the tiles have to be removed (unless the tiles are nibless), and each tile has to be secured with two nails. In slating, each unit has in any case to be secured with two nails, unless the slates are 12 in. by 6 in. or smaller, when one nail per slate is used.

Methods (3) to (6) are all better than (1) and (2), and one or other should be adopted where cost will permit it.

Holing and Sorting

The nail holes are usually made by the slater, but holing is undertaken by some quarries. The holes are punched on the under side of the slate, at about 1½ in. from each edge. By this method a slight countersinking is formed on the back of the slate—the surface which is uppermost when on the roof—into which the head of the nail fits when the slates are fixed. Without this countersinking the head of the nail would remain above the surface, and the slate above would not " sit down." The position of the nail holes is shown in Fig. 5, from which it will be seen that the position of the holes depends entirely upon the gauge.

Centre nailing, as Fig. 5, is adopted for all except small slates or peggies, which are nailed with one nail at the head. Head-nailing is not safe where the slate is over 12 in. long, as there is risk of lifting in a high wind.

While being holed, the slates should, if necessary, be sorted for thickness. The heaviest slates should be used near the eaves, and the lightest in the top courses.

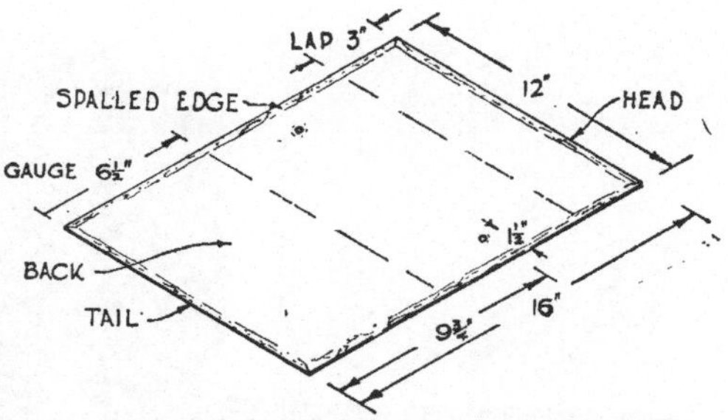

Fig. 5.—POSITION OF NAIL HOLES IN SLATE FOR CENTRE-NAILING

Eaves

The eaves course in slating must be formed as in plain tiling, with a double course. Fig. 6 shows the method.

Verges

Ordinary practice in slating is merely to bed and point the verge, but not to fit an undercloak. The use of an undercloak (Fig. 8) is, however, recommended as giving a better appearance from the ground, and a more secure finish. Wide slates should be used at verges and abutments in preference to cutting down an ordinary slate in width. The use of wide slates is, in fact, essential where the roofing slate is 8 in. wide or under (see Fig. 10).

Ridges

The plain angle ridge, or some variation of it, suits a slated roof very well. The angular character of the slate seems to demand an angular finish at ridges and hips. The slates should be brought well up to the ridge tree. Half-round ridge (Fig. 7), either red or blue, may be used, and lead roll is also still popular.

Hips

Angular or other ridge tiles are, in modern practice, widely used on hips. They give excellent cover on both sides, and are not liable to removal in high winds. Lead roll may also be used.

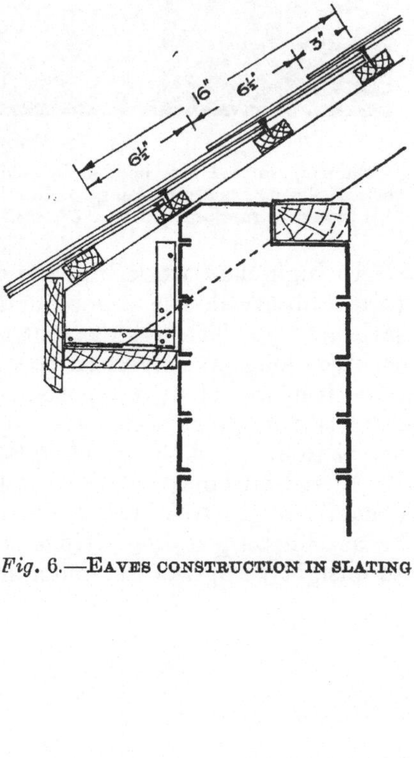

Fig. 6.—EAVES CONSTRUCTION IN SLATING

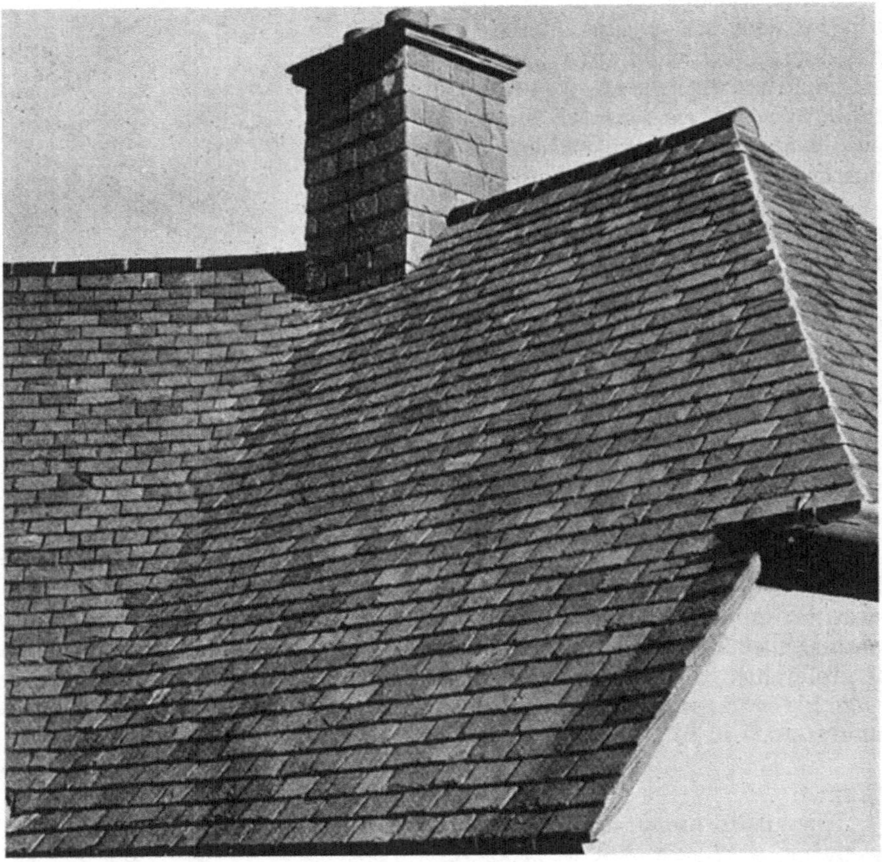

Fig. 7.—Modern slating practice

Showing mitred hip, bedded in coloured cement; half-round ridge; swept valley; vertical slating; slate capping to chimney. The slates are Old Delabole No. 2 grading, 14 in. long, in random widths. (*Setchell & Sons Ltd.*)

In high-class work hips are often mitred, but unless extraordinary care is observed, and a good craftsman employed, the result may be unsatisfactory. The weakness of the mitred hip is that fixing can only be secured along a relatively narrow section of the slate, while the broad base of each mitred slate is exposed. The stripping of a mitred hip in a high wind is a frequent occurrence, particularly where the pitch of the roof is less than 45°, and the building is in an exposed position.

Mitred hips may be either soakered or bedded. The soakers should be of sufficient size to ensure an adequate lap at the head and side, and should be as thin as possible. Thick soakers tend to raise the hip slates, give an unsightly appearance, and assist the wind in its efforts to lift the slates.

Lead soakers are here, as in all other cases, preferable to zinc. It is a good general rule to assume that zinc is satisfactory only where it is completely exposed to the weather. Contact with mortar produces conditions favourable to the disintegration of zinc.

Bedded mitres are preferable, provided that the bedding material is not squeezed out over the face of the slate below. A batten should be fixed on the common rafters along each side of the hip tree to take the edge of the mitred slate. Ordinary glazier's putty may be used for bedding, but there is a number of suitable mastics now available, and coloured cement (Fig. 7) is also used. Too much bedding material is fatal to the appearance of the hip.

Hips may alternatively be flashed, which means, in effect, that the soakers are left exposed instead of being covered by a slate. Seating on turret or similar roofs must be " swept " round, as in Fig. 9. This is best done in small slates.

Valleys

Valleys in slating may be (*a*) mitred, (*b*) open, or (*c*) swept. The mitred valley (Fig. 9) is excellent in appearance and satisfactory in use, provided that the gutter beneath it is properly formed.

Open metal valleys are usual in all but high-class work. It is better to have a fairly wide valley, say 3 in. to 4 in., than a narrow, almost secret, gutter. Secret gutters are usually to be avoided, because of the danger of clogging with dead leaves. The wide valley ensures always a clear passage for water. Open valleys may be " left dry," or an undercloak may be fitted: the latter method is preferable. An undercloak $4\frac{1}{2}$ in. wide is ample.

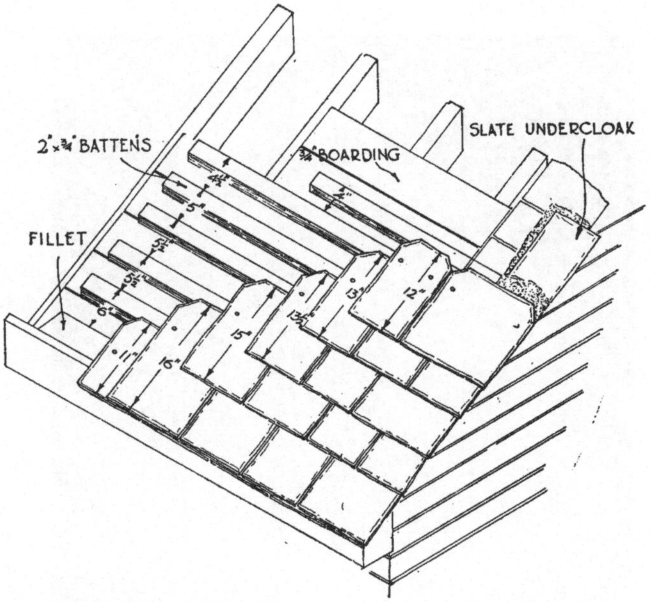

Fig. 8.—BOARDING, BATTENING, AND RANDOM SLATING; SLATE UNDERCLOAK AND WIDE SLATES IN ALTERNATE COURSES AT VERGE

Swept valleys in slating (Fig. 7)

are unusual and expensive. They can be gracefully formed only in slates of narrow width, as wide slates come round the valley in, as it were, a series of jerks, with wide spaces between the slates. With small slates a smooth curve can be formed. Large slates, again, require that the valley shall have a very wide sweep; with small slates the curve may be more restricted. The wide curve necessary with the large slate creates a difficulty at the top of the valley, and the junction with the ridge is likely to be ungainly.

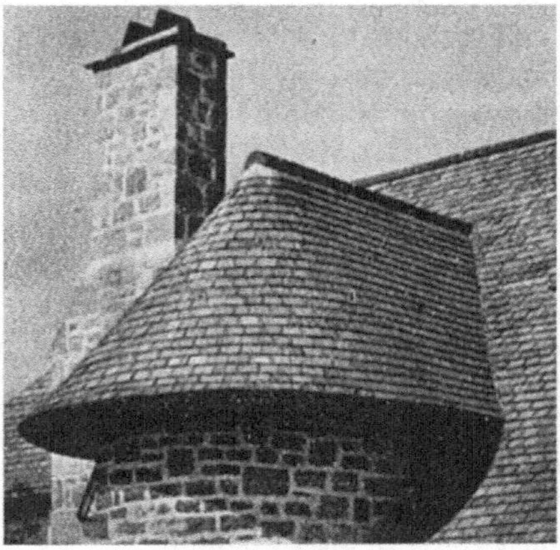

Fig. 9.—12-IN. BY 6-IN. OLD DELABOLE SLATES ON A CIRCULAR TURRET ROOF; MITRED VALLEY

Abutments

Soakers must always be used at abutments, and the width along the roof must always be sufficient to give the proper side lap. The turn-up against the wall must also be enough to ensure adequate cover by the stepped or other flashing.

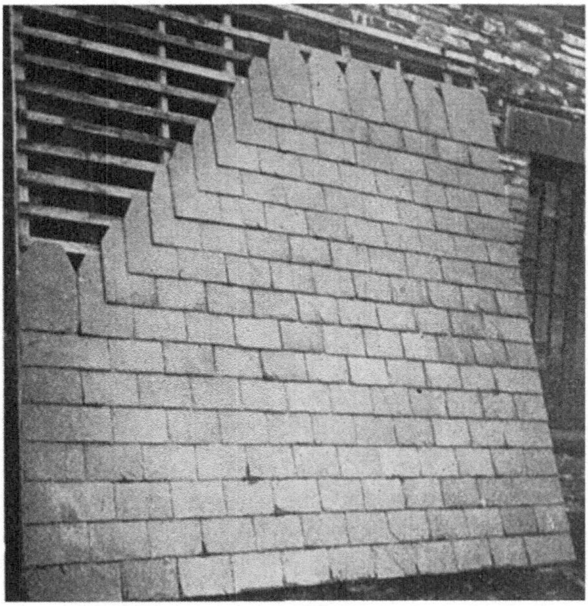

Fig. 10.—USE OF WIDE SLATES AT VERGES OR ABUTMENTS

Nailing

The question of nails for both slating and tiling is discussed in the next chapter. Here we need only remind the reader that the life of a slated roof is only as long as the life of the nails. Galvanised nails should not, therefore, be used on any slated roof.

Roof Pitches

The pitch of the rafters may generally be less for a slated than for a plain-tiled roof, but the size of slate must be taken into account. Large slates may be laid on a slower pitch than small slates, and the reasons are worth remembering. There is always a certain spread of moisture on either side of the vertical joints between adjacent slates in the same course, and the slower the pitch the greater the spread. The side lap in slating is equal to half the width of the slate, and if a small slate is used on a roof of slow pitch the moisture may spread until it finds its way between the vertical joints that are covered, and so into the roof.

A further reason for using large slates only on slow-pitched roofs is that the weight to be borne by the nails is reduced to a minimum. A 24-in. by 12-in. slate may weigh up to 7 lb., and this is too great a weight to be borne by two nails on a slope of 50° or 60°

Random Slating

Fig. 8 is an illustration of random slating on boards and battens. Nearly all random slates are shouldered at the quarries, on account of the difficulty of ensuring trueness to width in this class of slate. The slates shown diminish from 16 in. to 12 in., and the gradual decrease in the gauge to give a 3-in. lap throughout should be noted.

Chapter VI

HOW TO TILE ROOFS

Clay Tiles

CLAY suitable for the manufacture of roofing tiles is widely distributed over England, the largest deposits being in the Broseley district of Shropshire, North and South Staffordshire, Berkshire, the Bridgwater district of Somerset, and the south-east corner of England. The clays vary in their mineralogical and chemical compositions, and it is these variations that account for the different characteristics of the tiles produced. The Midland clays, those of Broseley and Staffordshire, for example, contain a high percentage of iron, and the tiles made in those districts can be naturally burnt to purple, brown, and blue colours that cannot be approached in tiles made in some other parts of the country, except by the application of artificial colouring.

Again, some clays are eminently suitable for the manufacture of only plain tiles, and others can be used as well for the production of larger units such as pantiles, Roman tiles, and single-lap tiles generally. It is, in fact, considered that tiles such as the Bridgwater Double Roman, Marseilles, and other types that depend for their effectiveness upon the roof on trueness to shape, can be made only from alluvial clays of recent deposit. However that may be, it is true that such tiles are successfully made only from those clays.

A discussion of the technicalities of clay, and the suitability of each kind for the manufacture of either bricks or tiles or both, is outside the scope of this book, but the reader should remember that there are nearly always very good reasons for the production of one kind of tile instead of another in any particular district. These reasons are usually technical, but often they form part of the fascinating history of the development of the English roofing tile.

Qualities

When taken from the kiln, clay tiles are sorted into best, second, and third qualities. Best tiles should be without a fault of any kind ; seconds tiles, as sent out by most works, are those which have some fault which precludes their ranking as best tiles, but which is not detrimental to the tile as a roof covering. Tiles that are slightly out of true, or have an unsightly " flash " or other blemish on their surface, are classed as

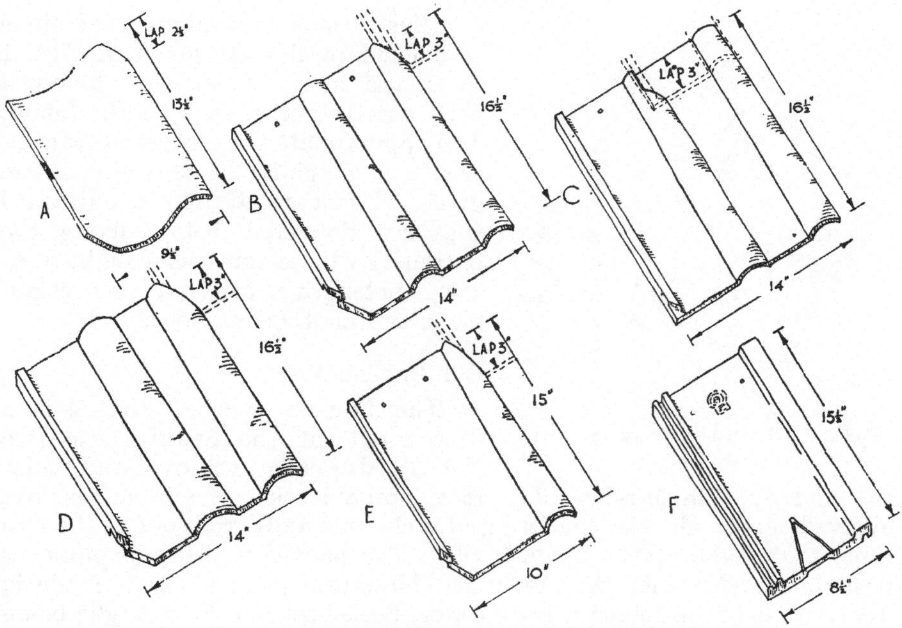

Fig. 1.—A FEW POPULAR FORMS OF ENGLISH SINGLE-LAP TILE

A. Old English pantile. B. Double Roman tile—straight joint. C. Double Roman tile—broken joint. D. Reynardo tile. E. Single Roman tile. F. Somerset interlocking tile—No. 13.

seconds. Third-quality tiles are usually either badly twisted or fire-cracked " above the gauge line," as the tiler says.

Classification of Clay Tiles

For practical purposes, tiles are most conveniently classified as single-lap and double-lap or plain.

In single-lap tiling each tile overlaps or is overlapped by the tiles on either side of it in the same course, and the tiles in the courses above and below. There is thus only one thickness of tile in most parts of the roof, and two thicknesses in some parts. Single-lap tiles may have a simple overlap, as in the case of the English pantile (Fig. 1), or there may be an interlock at the head or at the side and head. The Somerset interlocking No. 13 (Fig. 1) has a side lock. The imported interlocking improved pantile (Fig. 4) has both side and head locks.

In double-lap or plain tiling, each tile overlaps the tile in the next course but one below it, but there is no overlap at the side. The length of tile exposed on the roof is called the gauge, and the amount by which one tile overlaps the tile in the course next but one below it is called the lap. In plain tiling, it will be noted, there are at least two thicknesses of tile in every part of the roof, and three thicknesses in most parts.

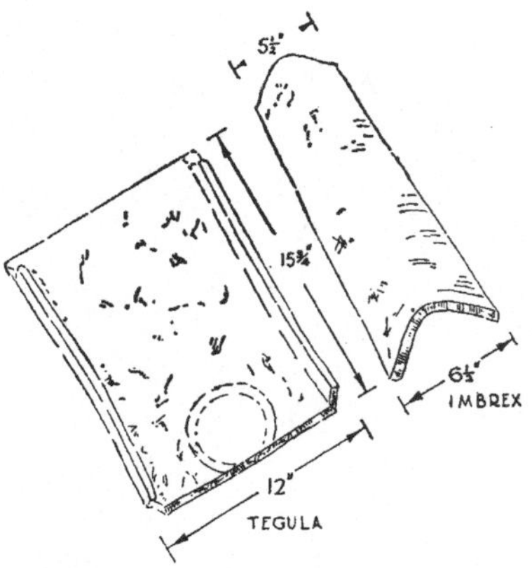

Fig. 2.—Roman Tegula and Imbrex

Illustrations of a number of kinds of single-lap tiles are given in Figs. 1 to 5, and in the notes that follow a brief description of each will be found. The approximate sizes, covering capacities, and gauge for battens of each are given. Users are advised to wait until tiles are delivered before fixing the battens, as in certain cases slight variations in length as between one consignment and another may occur.

Old English Pantile

The English pantile (Fig. 1) is a descendant of the Spanish tile (see Fig. 3), also called the over-and-under tile and Spanish Mission tile. It is probable that the Flemings first evolved this single tile, consisting of a channel and a roll, out of the two units that make up the Spanish tile. The pantile is justly popular, as it fits admirably into the modern architectural picture. It is made in many parts of the country, Bridgwater, Berkshire, and East Anglia being the largest centres of production.

The following data are subject to much variation, as the pantiles made by different works are dissimilar in both length and width.

Size : 13½ in. by 9 in. Cover : 150 per square. Gauge for battens : 12 in.

Double Roman Tile

The Double Roman tile (Fig. 1) is a product of the Bridgwater district of Somerset, and is the largest tile in use in England. It is a descendant of the Roman *tegula* and *imbrex* (Fig. 2), which the Romans used extensively in England for their villa roofs. In the Double Roman tile, two *tegulæ* and two *imbrices* are combined into one unit.

Technical Data.—Size : 16½ in. by 14 in. Cover : 85–90 per square. Gauge for battens : 13½ in.

Single Roman Tile

This is the smaller, and not so popular, brother of the Double Roman tile, and is a little closer to the line of descent from the *tegula* and *imbrex*. It also is a product of Bridgwater, although a nearly similar type is made in Lincolnshire. A larger type, equal in size to the Double Roman, is also made.

Technical Data.—Small Pattern. Size : 15 in. by 10 in. Cover : 125 per square. Gauge for battens : 12 in. *Large Pattern.* Data as for Double Roman.

Double Roman Interlocking

This tile has the same appearance as the ordinary Double Roman tile on the roof, but is laid with a broken joint. The ordinary Double Roman is laid with a straight joint. (See Fig. 1.) The practical advantage of the broken joint is that the water running down the side channel of any one tile is discharged on to the face of the tile below, and not, as in the case of the straight-joint tile, into the side channel of the tile below.

Technical Data as for Double Roman tile.

Somerset Interlocking Tile No. 13

A very effective tile (Fig. 1), manufactured expressly for cheap domestic or industrial roofing. It is of adjustable lap, and has been used without felt on roofs as low as 30° of pitch at the eaves. This tile is produced by the Somerset Trading Co. Ltd., Bridgwater.

Technical Data.—Size : 15½ in. by 8 in. Cover for 3-in. lap, 155 tiles per square. Gauge for battens for 3-in. lap : 12½ in.

Reynardo

The Reynardo (Fig. 1) is essentially a Double Roman tile, but it has a bolder roll, and on the roof an appearance somewhat similar to that of the Spanish tile. The Reynardo tile is an exclusive product of Messrs. Colthurst, Symons & Co. Ltd., Bridgwater.

Technical Data as for Double Roman tile.

Spanish Tile

The tiles are laid alternately concave and convex in courses, and there is a lap at both sides and at the head of each tile (Fig. 3).

Technical Data.—There are many makes of Spanish and Italian tile, all of different size and covering capacity, and users should obtain information from the manufacturers concerned.

Italian Tiles

Similar in type to the Spanish tile, with this difference—that the under tile is flat instead of concave. This distinction between Italian and Spanish tiles is not generally understood, and cases have occurred where a specification has called for Spanish tiles when Italian tiles were meant.

Both kinds are expensive, but eminently suited to buildings where a bold, vertical roll on the roof is required to heighten the effect of the general elevation.

Courtrai-du-Nord Tile

This tile, shown in Fig. 5B, was once known in England only as a cheap but effective roof covering. It is now made in a great variety of colours, both matt and glazed : meadow green glazed, bluish green glazed, tea-

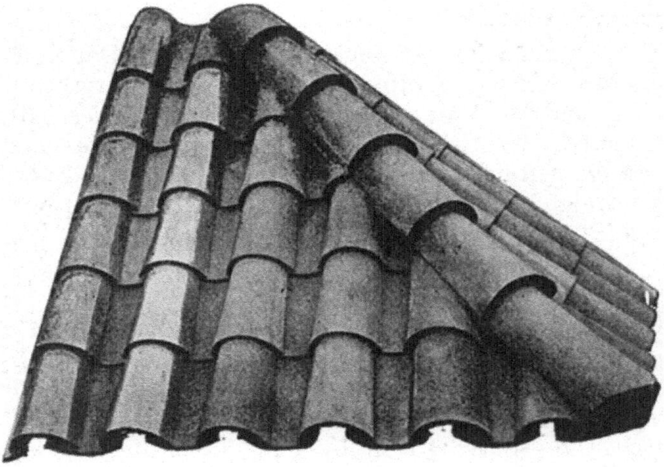

Fig. 3.—SPANISH TILING—SHOWING USE OF TAPERED HIPS. (*Colthurst, Symons & Co. Ltd.*)

pot brown glazed, autumn leaf glazed, moss green, and lichen green are a few of the colours listed by the importers, Messrs. Langley London Ltd.

Technical Data.—Size : 11½ in. by 8½ in. Cover : approximately 208 tiles per square. Gauge for battens : approximately 9⅜ in.

Improved Interlocking Pantile

This (Fig. 4), like the Courtrai-du-Nord tile, is of Continental make, and obtainable in a variety of colours, both matt and glazed. Comparison with Fig. 2 shows that it differs from the ordinary English pantile principally in the fact that the interlocking improved pantile has a side and head lock. For technical reasons this type of pantile has not so far been made in England.

Technical Data.—Size : 13¼ in. by 9¾ in. Cover : approximately 147 tiles per square. Gauge for battens : approximately 11½ in.

The Cloister Tile

This is designed to give on the roof an effect somewhat similar to that of Spanish or Italian tiling (Fig. 5A).

Technical Data.—Size : 11¾ in. by 8½ in. Cover : approximately 200 tiles per square. Gauge for battens : approximately 9⅞ in.

Plain Tiles

Fig. 6 illustrates the ordinary two-holed, two-nibbed plain tile, and the fittings that are used with it for roofing and vertical tiling. Two sections of half-round ridge are shown : 90° pitch for main ridges, and 105° for hips. The 90° ridge is too bold for use on hips, and its use for that purpose makes an awkward intersection at the point where the main ridge and hip meet.

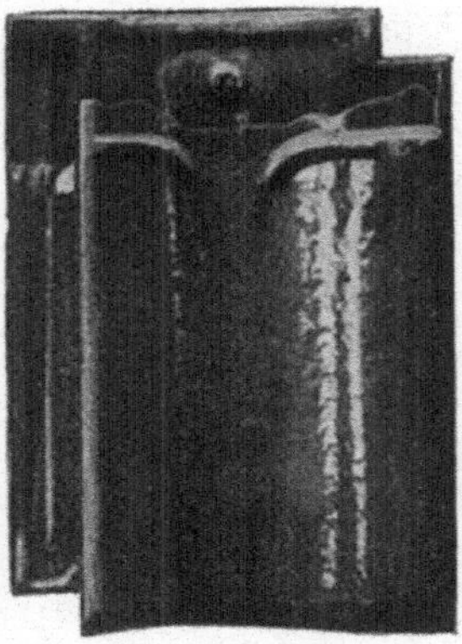

Fig. 4.—Improved Interlocking Pantile

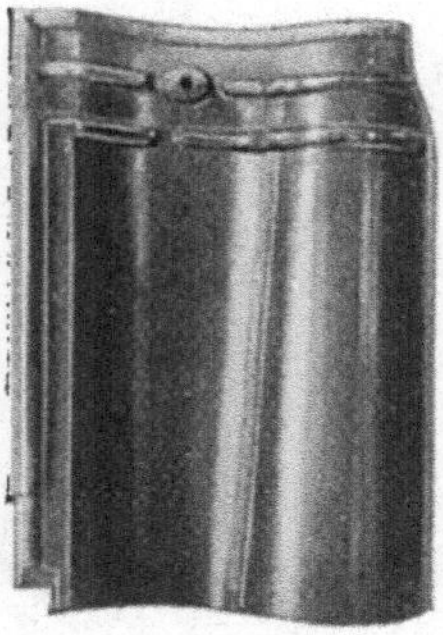

Fig. 5A.—Cloister Tile

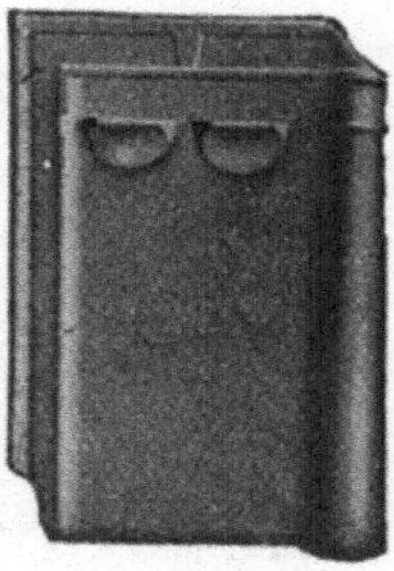

Fig. 5B.—Courtrai-du-Nord Tile (*Langley London Ltd.*)

CALCULATIONS

Plain Tiling

It is commonly said that a square of tiling requires 600 plain tiles, and although this is a good approximate figure, it is rarely accurate. The standard size of plain tiles is 10½ in. by 6½ in., but in practice sizes vary from 10 in. by 6 in. up to 11 in. by 7 in., and to calculate accurately the number of tiles needed to cover one square we must know (*a*) the size of tile, and (*b*) the lap, or gauge.

The length of each tile when laid on the roof may be considered as made up of twice the gauge plus the lap, and a 10½-in. by 6½-in. tile laid to a 2½-in. lap shows a gauge of 4 in. The number of tiles required to cover one square is clearly the number of times that the exposed area of each tile divides into one square. Thus :—

$$\frac{1 \text{ square}}{6\tfrac{1}{2} \text{ in.} \times 4 \text{ in.}} = \frac{14{,}400 \text{ sq. in.}}{6\tfrac{1}{2} \text{ in.} \times 4 \text{ in.}}$$

$$= 554 \text{ tiles.}$$

Similarly, an 11-in. by 7-in. tile laid to a 3½-in. lap (3¾-in. gauge) will require :—

$$\frac{14{,}400}{7 \text{ in.} \times 3\tfrac{3}{4} \text{ in.}} \text{ or } 549 \text{ tiles.}$$

An 11-in. by 7-in. tile laid to a 2-in. lap (4½-in. gauge), as for vertical tiling, will require only 457 tiles per square.

The following Table gives the number of plain tiles per square required for three sizes of tile laid to various laps. A minimum lap of 2½ in. is recommended for roofing, but 1½ in. is usually sufficient for vertical tiling.

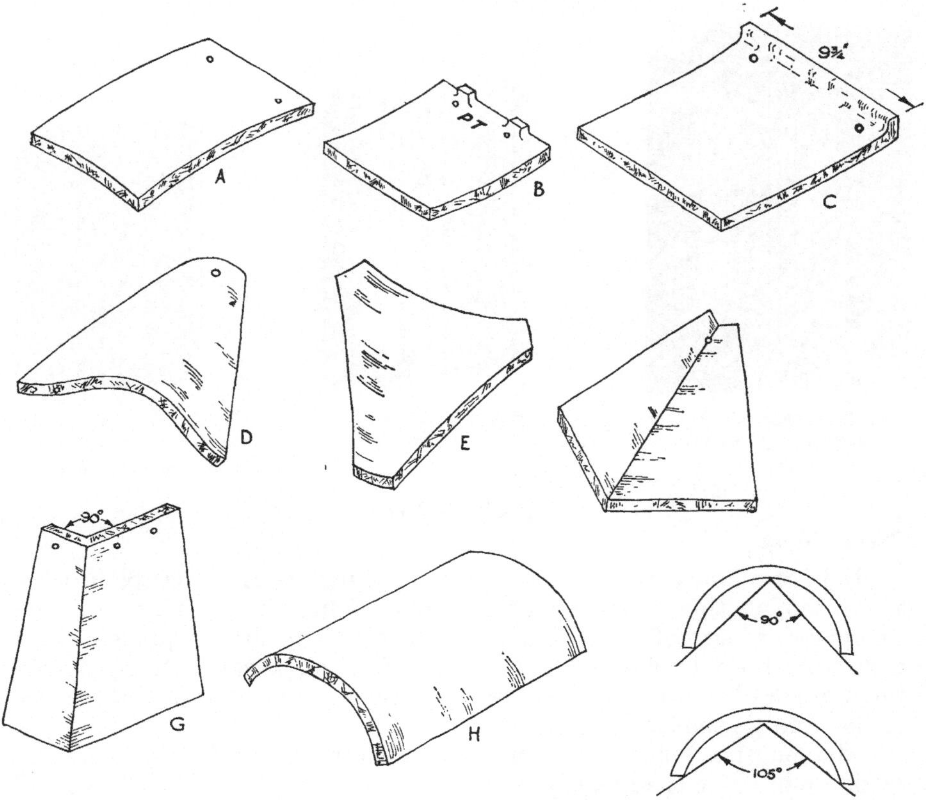

Fig. 6.—PLAIN TILE AND FITTINGS

A. Plain tile. B. Under side of eave tile. C. Under side of tile-and-half tile (continuous nibbed, machine made). D. Bonnet hip tile. E. Valley tile. F. Close-fitting hip tile. G. Angle tile handed, external. H. Half-round ridge tile.

Size of Tile	*Lap in Inches and No. per Square*					
	1½	2	2½	3	3½	4
11 in. by 7 in.	433	457	484	514	549	588
10½ in. by 6½ in.	492	521	554	591	633	682
10 in. by 6 in.	565	600	640	686	738	800

Ridge Tiles

These are usually made in 12-in. or 18-in. lengths, although odd lengths do sometimes occur. The required number is easily obtained.

Bonnet Hips, Hip Tiles, and Valley Tiles

A rough and ready method of calculating the number of these is to take 3 per foot run of hip or valley, but this figure in many cases will allow rather too many for waste. In Fig. 7 the length of the common rafter is 16 ft., and of the hip, 20 ft. The tiles are laid to a 4-in. gauge. If we allow 3 hip tiles per foot, the number ordered would be 60, or 240 for the four hips. The actual net number required for each hip would be 48 or perhaps 49. This is estimated as follows: the number of hip tiles will be the same as the number of courses of tiles on the main slope: a rafter length of 16 ft. gives us, at 4-in. gauge, 48 courses of tiling, and this is the number of hip tiles that will be needed. For the four hips the number would be 49 by 4, or 196, and the tiler would order, say, 204.

The calculations for valley tiles are made similarly.

Angle Tiles

The number of these is estimated similarly by finding the number of courses of plain tiles.

Single-lap Tiling

Here the principle is the same as for plain tiling: divide 100 sq. ft. by the exposed area of each tile, but it must be remembered that the length of each single-lap tile is made up of the gauge plus the lap.

Example.—A single-lap tile measures $16\frac{1}{2}$ in. by 14 in., and has a vertical lap of 3 in., and a side lap of $1\frac{1}{2}$ in. The number of tiles required per square is :—

$$\frac{14{,}400}{13\frac{1}{2} \times 12\frac{1}{2}} \text{ or 85 tiles.}$$

These figures are, in fact, those applicable to one of the best known of the English single-lap tiles: the Bridgwater Double Roman tile. The technical data given in the preceding pages for each kind of single-lap tile named have been similarly calculated. Makers or importers will always give this information to customers: the figures are, in fact, almost invariably given in their catalogues.

Weights

The weights of plain tiles are approximately as under :—

10 in. by 6 in.	19–21 cwts. per 1,000
$10\frac{1}{2}$ in. by $6\frac{1}{2}$ in.	20–23 cwts. ,, ,,
11 in. by 7 in.	21–25 cwts. ,, ,,

but it is advisable always to get the correct weight from the makers.

Bonnet hips weigh about $3\frac{1}{2}$ cwts. per 1,000; angle tiles about 4 cwts. per 1,000; and ridge tiles, 12 in. long, about $8\frac{1}{2}$ lbs. each.

CHOOSING A TILE

In choosing a tile, the architect has to decide (*a*) the type of tile, whether plain or single-lap, and sometimes (*b*) the kind of tile, whether hand- or machine-made. The following hints may be of assistance to those who have to decide how the roof, the most important single element in an elevation, is to be covered.

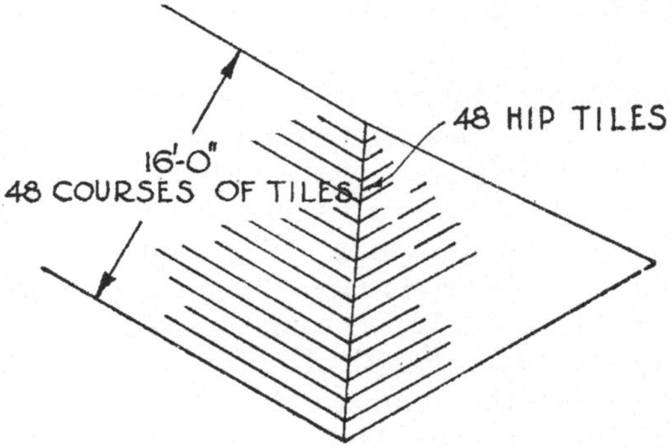

Fig. 7.—ILLUSTRATING METHOD OF CALCULATING NUMBER OF HIP TILES

(1) In single-lap tiling the unit is large, and usually shows a series of well-defined vertical and horizontal lines on a roof. Single-lap tiles are therefore suitable for large and high buildings.

(2) The plain tile is suitable for complicated roofs, having hips, valleys, dormers, and small projections.

(3) Concrete tiles are usually cheaper than machine-made clay tiles of comparable quality, and the latter are cheaper than hand-made tiles.

(4) For slow-pitched roofs the single-lap tile is to be preferred.

(5) Care should be taken to ensure that the tile used is one that can at any time be repeated. Do not, for example, use an imported single-lap tile of which future supplies are not assured.

(6) Remember that if a hand-made tile is chosen, it will " weather " on the roof, but not on the vertical tiling. Machine-made tiles, unless sand-faced, do not usually weather.

(7) If a machine-made clay tile is chosen, one that has been burnt naturally to a dark or brindled shade is preferable to a light-red tile. The latter may laminate ; the former will not. It is not, however, possible to be dogmatic on this point, for the products of some works are light red, however long the period of burning may be.

(8) A well-cambered plain tile should be chosen in preference to a tile that is straight in its length (Fig. 8). The camber not only helps the tail of each tile to sit snugly on the course below, but it provides an air space for ventilation among the tiles and battens. Lamination is hastened by the close bedding of one tile on another for the greater part of its length : capillary action tends to keep the upper surface of one and the lower surface of the other damp for long periods. The circulation of air among plain tiles is assisted if the tile is slightly cambered in its width. Fig. 8 shows a plain tile cambered only in its length, and two kinds of tiles cambered in their length and width.

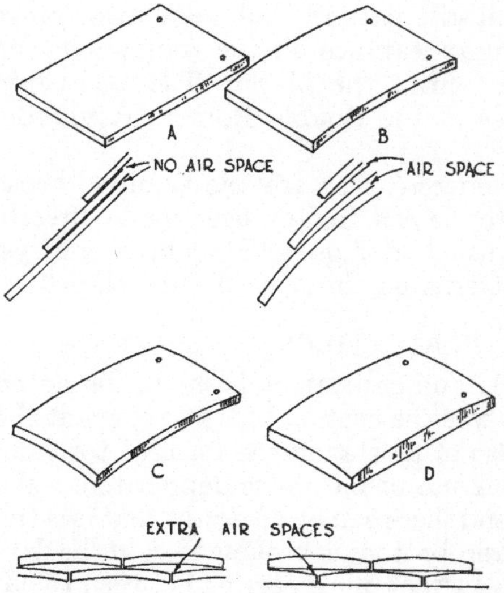

Fig. 8.—A WELL-CAMBERED PLAIN TILE SHOULD BE CHOSEN IN PREFERENCE TO A TILE STRAIGHT IN ITS LENGTH

A. Plain tile straight in its length and width. B. Plain tile cambered in its length only. C. " Full " double-cambered tile. D. " Half " double-cambered tile.

Special Tiles

It often happens that certain fittings—bonnet hips or angle tiles, for example—have to be made to a special pitch for a particular job. In such cases it is advisable to give the works as long notice as possible. Special fittings cannot usually be produced in less than eight weeks from the date of order, and contracts are frequently delayed because the order for the tiles is placed shortly before the roof is ready. It may even happen that, particularly in single-lap tiling, the tiles for part of the roof have to be purposely made. Fig. 9 shows a roof, circular on plan, to be covered with hand-made pantiles: on each slope there have to be the same number of tiles at the eave as at the ridge. Hence, on the outer slope the pantiles have to be wider at the tail than at the head, and vice versa on the inner slope. Special moulds have had to be made for each course—sixteen on each slope.

Concrete Tiles

The concrete tile has taken its place beside the other and longer-established roofing materials. The quality of the best-known makes is high, the permeability is negligible, and the colours, although not yet permanent, do not bleach out and disappear entirely.

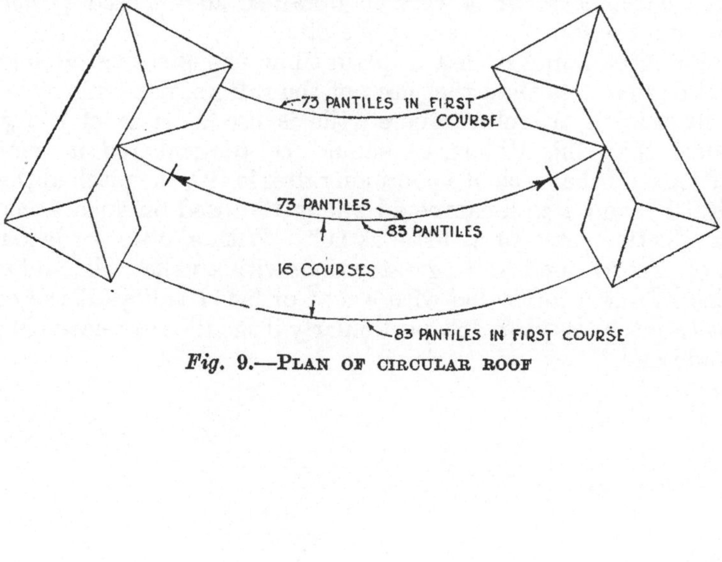

Fig. 9.—PLAN OF CIRCULAR ROOF

Most concrete tiles are of the plain-tile pattern, but some firms make a form of interlocking tile that is, in appearance on the roof, similar to the Somerset No. 13 tile, while one firm, the Marley Tile Company, manufactures concrete single-lap tiles of the Double Roman, Reynardo, pantile, and Spanish patterns.

The methods of application of concrete tiles are the same as those described for clay tiling : the concrete tile has, in fact, been made directly in imitation of the clay tile. The usual fittings—ridges, hips, valleys, angle tiles—are all of the same patterns as those used with clay tiles.

TILING WITH PLAIN TILES

One striking difference between old and new methods should be noted at the outset. Until recent years it was the custom to try to prevent the penetration of water by the lavish use of mortar in the form of torching and bedding. In modern practice the use of mortar is deprecated. We ventilate, rather than seal, our roofs, and there can be no doubt that it is the better practice. The life of the tiles and battens is prolonged, and the drying out of wet tiles is accelerated, by a current of air passing between them.

Roof Pitches

The question of rafter pitch for plain tiling must always be considered in conjunction with the other factors involved : permissible cost, position and exposure of building, and kind of tile.

The cost of all items increases as the pitch is raised, and this is a factor to which architects have to give consideration. A sheltered roof can safely have a slower pitch than could be used for one in a very exposed position. In general, plain tiling demands a steeper pitch than does any form of single-lap tiling, but that is not to say that the appearance of a house with a single-lap tiled roof will not be improved by having a roof of fairly steep pitch rather than one of 30°

Experience has shown that in England a pitch of 45°, there or thereabouts, is satisfactory for a plain-tiled roof under ordinary conditions of exposure. Greater security can be obtained in exposed positions by (*a*) increasing the lap or (*b*) raising the pitch.

A point to be noted is that in plain tiling the effective pitch (Fig. 10) is several degrees less than the pitch of the rafters, particularly when, as in the illustration, a well-cambered tile is used. It is of the greatest importance that this difference should be remembered in connection with valleys. If the pitch of a common rafter is 40°, the pitch of the valley rafter is 31°, and a well-cambered valley tile used on such a roof may have an effective pitch of as little as 20° With a swept or laced valley the risk of penetration is even greater than with a valley tile, and a generous width of felt is advisable with swept or laced valleys if the common rafter has a pitch less than 45°, particularly if the tile is a relatively porous, hand-made one.

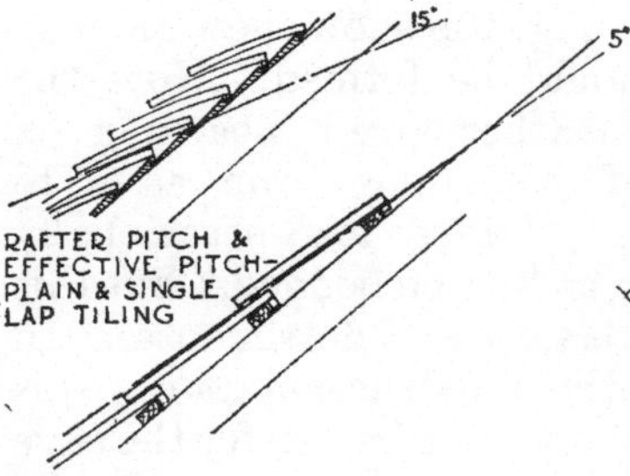

Fig. 10.—Rafter pitch and effective pitch

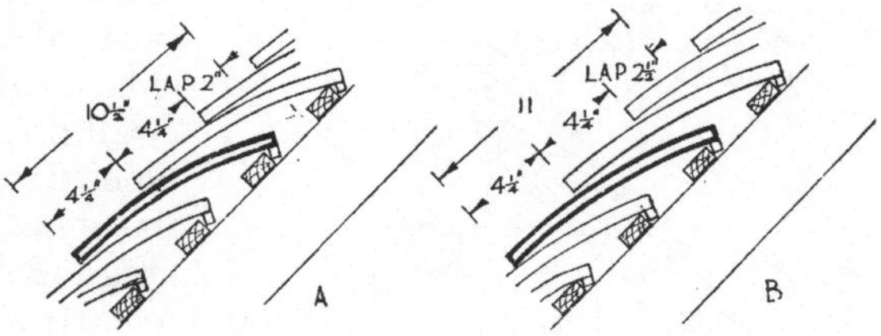

Fig. 11.—Gauge and lap—11-in. and 10½-in. plain tiles

Gauge and Lap

The lap should always be mentioned in any specification, since tiles vary in length, and to specify only the gauge is to run the risk of getting insufficient lap. Two and a half inches is the minimum lap for plain tiling, and, as Fig. 11 shows, while this lap is obtained with a 4¼-in. gauge where a tile 11 in. long is used, a 10½-in. tile would give only a 2-in. lap.

Roof Preparation

The following are the alternative forms of roof preparation adopted in modern practice :—

(*a*) Open battens : ideal from the point of view of roof ventilation, but obviously unsuitable where use is to be made of the roof space.

(*b*) Feather-edged boards : less ventilation and less dust and soot in the roof space than with (*a*), and rather better "tying-in" value ; should never be used with a relatively porous, hand-made plain tile.

(*c*) Plain boards and battens : better than either (*a*) or (*b*), and giving, with good boarding, a practically dustproof roof space. The addition of counter-battens is well worth the small extra cost.

(*d*) Untearable felt and battens : comparable in value with (*c*), but the felt must be untearable (that is, a bituminous felt with a strong canvas or other base), or the tilers will put their feet through it.

(*e*) Plain boards, felt, counter-battens, and battens : the ideal roof preparation from all points of view, but the most costly.

Sizes of Battens

For plain tiling, battens may be of any scantling from 1 in. by ¾ in. up to 2 in. by 1 in. A good ordinary size is 1¼ in. or 1½ in. by 1 in. In plain tiling, the gauge should be taken from top to top of battens, not from centre to centre.

Eaves

A section through the eaves in a plain-tiled roof is shown in Fig. 12A. This also illustrates a normal method of closing the soffit of overhanging

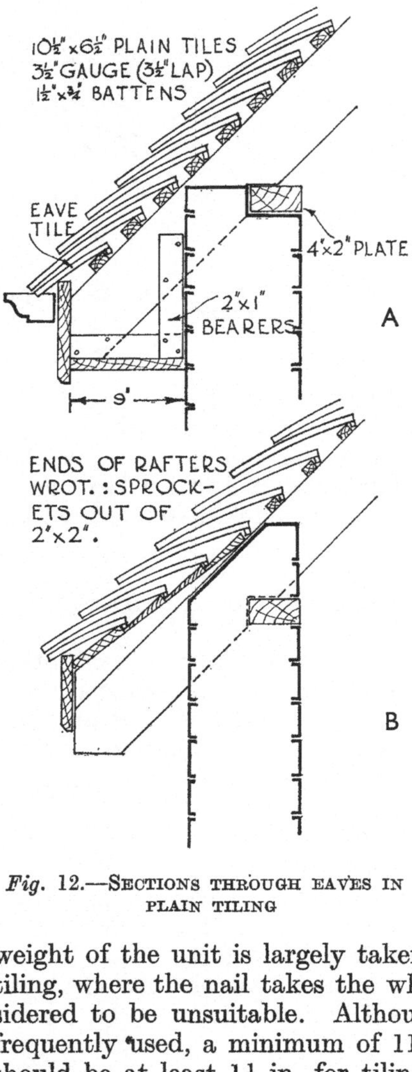

Fig. 12.—SECTIONS THROUGH EAVES IN PLAIN TILING

rafters. Fig. 12B shows how an open soffit should be formed. Note the use of feather-edged boarding in place of battening from eave to wall-line. Eaves are occasionally specified as "to be bedded," but this is unnecessary and detrimental. In Fig. 13 the construction at eaves is clearly shown, the batten for the eave tile being the first above the fascia. The tiler's method of loading the roof is also seen: a tiler's mate will carry up a ladder as many as forty to forty-five plain tiles on his head, a weight of perhaps 100 lbs. or more.

Sprocketed eaves improve the appearance of a roof, but care should be taken that the sprocketed part is not of too slow a pitch. No part of a plain-tiled roof, excepting, of course, hips and valleys, should be of less than 40° pitch.

Nails and Nailing

Nails for tiling and slating may be conveniently considered under one heading.

The kinds ordinarily in use are of galvanised iron or steel, zinc, yellow cast composition, and copper.

Galvanised nails are used for ordinary tiling work, where the weight of the unit is largely taken by the nibs. For slating or nibless tiling, where the nail takes the whole weight, galvanised nails are considered to be unsuitable. Although gauges as fine as 12 and 13 are frequently used, a minimum of 11 gauge is recommended. The length should be at least 1½ in. for tiling: a nail 1¼ in. long, if used with a thick tile, will not give sufficient fixing into the battens.

Zinc nails are cut, not cast, and are satisfactory on all jobs excepting those where the nails may be exposed to fumes that are injurious to zinc. A minimum length of 1¼ in. for small slates, and 1½ in. or 2 in. for large slates, is recommended. Average weights of zinc nails are :—

1½ in.	4½–5 lbs. per 1,000
1¾ in.	6½–7 lbs. ,, ,,
2 in.	10–11 lbs. ,, ,,

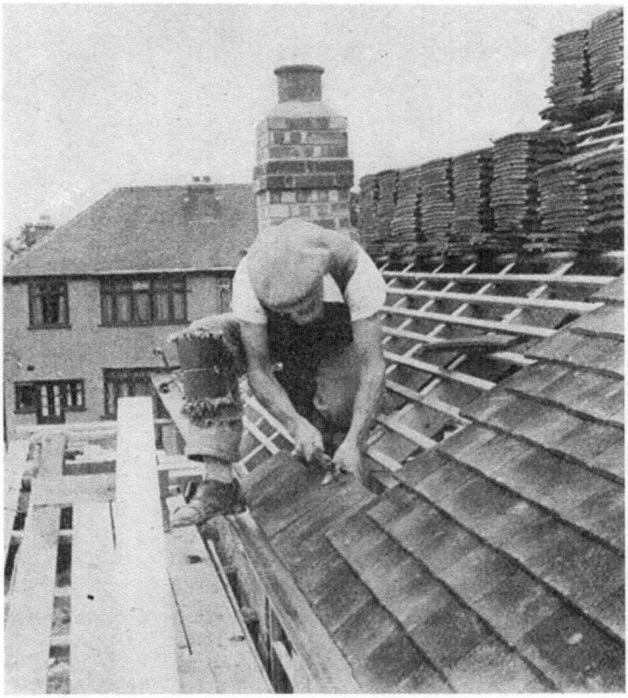

Fig. 13.—CONSTRUCTION AT EAVES IN PLAIN TILING

Yellow cast-composition nails are made of an alloy of copper, zinc, and tin. They are practically indestructible under all conditions, and have the advantage over copper that they are harder and more readily driven. Composition nails are used for all kinds of slating and tiling, but are costly: about 2*d*. per pound more than copper nails, and about four times as much as galvanised. Composition nails are about 10 per cent. heavier than copper.

Copper nails are generally used for slating, and for this purpose are unequalled. Of the many slated roofs that have to be stripped and re-slated, in probably 95 per cent. of the cases the trouble is due to defective nails rather than to any defect in the slates themselves. Galvanised nails should never be used in slating: copper, zinc, or composition are safer. Average weights of cut copper nails are:—

$1\frac{1}{2}$ in. . .	$4\frac{1}{2}$ lbs. per 1,000
2 in. . .	10 lbs. ,, ,,

Cast copper nails are lighter than the cut variety.

Cost of Nailing

It is not possible to give costs per square for nailing: each class of work requires a different number of nails per square. Plain tiling is ordinarily nailed at every fourth or fifth course, with two nails to each tile. Fifth-course nailing laid to a 4-in. gauge thus requires $554 \times 2 \div 5$,

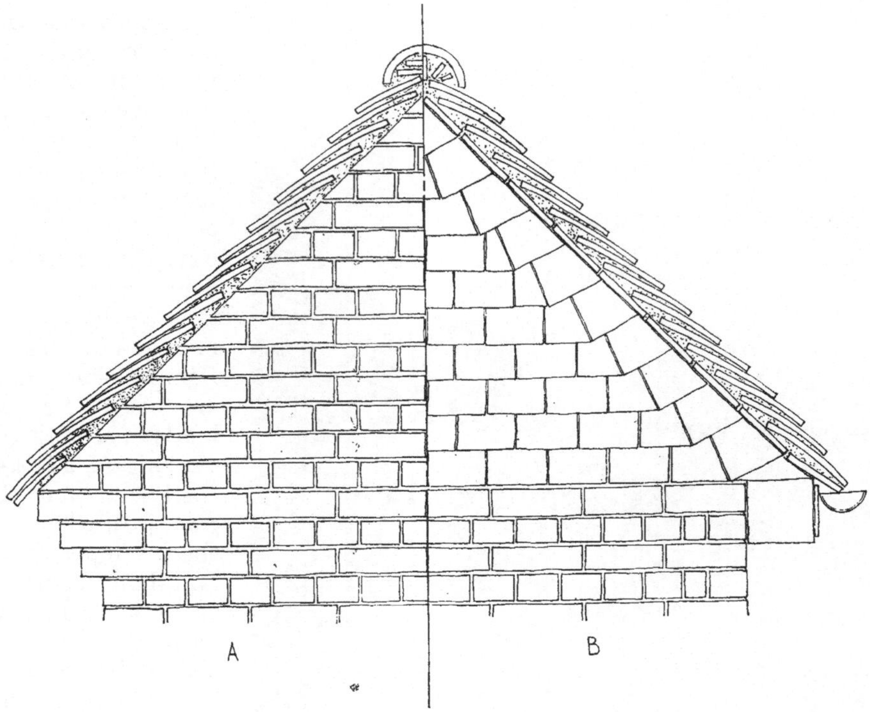

Fig. 14.—VERGES IN PLAIN TILING

A. Verge bedded and pointed. B. Bedded and pointed, with course of plain tiles a undercloak. Note Winchester cut of vertical tiling against undercloak.

or 222 nails per square net, and if the nail used is a copper nail 1½ in. long, weighing 4½ lbs. per thousand, and costing 10*d*. per pound, the cost per square for nails would only be about 11*d*. This would allow a reasonable percentage for waste. The 554 in the above calculation is the number of tiles per square. Other examples are worked out by the same method.

Verges

Verges ordinarily project 2 in. over a brick wall or barge board, but on high buildings this should be increased. Verges may be bedded and pointed only (Fig. 14A), or bedded and pointed with the addition of one or more courses of plain tiles laid flat as undercloak (Fig. 14B). The latter method is preferable for two reasons : the appearance is improved, and the verge is given a slight tilt, which helps to prevent water from dripping over the edge of the verge.

Where vertical tiling occurs under a verge, as in Fig. 14B, the undercloak is essential if a neat finish is to be made between the vertical tiling and

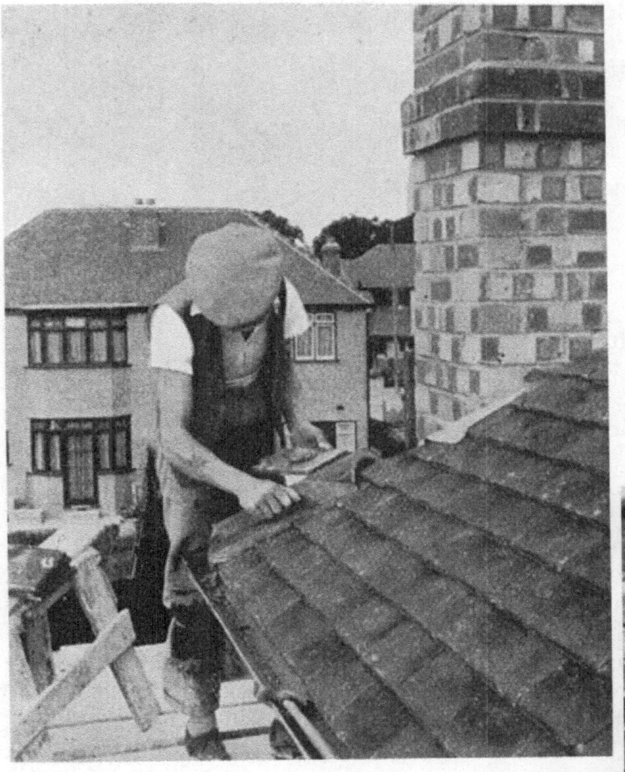

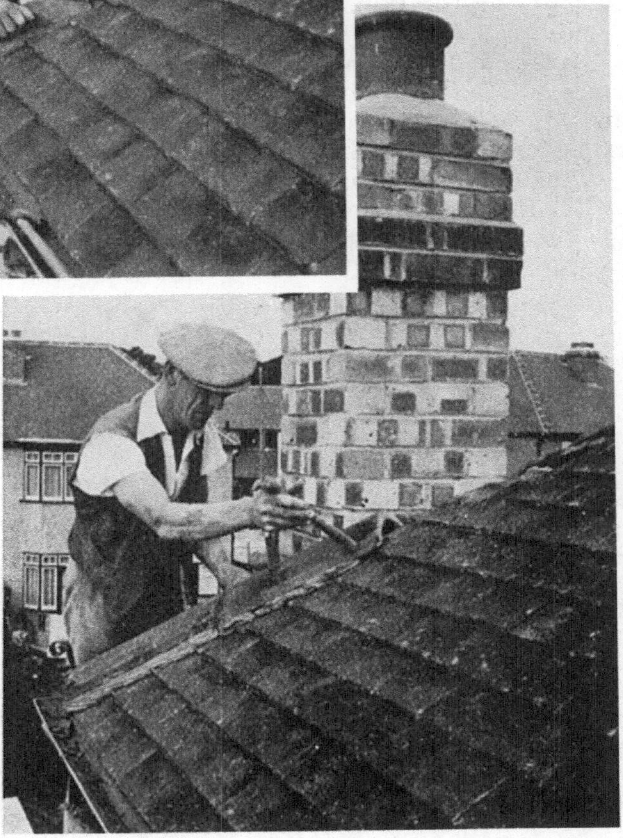

Figs. 15 *and* 16.—HIP COVERED WITH HALF-ROUND RIDGE

Note use of lead where hip passes near chimney stack.

undercloak. This illustration also shows the method of splay-cutting known as Winchester cut, a finish that is becoming increasingly popular. It is, of course, more expensive than the continuation of the courses of vertical tiling in a straight line until they meet the under side of the verge.

Ridges

Ornamental ridges are now rarely used in tiling: nor, for that matter, in slating either. Most architects favour, for tiling, the half-round ridge, bedded and pointed in cement mortar. The practice of bedding ridges, hips, etc., in lime and hair mortar, and pointing in cement mortar, is also dying out. It had no practical advantage, and was rarely carried out to specification.

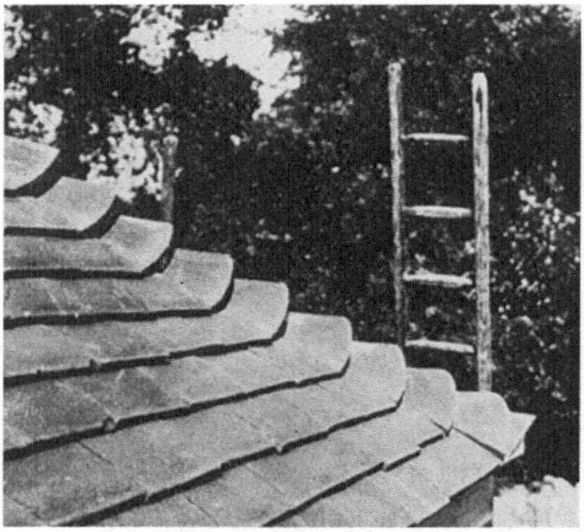

Fig. 17.—BONNET HIP TILING

Hips

Hips may be :—

(*a*) Covered with half-round or other ridge tiles (Figs. 15 and 16).

(*b*) Of bonnet hips (Fig. 17).

(*c*) Of hip tiles (Fig. 18).

(*d*) Mitred (Fig. 19).

Half-round ridge may be used with either hand-made or machine-made tiles. Bonnet hips are usual in good-class hand-made tile work, and hip tiles are associated with machine-made tiles. Mitred hips are commoner in slating than in tiling.

Here are a few points to be noted :—

(1) Hip irons are needed with a ridge on the hip. Their function is to prevent the whole length of hip ridge from slipping.

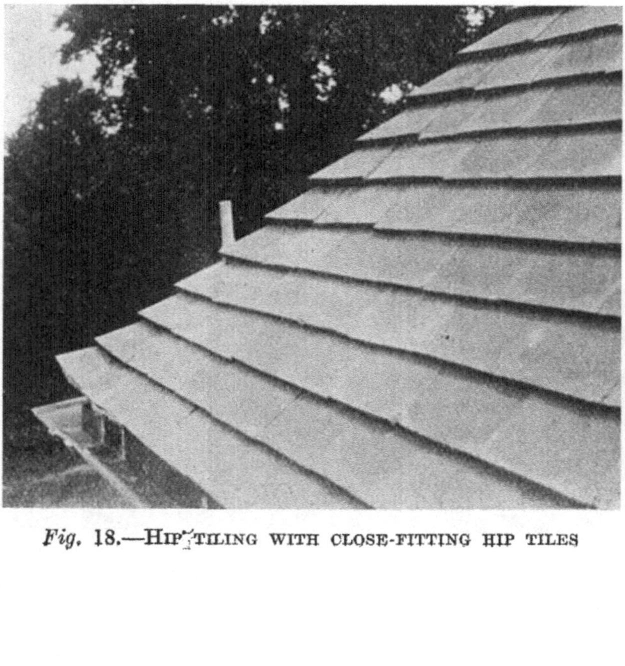

Fig. 18.—HIP TILING WITH CLOSE-FITTING HIP TILES

(2) Every bonnet hip or hip tile has to be nailed, and there is thus no necessity for hip irons.

(3) There is one bonnet hip or hip tile to each course of tiles on either side of the hip. If the two pitches coming into a hip are different, the longest common rafter on the steeper pitch will be shorter than that on the slower pitch, but the number of

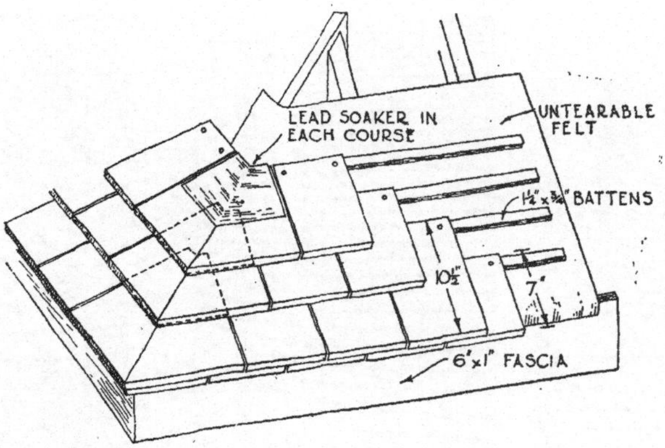

Fig. 19.—MITRED HIP IN PLAIN TILING

courses of tiling remains the same. Therefore, on the steeper pitch the gauge is shorter, and provision must be made for this when battening. The rule is: where bonnet hips or hip tiles are used, the battens must intersect at the hip.

These remarks apply also to valley tiling and mitred valleys and hips. Where ridge tiles are used on a hip, or valleys are of metal, the courses need not "follow round."

Valleys

The valley is the most vulnerable part of a roof, and needs extra care on the part of the tiler. The usual forms of valley are (*a*) valley tile, (*b*) mitred valley, (*c*) laced valley, (*d*) circle or swept valley, and (*e*) metal valley.

The valley tile (Fig. 21) is the commonest and most serviceable form for use with plain tiling. Valley tiles are not nailed, as the tiles on either side keep the valley tile in place.

The mitred valley is not much used in modern practice, and the open valley only in cheap work. Both involve the co-operation of another trade, and both are less satisfactory than the tiled valley.

Laced and swept valleys are pleasing in appearance, but expensive in both labour and material, as so many tiles have to be cut. A laced valley is shown in Fig. 22. Note the characteristic upward sweep of the courses as they approach the valley, and compare with the tiled valley of Fig. 21.

Abutments

The best finish at abutments is without doubt provided by soakers and lead flashings. Architects prefer, however, to have as little lead as possible visible on the roof,

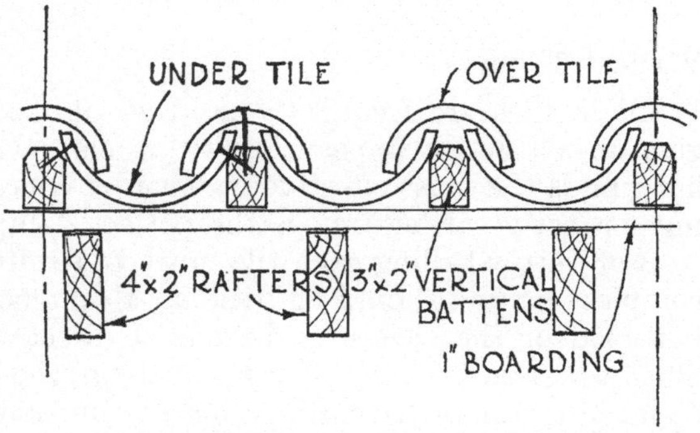

Fig. 20.—SECTION THROUGH SPANISH TILING

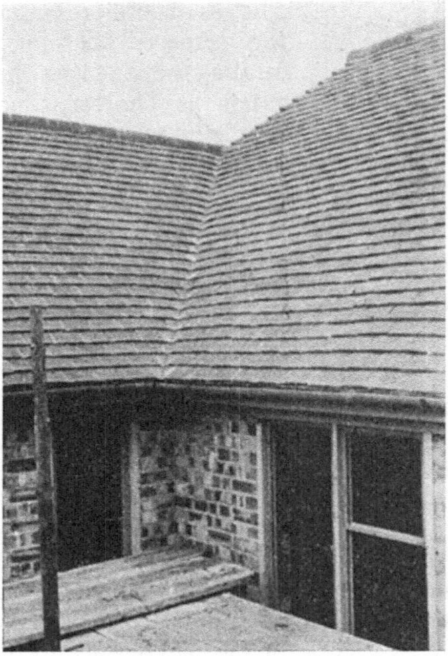

Fig. 21.—Valley tiling

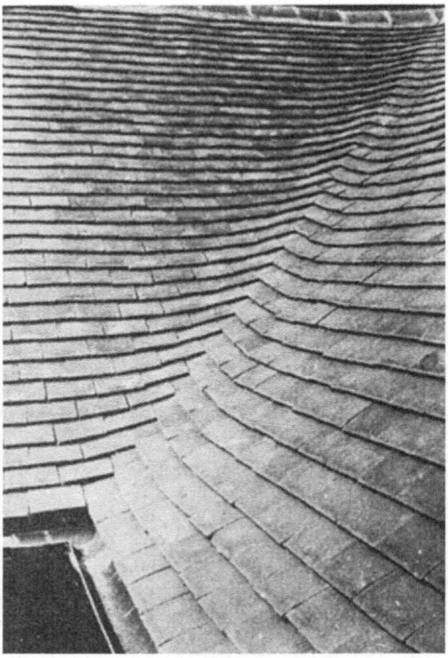

Fig. 22.—A laced valley

and the fashion has spread of having a tile flaunching or tile flashing instead of the stepped flashing. Where this form of construction is adopted the tile flashing must be let into a chase : if this is not done, and roof settlement occurs, the tile fillet will come away from the wall, and water will penetrate the gap so left.

Soakers and lead flashings are best from a constructional point of view : in all cases soakers must be inserted, whether a lead flashing, tile flashing, or cement fillet is used. Cement fillets are not recommended.

Vertical Tiling

Plain tiles are frequently used as tile hanging, partly because they give an attractive appearance to an elevation, and partly because tile hanging is the most effective waterproof covering for a wall. Tile hanging, properly carried out, is the perfect damp-resister.

For vertical tiling each tile must be secured with two nails : in fact, complete nailing should be done on all pitches over 55° Walls may be battened or the tiles may be nailed direct to the joints of brickwork. Since water runs easily off vertical tiling, the lap is not important, and a $4\frac{1}{2}$-in. gauge may be used. This is convenient where the tiles have to be fixed directly to the joints of brickwork on edge.

SINGLE-LAP TILING

The kinds of single-lap tiles are so numerous that it is not possible here to do much more than mention the general principles underlying the covering of a roof with any kind of single-lap tile.

Roof Pitches

For single-lap tiling, roof pitches in general may be slower than for plain tiling, owing to the larger size of the units and the more effective lapping at side and head. A minimum of 35° is recommended, even though in practice slower pitches are seen.

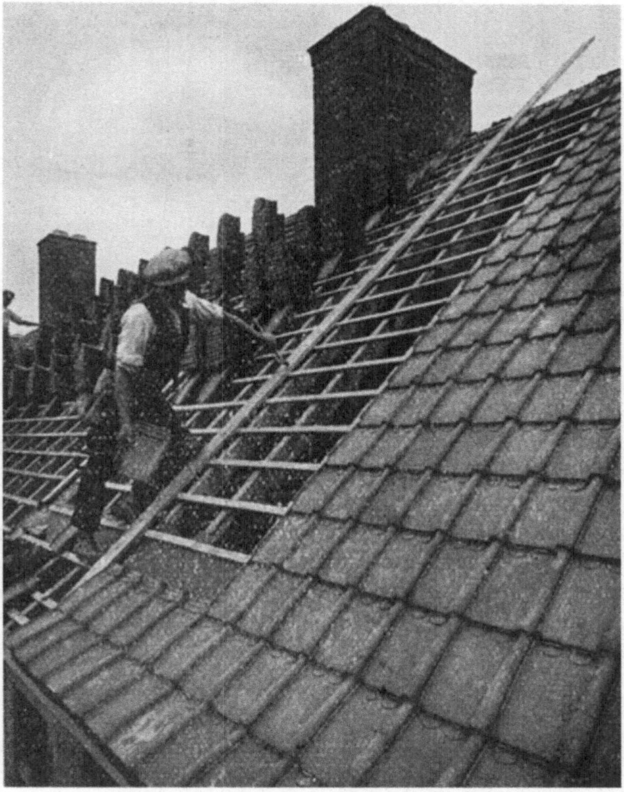

Fig. 24.—Courtrai-du-Nord tiling on open battening

Showing method adopted to ensure that the rolls of the tiles run in straight lines from eaves to ridge. (*Langley London Ltd.*)

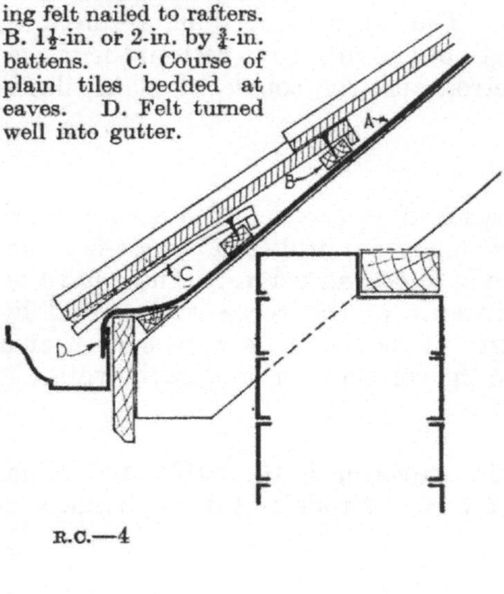

Fig. 23.—Construction of eaves in single-lap tiling

A. Untearable roofing felt nailed to rafters. B. 1½-in. or 2-in. by ¾-in. battens. C. Course of plain tiles bedded at eaves. D. Felt turned well into gutter.

Roof Preparation

Nearly all forms of single-lap tile require a continuous covering—boards or felt—between them and the rafters.

The ideal roof preparation is that recommended for plain

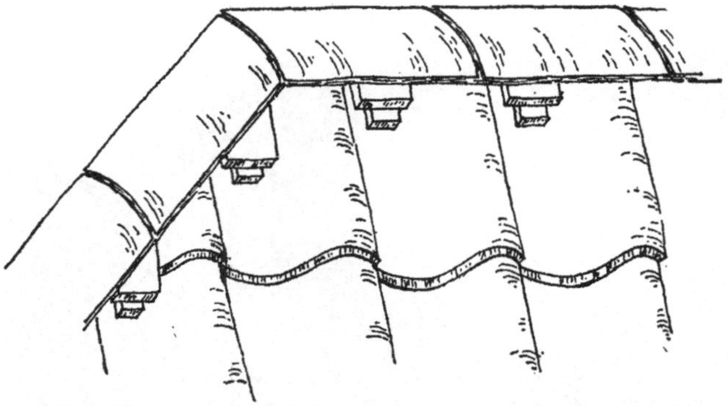

Fig. 25.—TILE LAMINATIONS FITTED BETWEEN ROLLS AT RIDGES AND HIPS

tiling, namely, plain boards, felt, counter-battens, and battens. When for reasons of cost this is impossible, then a satisfactory and reasonably inexpensive substitute is provided by untearable felt and battens. The felt should be allowed to sag slightly, but only slightly, between the rafters, and must always be carried well over the fascia and turned into the gutter. The sagging provides a series of channels down which any water that may penetrate the joints of the tiles can run to the eaves.

For Spanish and Italian tiling special preparation is necessary. The size and spacing of the vertical battens vary in different makes, and the maker's instructions must be followed. Fig. 20 is a typical section through a roof covered with Spanish tiles. The under tiles are nailed to the sides of the vertical battens, and the upper tile is fixed by a nail driven through the hole provided at the head of the tile.

Eaves

The general construction at eaves in single-lap tiling is illustrated in Fig. 23. A course of plain tiles is usually fixed over the fascia, and the first course of tiles bedded on it. No course of plain tiles is fitted at the eaves of the roof shown in Fig. 24. The tile used, a Courtrai-du-Nord, has only a small roll, and a good length of flat surface to rest on the fascia. With a pantile, or any other large-roll tile, the course of plain tiles is essential.

Verges

An undercloak should always be fitted at verges: this is even more necessary than in plain tiling. With certain makes of single-lap tile, double-roll tiles are provided for use at left-hand verges. These have no constructional value, but the appearance of the verge is improved by their use. Unfortunately, the length of roof is not always such that a double-roll tile can be used and give the correct overhang at the verge.

Ridges and Hips

The normal type of ridge and hip covering is the half-round ridge. Where a single-lap tile that shows a series of rolls and deep channels is

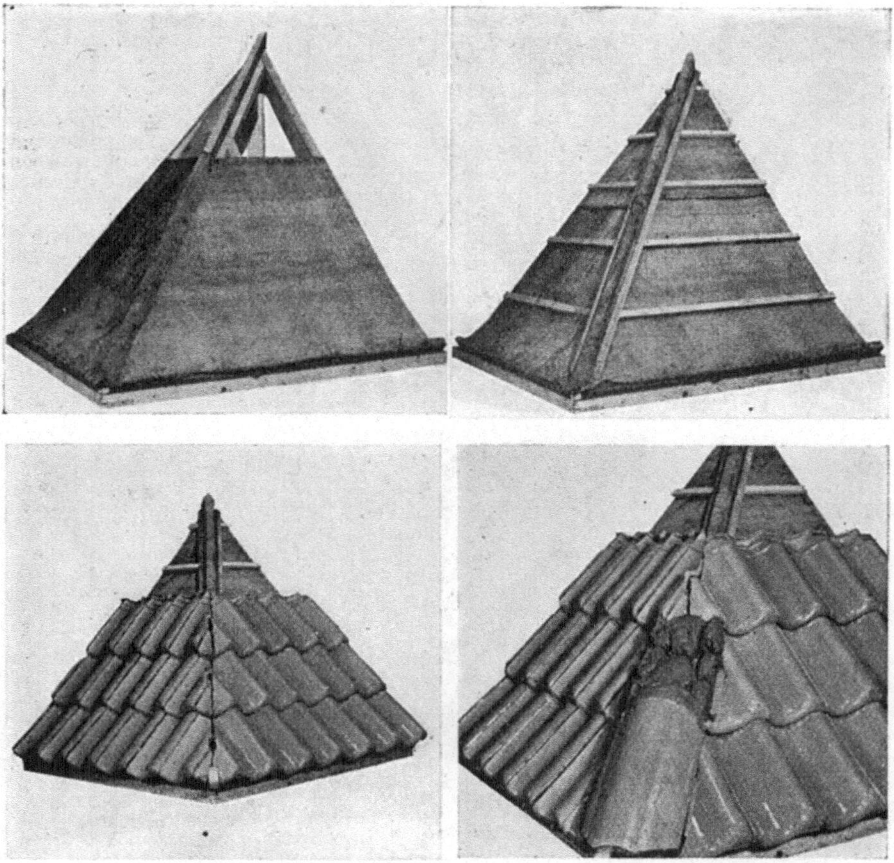

Fig. 26.—FOUR STAGES IN THE COVERING OF A HIP IN SINGLE-LAP TILING (*Langley London Ltd.*)

used (for example, a pantile, or Spanish or Italian tile), tile laminations are inserted at ridges and hips to avoid the showing of large masses of mortar (Fig. 25). With pantiles only two laminations are possible, but with Spanish and Italian tiling three or more may be used. Fig. 26 shows the four stages in the completion of a hip in single-lap tiling. Note that the felt is well lapped at the hip, that it is turned over the fascia so as to come well into the gutter, and that battens run parallel to the hip on each side to give a good fixing for the splay-cut tiles.

Valleys

Where single-lap tiles are used it is better to avoid valleys altogether. The single-lap tile does, in fact, appear at its best on large four-hipped or

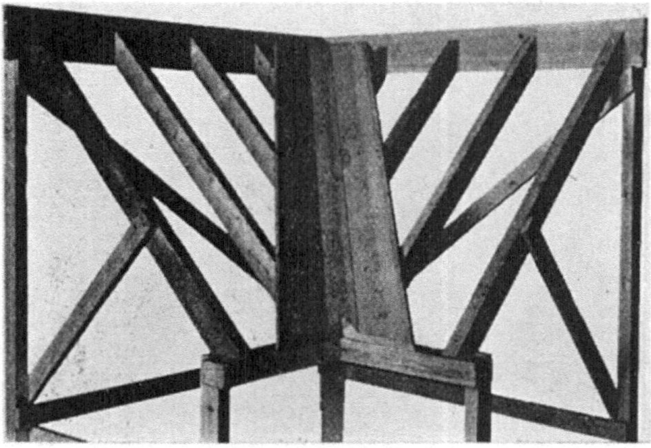

Fig. 27 (*Left*).—VALLEY CONSTRUCTION IN IMPROVED INTERLOCKING PANTILES —FIRST STAGE

Valley boards fixed. (*Langley London Ltd.*)

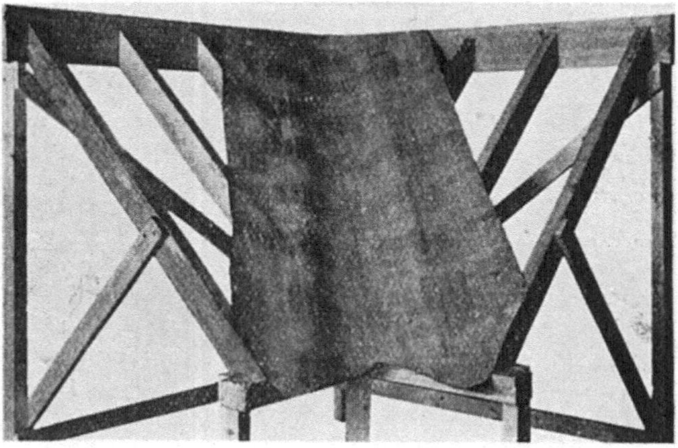

Fig. 27A (*Right*).—VALLEY CONSTRUCTION IN IMPROVED INTERLOCKING PANTILES—SECOND STAGE

Untearable roofing felt nailed to rafters. (*Langley London Ltd.*)

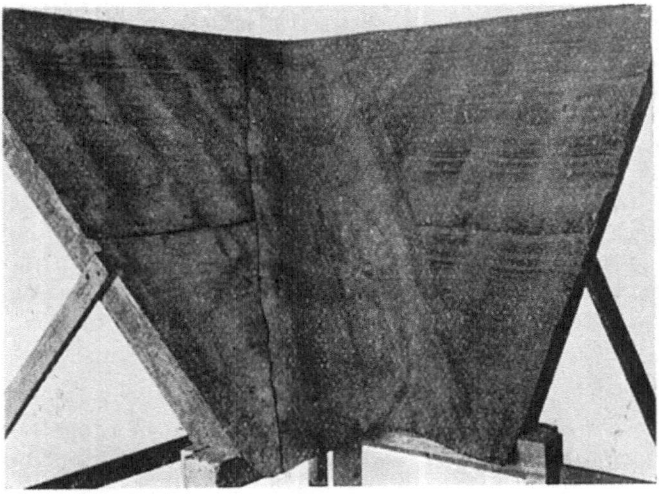

Fig. 27B (*Left*).—VALLEY CONSTRUCTION IN IMPROVED INTERLOCKING PANTILES —THIRD STAGE

Felting in valley completed. (*Langley London Ltd.*)

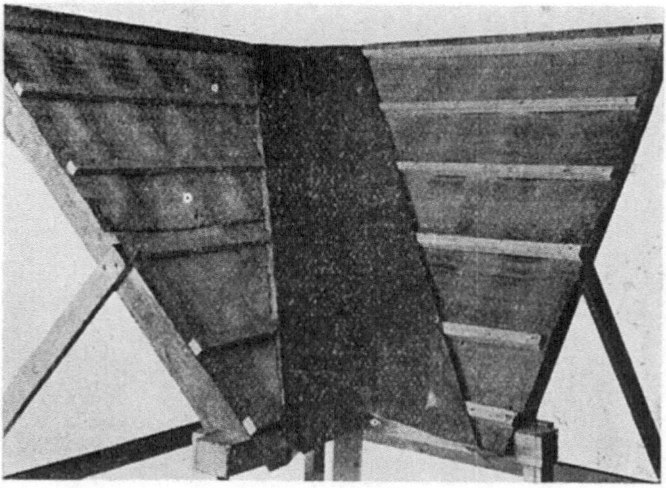

Fig. 27c.—VALLEY CONSTRUCTION IN IMPROVED INTERLOCKING PANTILES — FOURTH STAGE

Battens fixed on felt and lead valley fitted. (*Langley London Ltd.*)

plain-gabled roofs. Complicated roof plans, and roofs having dormers, are best covered with plain tiles.

Valleys in single-lap tiling are usually of metal, lead being the best material to use. Fig. 27 shows stage by stage the construction of a valley in improved interlocking pantiles.

A good craftsman should be employed for valleys in single-lap tiling: nothing in tiling is more difficult than to make such valleys watertight.

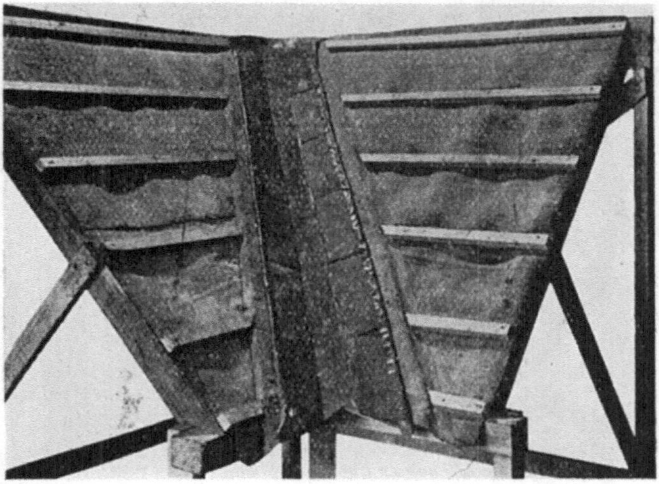

Fig. 27d.—VALLEY CONSTRUCTION IN IMPROVED INTERLOCKING PANTILES—FIFTH STAGE

Battening to valley completed. Slate undercloak fitted to valley. (*Langley London Ltd.*)

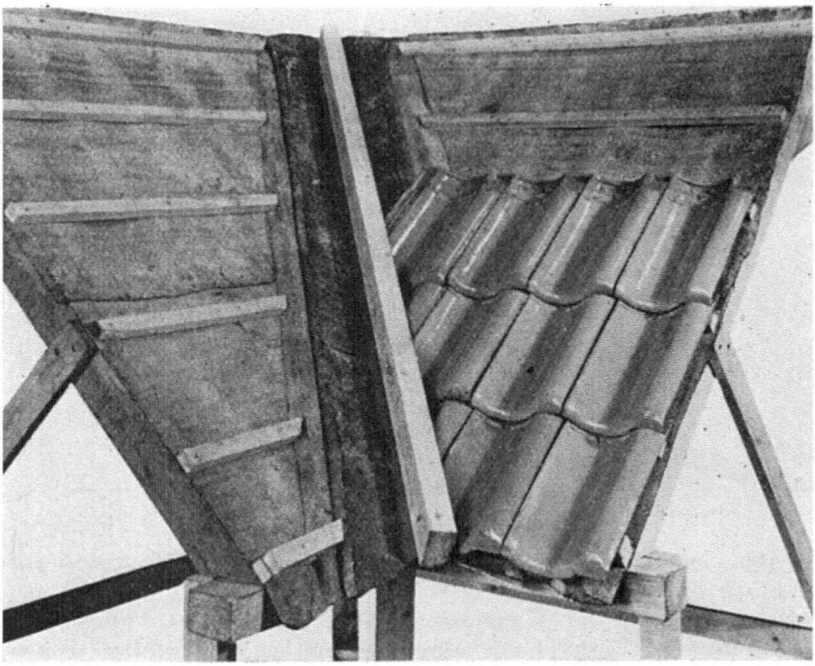

Fig. 27E.—Stage 6—tiling to valley
Note precaution to keep edges of valley straight. (*Langley London Ltd.*)

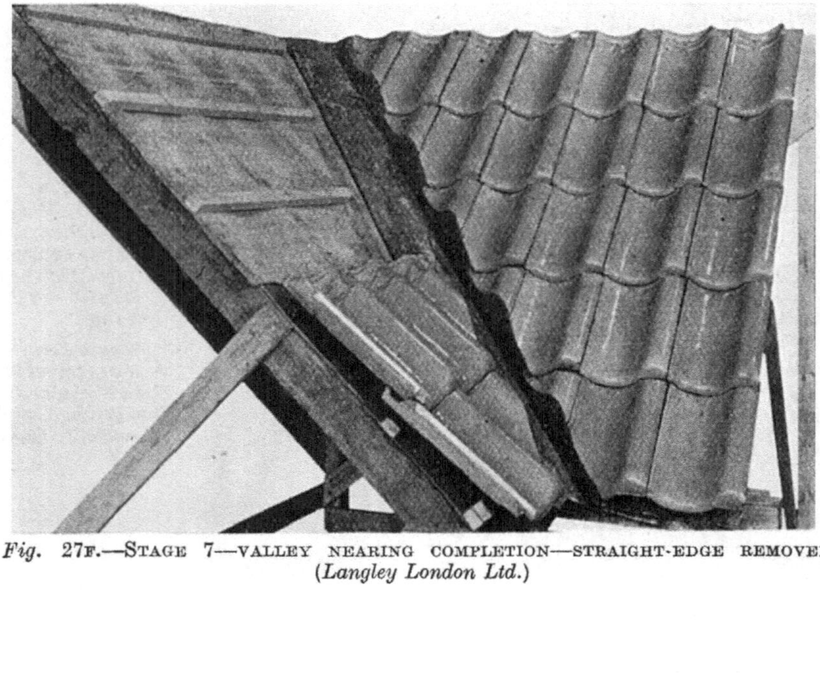

Fig. 27F.—Stage 7—valley nearing completion—straight-edge removed
(*Langley London Ltd.*)

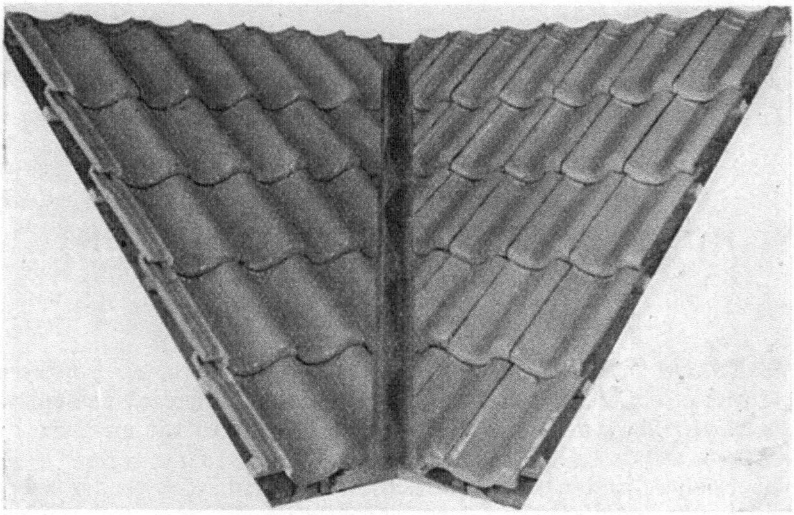

Fig. 27G.—VALLEY CONSTRUCTION IN IMPROVED INTERLOCKING PANTILES—THE COMPLETED VALLEY. (*Langley London Ltd.*)

The photographs in Figs. 27 to 27G illustrate the various step-by-step stages in tiling a valley.

Chapter VII

ROOFING WITH ASBESTOS-CEMENT MATERIALS

ASBESTOS-CEMENT is a non-permeable, strong, fire-resisting, durable concrete, composed of asbestos fibre and cement; the asbestos fibre, unlike most aggregates, adds to the strength of the cement.

The fineness and fibrous character of the asbestos render asbestos-cement easily moulded into very thin sheets of large size, making it eminently suitable for roofing slates, tiles, and corrugated and flat sheets.

Roofing Materials

The standard forms of asbestos-cement roofing materials are :—

Diagonal or diamond-pattern slates 15¾ in. by 15¾ in.

Straight-cover slates.

Small-section corrugated sheets.

Large-section corrugated sheets.

Angular-section corrugated sheets.

Pantiles.

The dimensions and specifications of each of these types have been standardised by the British Standards Institution in *Specification No.* 690–1936, *Asbestos-cement Sheets and Unreinforced Flat Sheets and Corrugated Sheets.*

ASBESTOS-CEMENT SLATES

Diagonal-pattern Slates

Asbestos-cement as a roofing material was first known in this form. Its appearance on the roof and method of fixing are shown in Fig. 1, where also the terms used in connection with diagonal slating are illustrated. It should be noted that the lap is the amount by which one slate overlaps the ones beneath, measured at right angles to the top edge of the slate that is covered.

The slates have to be specially holed by the makers to give the desired lap—2¾, 3, 3½, or 4 in. Each slate is secured with one copper disk rivet and two slate nails; copper slate nails are recommended, particularly in acid-laden atmospheres. The slates may be laid on battens or close boards. If the latter method is adopted, care is necessary in the coursing of the slates: true lines and uniform lap are essential to the avoidance of leaks.

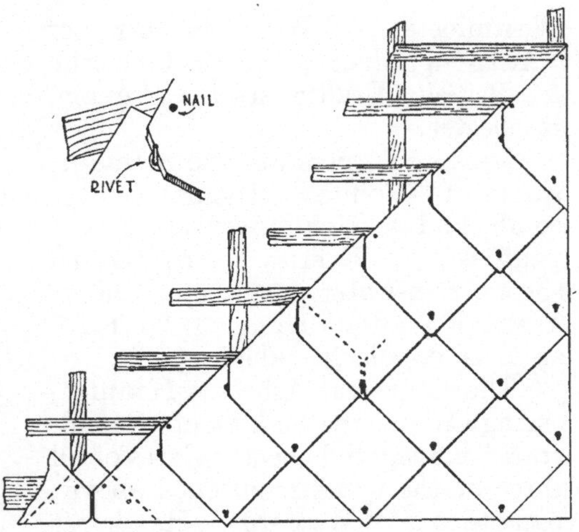

Fig. 1.—DIAGONAL-PATTERN ASBESTOS-CEMENT SLATES, 15¾ IN. BY 15¾ IN.

A variation of the diagonal pattern is the honeycomb-pattern slate, Fig. 2, in which the "drop-point" is eliminated. The method of fixing is similar to that of diagonal-pattern slates, but the honeycomb type is made only for 2¾-in. and 3½-in. laps.

Technical data for these and all other asbestos-cement materials are given in detail by the manufacturers, and the figures given in these pages have been taken from the catalogues of Messrs. Turner's Asbestos Co. Ltd., Asbestos House, Southwark St., S.E.1, and the Universal Asbestos Manufacturing Co. Ltd., 43–46 Southampton Buildings, Chancery Lane, W.C.2.

Other large makers are The Atlas Stone Co. Ltd., 15 Victoria Street,

TECHNICAL DATA FOR 15¾-IN. BY 15¾-IN. DIAGONAL AND HONEYCOMB SLATING

Method of Laying	*Lap in In.*	*No. of Slates per Square*	*Batten Gauge in In.*	*Feet of Battens per Square*	*Weight of Slates per Square in Lb.*
Honeycomb	2¾	86	8⅛	149	224
"	3½	99	7⅜	164	257
Diamond	2¾	86	8⅞	136	250
"	3	89	8½	142	261
"	3½	96	8¼	146	282
"	4	105	7⅝	158	308

These figures are net and include no allowance for waste. The weights vary slightly as between different makes.

Westminster, S.W.1, makers of "Atlas" products; and the Cellactite & British Uralite Ltd., Higham, Rochester.

Messrs. Turners are the manufacturers of "Poilite" diagonal, honeycomb, and straight-cover slates and pantiles; "Everite" corrugated sheets, rain-water goods, etc., and of Turner's Trafford Tiling, or "T.T.T." as it is popularly called.

The Universal Asbestos Manufacturing Co. are the makers of "Handcraft" corrugated sheets; slates of all three of the types mentioned above; pan tiles; "Watford" Handcraft tiles, and other materials.

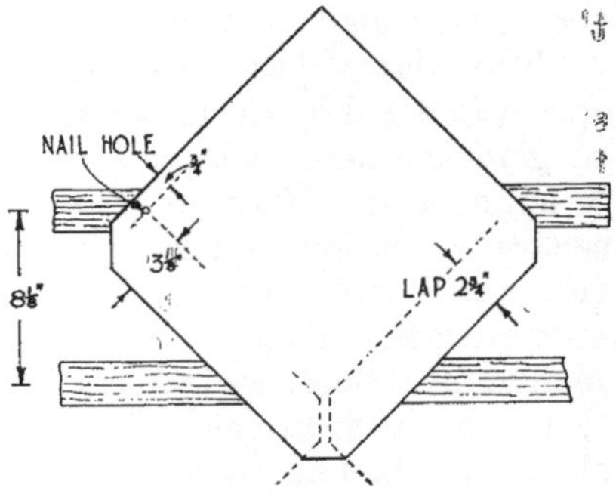

Fig. 2.—HONEYCOMB-PATTERN ASBESTOS-CEMENT SLATE, 15¾ IN. BY 15¾ IN.

Showing dimensions required by British Standard Specification No. 690–1936.

The roof pitches and their respective recommended minimum laps are as under:—

Pitch of Roof	*Minimum Lap*
40°	2¾ in.
35°	3 in.
30°	3½ in.
25°	4 in.

Straight-cover Slates

These are made in sizes 24 in. by 12 in.; 20 in. by 10 in.; 15¾ in. by 7⅞ in.; and 11¾ in. by 5⅞ in. They are laid in the same way as ordinary, natural slates, with the addition of one copper disk rivet near the tail of each slate, except in the case of the 11¾-in. by 5⅞-in. slate, which does not need a rivet. The slates are holed by the makers to give the correct lap.

TECHNICAL DATA

Size of Slate in In.	*Lap in In.*	*No. of Slates per Square*	*Spacing of Battens in In.*	*Linear Feet of Battens per Square*	*Weight of Slates per Square in Lbs.*
24 by 12	3	115	10½	114	398
24 by 12	4	121	10	119	418
20 by 10	3	170	8½	141	423
15¾ by 7⅞	3	289	6⅜	189	404
11¾ by 5⅞	2¾	519	4⅝	260	422

These figures are net, and include no allowance for waste. The weights vary slightly as between different makes.

CORRUGATED SHEETS

Two kinds of corrugated sheets are manufactured—the small section and the large. Sheets produced by any one maker are not necessarily identical in all respects with those made by any other firm, but the information given below may be taken as fairly representative of the products of all firms.

The small, or standard, section corrugated sheet is stocked in 4-ft. to 10-ft. sheets, in lengths which are multiples of 6 in. The standard width is 30 in., the pitch of corrugations is $2\frac{7}{8}$ in., the over-all depth of corrugations is $2\frac{7}{8}$ in., the reputed thickness of the sheets is $\frac{1}{4}$ in.

The end lap recommended for pitches down to about 30° is 6 in. For lower pitches, or in very exposed positions, the end lap should be increased or sealed with mastic or other suitable material. With a 6-in. lap and a side lap of $1\frac{1}{2}$ corrugations, the actual cover of a 9-ft. sheet is 8 ft. 6 in. by 2 ft. $1\frac{1}{2}$ in. The weight of 100 sq. ft. as laid is 270 lbs. to 330 lbs., according to the make and size of sheet. (The larger the sheets, the smaller the area that is covered twice.)

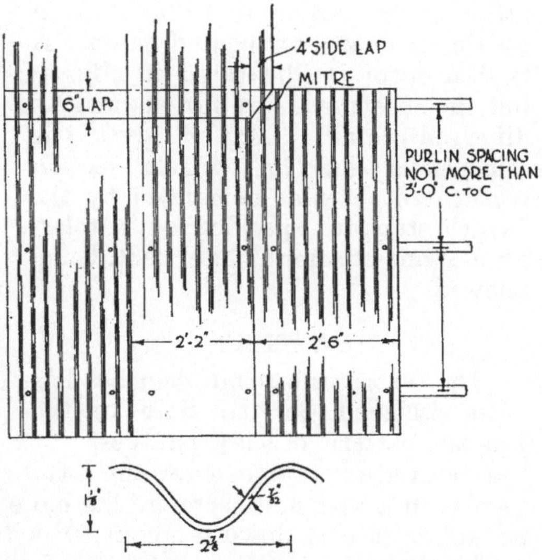

Fig. 3.—STANDARD-SECTION ASBESTOS-CEMENT CORRUGATED SHEETS FIXED TO WOOD PURLINS

Dimensions required by Specification No. 690–1936.

Fixing Corrugated Sheets

Fig. 3 shows in plan the method of fixing to wood purlins. Three-inch by $\frac{1}{4}$-in. galvanised iron screws, with lead cupped and fibre washers, are used, and it is important that the side laps should not be bolted together; nor should the sheets be fixed more tightly than is necessary to attach them securely. The purlin spacing should not exceed 3 ft. Detailed instructions for fixing are issued by each manufacturer.

For fixing to iron purlins, galvanised hook bolts are supplied by the makers.

The large-section corrugated sheet, of which the Everite "Big-Six" and Handcraft "Super-Six" are typical examples, differs from the standard sheet in that it has larger corrugations and is slightly thicker. It is stocked in 4-ft. to 10-ft. lengths, in lengths which are multiples of 6 in. The width varies between 40 in. and 43 in., the pitch of corrugations is $5\frac{3}{4}$ in., and the depth 2 in. Purlins may be spaced up to 4 ft. 6 in., as compared with the maximum of 3 ft. with standard sheets. The weight per square as laid varies between 310 lbs. and 350 lbs. The general fixing details are as for standard sheets, but the makers' instructions must in all cases be strictly followed.

Angular-section Corrugated Sheets

Angular-section corrugated sheets were originally designed to provide a rather better-looking roof than is given by the ordinary corrugated sheet. A typical form is illustrated in Fig. 4, but the sheets made by various makers differ in details. Fig. 4 gives the dimensions for an angular-section corrugated sheet as demanded by the British standard specification, a tolerance of one-quarter of 1 per cent. being allowed.

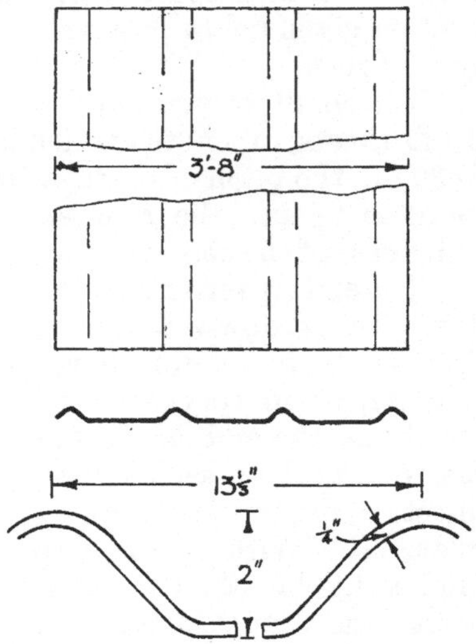

Fig. 4.—TYPICAL FORM OF ANGULAR-SECTION CORRUGATED ASBESTOS-CEMENT SHEET

PANTILES

The asbestos-cement pantile has been designed on the lines of the English pattern of clay pantiles. It has certain advantages over the latter: it is lighter in weight; more regular in shape, and therefore fits more closely on the roof; and it can be laid on pitches down to about 40° without felt or boarding.

Technical Data

	Large Pantile	*Small Pantile*
Size	$15\frac{3}{4}$ in. by $13\frac{1}{4}$ in.	$15\frac{3}{4}$ in. by $9\frac{7}{16}$ in.
Standard lap	4 in.	4 in.
No. of tiles per square (100 sq. ft.)	108	164
Centres of battens	$11\frac{3}{4}$ in.	$11\frac{3}{4}$ in.
Lin. ft. of battens per square (100 sq. ft.)	102	102
Approx. weight of tiles per square (100 sq. ft.)	362 lbs.	392 lbs.
Approx. weight of 1,000 tiles	29 cwts.	21 cwts.

Add 5 per cent. for cuttings to valleys, hips, etc.

Size of battens	2 in. by 1 in.
Colour	Russet-brown
Pitch of roof	Not less than 40° when laid on open battens. When boarding and/or felt is used under pantiles, a pitch of 30° can be adopted.

Method of Fixing

Fix pantiles with two galvanised nails per tile (one 2 in. by 10's gauge in the right-hand hole, and one $1\frac{1}{2}$ in. by 10's gauge in the left), driven

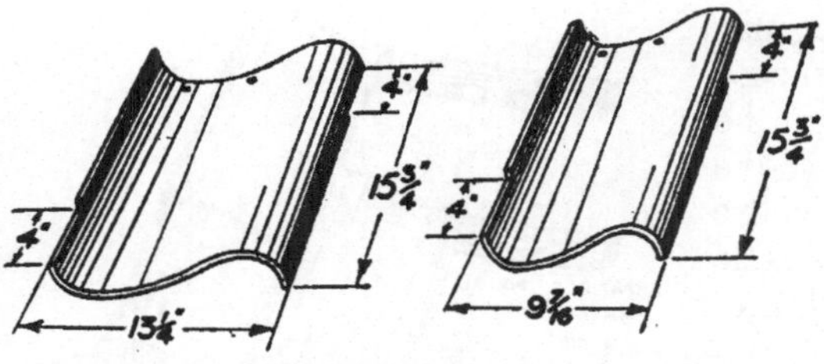

Fig. 5.—ASBESTOS-CEMENT PANTILES

at right angles to the surface of that portion of the tile through which they pass.

A proved method is to fix nail A first, 2 in. long, but driven only partly home. Next, drive nail B, 1½ in. long, fully home. Finally, return to nail A, which is just off that portion of the tile bearing on the batten, and drive it far enough to cause the roll of the tile to bind on the next tile under, as shown at point C.

There will be a tendency for the vertical lines of tiles up the slope to lean to the right, and to avoid this each pantile should be held firmly to the left while it is being nailed.

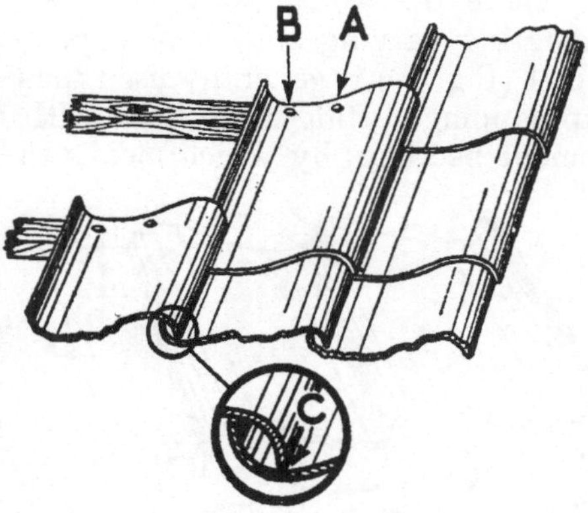

Fig. 6.—FIXING PANTILES

Eaves Finish

Stop-end pantiles are supplied, only in the large size, for use at eaves. These tiles are made with a closed end, which, when used in conjunction with an eaves strip, eliminates the gap over the back of the gutter.

In the case of the small pantiles, the eaves pantiles should be bedded on an asbestos-cement strip with expanded metal, nailed or stapled in position, used to assist keying. The ends of the pantiles should afterwards be pointed in cement.

Hips, Valleys, Verges, and Ridges

Twin pantiles have been specifically designed in both small and

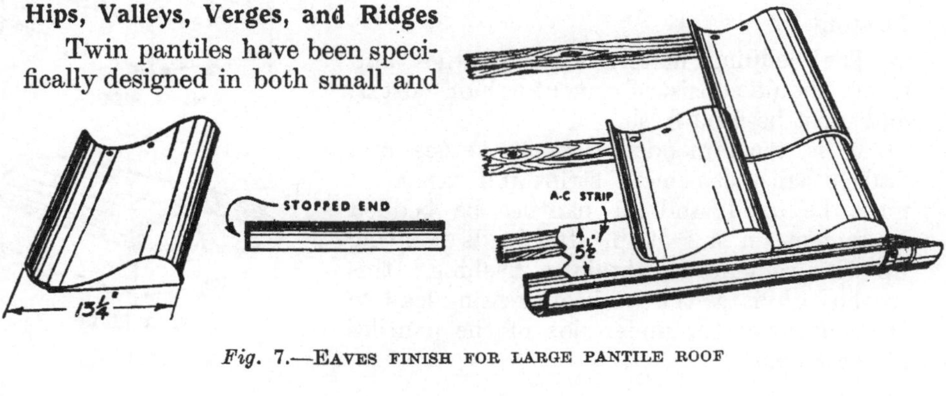

Fig. 7.—EAVES FINISH FOR LARGE PANTILE ROOF

large sizes to avoid small triangular pieces of tile which would otherwise occur at hips and valleys, and be difficult to fix securely. The above shows a typical instance where these twin pantiles are used. The illustrations below show the large-pattern twin pantile.

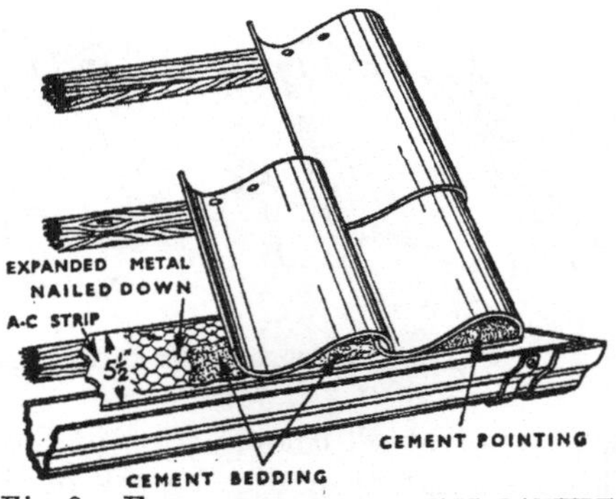

Fig. 8.—Eaves finish for small pantile roof

Double-roll pantiles, made in both small and large sizes, are for use on left-hand verges, and enable a roll finish to be given to a roof verge.

There are two ridges for accommodating varying angles of slope. No. 1 (Fig. 10) is generally used for ridge capping, and No. 2 pattern for hip capping. Ridges are lined with concrete to give a good key to the cement bedding, by which means the ridges should be fixed, afterwards

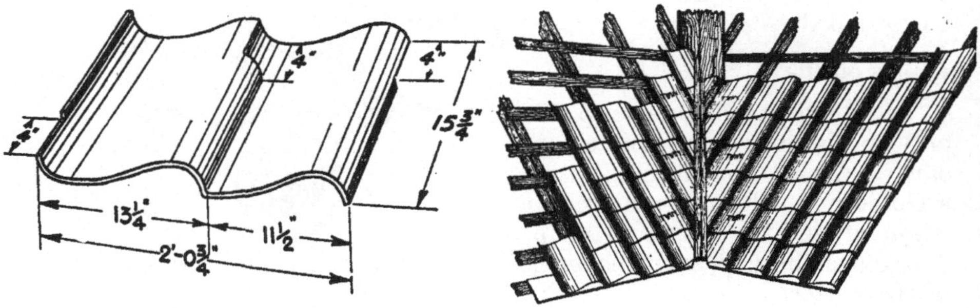

Fig. 9.—Twin pantile and its application at valley

being pointed to give a clean finish. Hip irons should always be used.

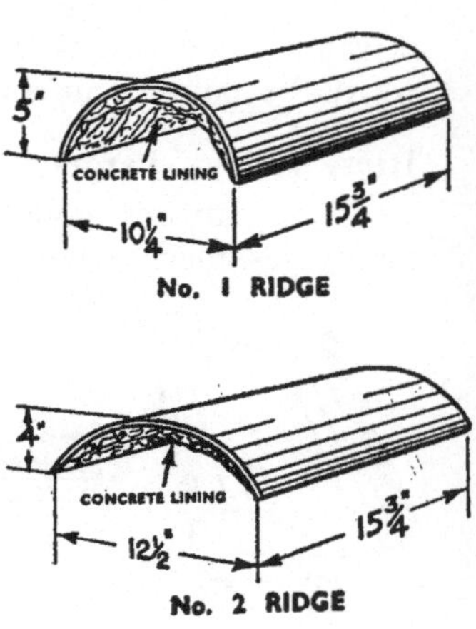

Fig. 10.—Ridges

Bedding

The bedding materials for pantiles and ridges should consist of cement or hair mortar, and must be used fresh.

It is recommended that at verges and valleys asbestos-cement strips and expanded metal be fixed, and the pantiles be bedded in cement on this strip, afterwards pointing up with cement, to obtain a flashing; this method obviates the work of dressing lead to the contour of the under side of the pantiles at these points.

Chapter VIII

COVERING ROOFS WITH ASPHALTE SHINGLES

ASPHALTE as used for roofing is well known for its durability, being impervious to water and providing an effective barrier to the passage of heat and cold. Its use as a covering for flat roofs has already been mentioned in Chapter III.

A form of asphalte shingle has been developed as a covering for sloping roofs and placed on the market under the name of Flextile ; this material consists of high-quality asphalte roofing covered with a layer of slate or tile chippings on the exposed surface. The roofing is cut into strips 36 in. × 10 in., these strips being further subdivided into four by a slot or " cut-out " 4 in. deep. The strips are laid with 4 in. exposed to the weather, giving a 6-in. overlap and 2-in. cover as in tiling. The appearance of the finished job resembles that of a slated or tiled roof, the " cut-outs " throwing a sufficient shadow to give an appearance of solidity. The shingles are made in two colours, rust-red and grey-green ; the colours are natural, since they are due to the chippings applied to the asphalte roofing, and weather similarly to slates or tiles.

The shingles are light, weighing only 200 lbs. per square, thus assisting economy in roof design. The light weight reduces the handling of the material and enables the shingles to be easily and quickly laid.

This type of roofing lends itself easily to awkward shapes, since the shingles can be cut with a knife to fit round dormers, curved soffits, valleys, etc.

Laying of Flextile Shingles

The shingles should be applied on top of close-jointed boarding, and the valleys and gutters should be constructed first. The valleys and gutters may be of lead or copper, but if desired may be formed with asphalte roofing strips in two layers. The roofing strips are supplied for the purpose in any width required, the recommended widths being 12 in. for the under strip and 18 in. for the upper, thus bringing the edge well under the shingles, as shown in Fig. 1.

The understrip is nailed to the boarding, and the upper strip cemented to it with mastic applied hot. The upper strip is nailed at the edges only, as shown in Fig. 1, thus leaving no nail heads exposed when the roof is completed.

A strip of asphalte roofing is next fixed at the verges as shown in Figs. 2

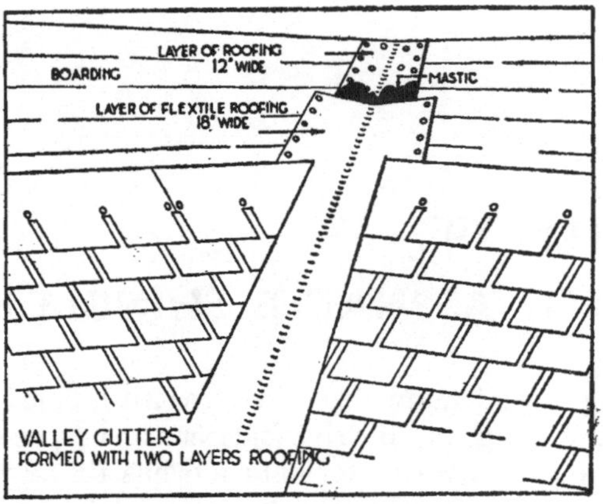

Fig. 1.—Showing double protection of Flextile roofing strips in valley (*D. Anderson & Son Ltd.*)

and 3. The eaves course should be a row of shingles reversed (see Fig 2), or alternatively a strip of asphalte roofing not less than 9 in. and preferably 18 in. wide may be used as shown in Fig. 3.

The laying of the shingles then proceeds in the same manner as slating or tiling, starting at the eaves and working up the roof. Fig. 4 shows the first row of shingles in position. Each alternate row should begin by cutting off half of the first leaf, so as to bring the joints in each row midway between those in the next.

The first course proper should overhang the edge of the roof boarding by about $\frac{3}{4}$ in., with a similar overhang at the verges. The asphalte roofing strips should be bent over and nailed to the edges of the boarding as shown in the illustrations. If barge boards are used, the shingles are finished flush with the edge of the barge boards.

Lap

The width of the shingles being 10 in. and the depth of the slot 4 in., they are laid so that the bottom edge is in line with the top of the slot in the course below, thus giving the 6-in. overlap already described.

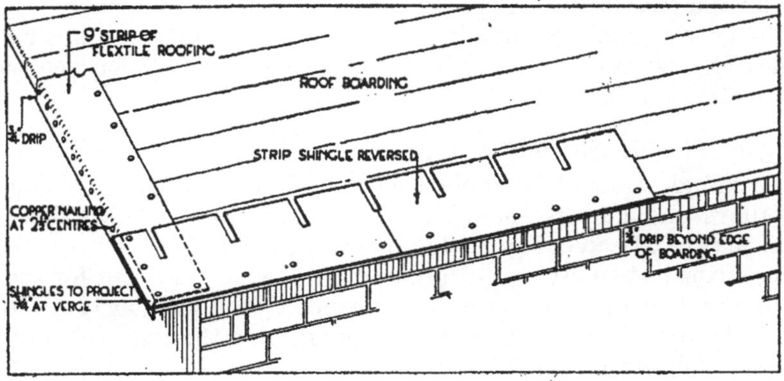

Fig. 2.—Showing 9-in. strip of Flextile roofing at verge and starting or eaves course of shingles reversed

This course is begun by cutting off half of the first leaf to ensure breaking joint when the first course proper is laid. (*D. Anderson & Son Ltd.*)

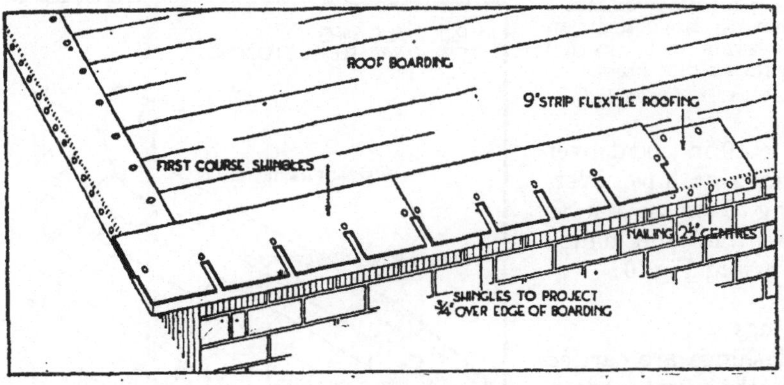

Fig. 3.—SHOWING STRIP OF FLEXTILE ROOFING AS STARTING OR EAVES COURSE WITH FIRST COURSE OF SHINGLES IN POSITION
Note the Flextile roofing bent over and nailed to edge of boarding.
(*D. Anderson & Son Ltd.*)

Nailing

One-in. galvanised clout nails are used, each course being nailed ½ in. above each slot as shown in Figs. 3 and 4. At projecting edges exposed to wind pressure some additional nailing should be provided, and care should be taken to avoid driving nails between the joints of the boarding.

Ridges and Hips

There are two alternative treatments for ridges and hips in this type of roofing. The first is to use asphalte roofing strips 9 in. wide, bent over the ridge or hip, lying 4½ in. on each side, and nailed along the edge at 2-in. centres ¾ in. from the edge as illustrated in Fig. 5.

Alternatively. the shingle strips may be cut into individual pieces

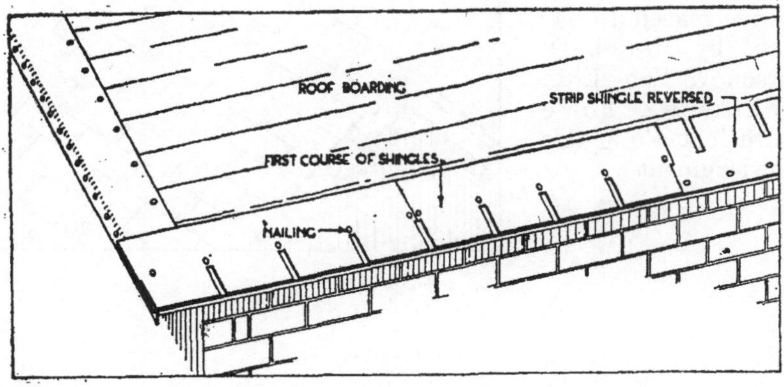

Fig. 4.—SHOWING FIRST ROW OF SHINGLES IN POSITION. (*D. Anderson & Son Ltd.*)

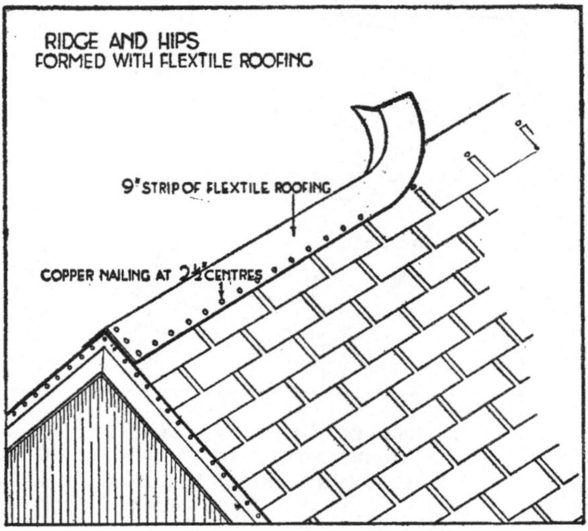

Fig. 5.—SHOWING ROOF BEING CLOSED IN AND COMPLETED WITH STRIP OF FLEXTILE ROOFING AT THE RIDGE (*D. Anderson & Son Ltd.*)

9 in. × 10 in., bent over the ridge or hips, overlapping to expose 5 in. to the weather and nailed as shown in Fig. 6.

Flashings

Flashings are carried out in the usual manner employed in slating. Upstands may be formed of asphalte roofing strips if desired, but metal is recommended for all counter flashings.

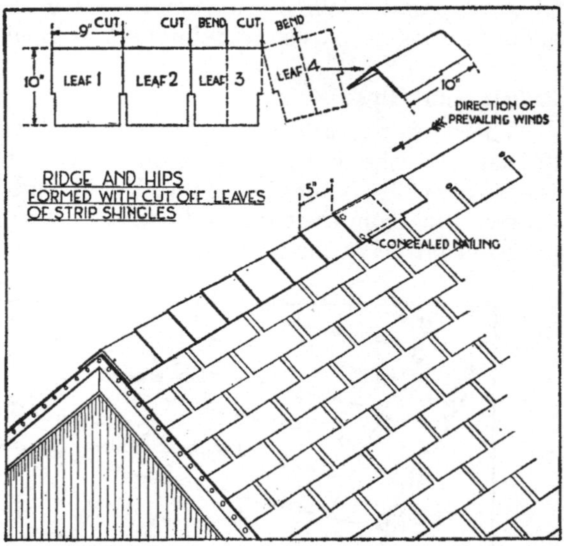

Fig. 6.—SHOWING METHOD OF CUTTING STRIP IN PIECES AND FIXING OVER THE RIDGE (*D. Anderson & Son Ltd.*)

The constructional details and technical data relating to the use of asphalte shingles which are given in this chapter have been based on information placed at our disposal by Messrs. D. Anderson & Son Ltd., to whom we have pleasure in making this acknowledgment.

Chapter IX

COVERING ROOFS WITH ASBESTOS-FELT

THE following information relates to the use of asbestos-felt roofing material.

STANDARD WEIGHTS AND MEASUREMENTS OF MATERIAL

Material	*Length of Roll*	*Width*	*Weight per Roll*
Asbestos-felt, standard weight (uncoated)	24 yds.	1 yd.	30 lbs.
Asbestos-felt, No. 1 ply coated	12 yds.	1 yd.	36 lbs.
Asbestos-felt, No. 2 ply uncoated	12 yds.	1 yd.	33 lbs.
Asbestos-felt, No. 2 ply coated	12 yds.	1 yd.	56 lbs.
Asbestos-felt (fire-resisting)	12 yds.	1 yd.	63 lbs.

Laying Felt

For convenience in handling, cut rolls into 18-ft. or 24-ft. lengths, stretch felt smoothly and evenly next to and along eaves, allowing it

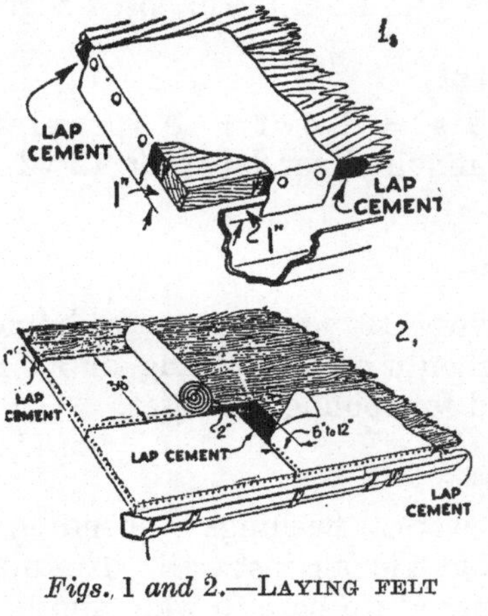

Figs. 1 *and* 2.—LAYING FELT

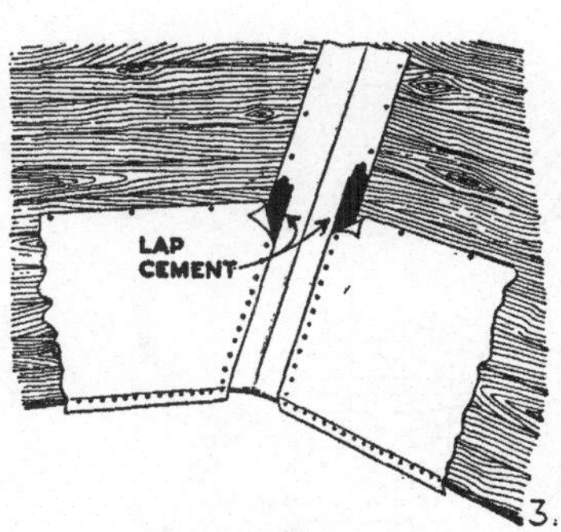

Fig. 3.—LAYING FELT AT VALLEY GUTTER

to project so that when turned down it will hang about 1 in. below edge of roof boards at eaves and gables, then drive a few clout nails about ½ in. from top edge to fasten temporarily. Lower edge of second piece should overlap top of first piece by 2 in. Secure temporarily along top edge as before. Raise lower edge of second sheet, and apply between this lap a thorough coat of bituminous solution or lap cement. Allow lower edge of upper sheet to fall back and embed it thoroughly in jointing cement. Side laps should be laid in a similar manner, but with a cover of from 6 in. to 12 in., and arranged in staggered formation. For nailing, use ordinary clout nails, ½ in. long when working on ¾-in. boards, and ¾ in. long when working on 1-in. or thicker boards. Drive nails through centre of lap 2½ in. to 3 in. apart. Coat all nail heads and exposed edges with jointing cement.

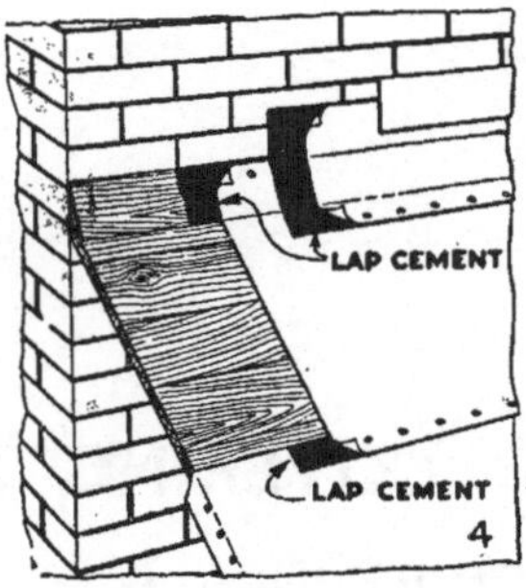

Fig. 4.—FINISHING AT LEAN-TO

Felt projecting over eaves and verges should now be turned down (edges of boards being coated with lap cement), and securely nailed.

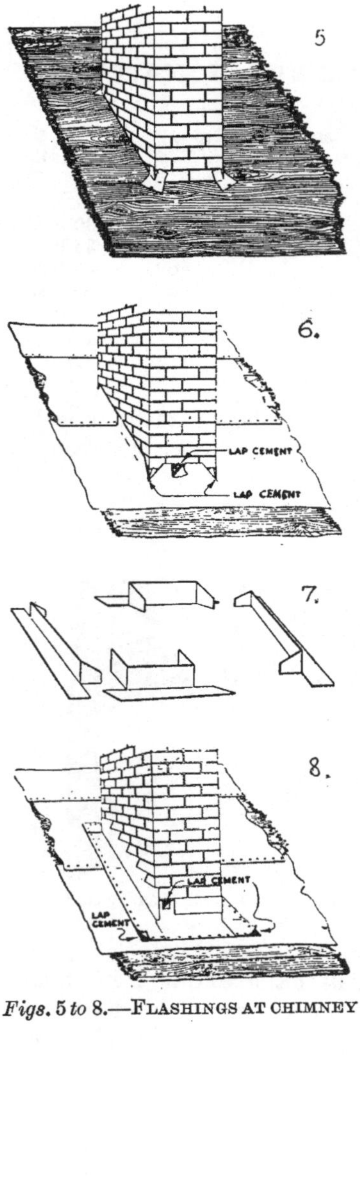

Figs. 5 *to* 8.—FLASHINGS AT CHIMNEY

Valley Gutters

(See Fig. 3.) Strip of roofing felt should be wide enough to underlap felting at sides by not less than 6 in. This lap should be cemented, and nailed every 2½ in. through the lap, at ¾ in. from the exposed edges.

Lap Cement

(11 gals. = 1 cwt.) Approximate quantity required for laps per 12-yd. roll is ½ pint.

Clout Nails

For every 12 yds., 100 nails should be allowed when used for sarking, or 300 nails when used for roofing purposes.

Flashings

Make vertical flashings by bending felting up about 4 in. against wall. Thoroughly cement turned-up part to wall, and nail at upper edges with nails about 9 in. apart. Fit strips of roofing felt 12 in. wide length-

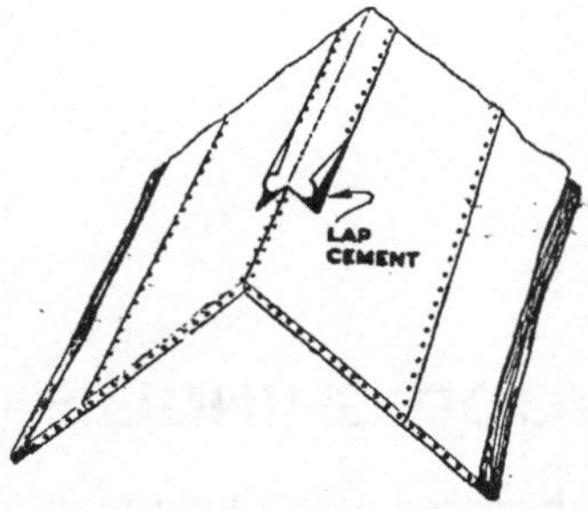

Fig. 9.—Ridge treatment

wise into angle over the turned-up edge, and cement to wall and roofing underneath. Nail lower edge of strip every $2\frac{1}{2}$ in. through cemented lap, about $\frac{3}{4}$ in. from bottom exposed edge. Upper edge of this strip may be flashed with a lead apron flashing, or, as an alternative where there is a coping, a strip of roofing felt may be cut, wide enough to extend under the coping and over the felting to roof level, where it should be cemented and nailed.

Flashings at Chimneys

Cut pieces of felt 4 in. square and fit them around corners of chimneys, as shown (Fig. 5). Then lay roofing in manner already described, cutting it so that it may be turned up, fitted, and cemented round chimney (Fig. 6) about 4 in. For each side of chimney, cut strip of roofing 12 in. wide, and 12 in. longer than side to be flashed. Also cut pieces to fit above and below chimney. Cut and fold as shown in diagram (Fig. 7) and thoroughly cement to chimney and roofing underneath. Step and apron flash the upper edge as shown in Fig. 8, the felt being stuck down with lap cement, and sealed into brick joints with bituminous cement.

Ridges and Hips

Use strip of roofing felt at least 9 in. wide, bending it over ridge as a capping. Thoroughly cement between laps, and nail as already described.

Sarking

For convenience in handling, when fixing asbestos-felt for sarking under slates, tiles, or corrugated sheeting, cut roll into 18-ft. or 24-ft. lengths. Lap 2 in. Use similar nails as for roofing. Drive nails through centre of lap, at about 9 in. apart.

If the sarking felt is to be applied over spars and under slate laths, it should be evenly stretched in position over spars and temporarily secured, allowing 2-in. overlap (see lower illustration). Fixing laths over felt will secure it. Where possible, it is advisable to nail felt to under side of laths, through the lap between the spars.

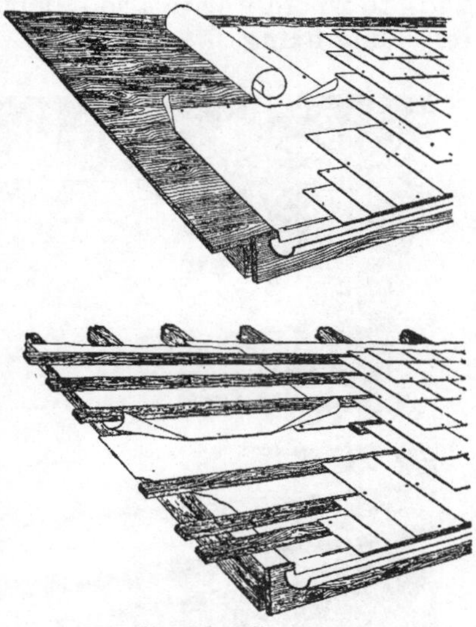

Fig. 10.—Sarking

Chapter X

COVERING ROOFS WITH WOOD SHINGLES

WOOD shingles are becoming increasingly popular in England, and this is not surprising, in view of their suitability for buildings in well-wooded country districts. Two objections are frequently raised when shingles are put forward as a suitable covering for domestic work : their non-durability, and their non-resistance to fire.

The durability of wood shingles is much greater than is popularly supposed ; there are many shingled roofs of oak or cedar in England and Wales that have stood for forty years and more, and are still perfectly sound. The risk of fire is also greatly exaggerated. In British Columbia, where red-cedar roofs are universal, fires that originate in the roof are exceedingly rare. If desired, the shingles can be coated with a fire-preventive paint.

Types

Shingles are commonly of English oak or imported cedar, the former being the more expensive. The photographs illustrating this chapter are of Canadian red cedar-wood shingling supplied by Messrs. W H. Colt Ltd., to whom we are also indebted for much of the following information regarding fixing.

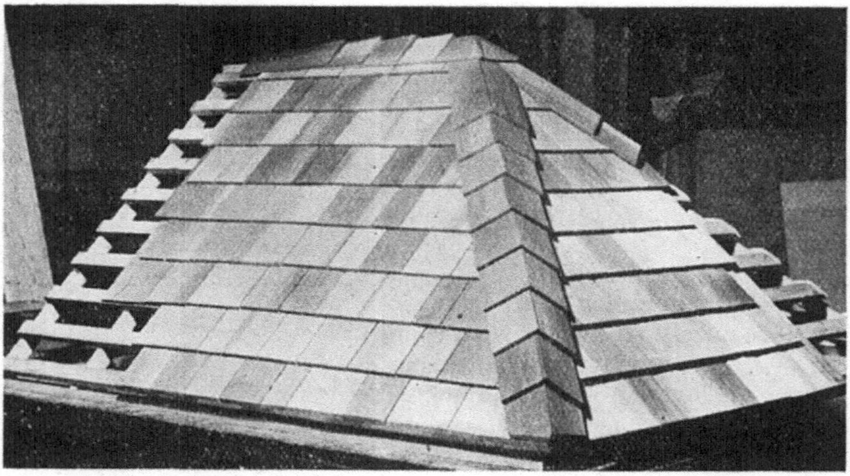

Fig. 1.—CANADIAN RED CEDAR SHINGLES ON OPEN BATTENING AT 5-IN. GAUGE, SHOWING FORMATION OF RIDGE AND HIPS. (*W. H. Colt Ltd.*)

Size

Cedar-wood shingles are 16 in. long; $\frac{2}{5}$ in. thick at the butt, tapering to the top. The widths vary from 4 in. to 12 in. A 5-in. exposure (or gauge) is satisfactory for all pitches down to 30° ; for slower pitches the gauge should be decreased.

Shingles are sold in bundles, the covering capacity being as follows :—

At $3\frac{3}{4}$-in.	gauge	one	bundle	covers	19·2	sq. ft.
,, 5-in.	,,	,,	,,	,,	25·7	,, ,,
,, $5\frac{1}{2}$-in.	,,	,,	,,	,,	28·3	,, ,,
,, $7\frac{1}{2}$-in.	,,	,,	,,	,,	38·5	,, ,,

The $7\frac{1}{2}$-in. gauge is recommended only for vertical shingling.

Weight

The weight of a square of shingling is approximately one-tenth of the weight of a square of plain tiling : an ordinary specification for a shingled roof calls for 2-in. by 3-in. rafters at 2-ft. centres, and 1-in. by 2-in. battens at 5-in. centres.

Nailing

Shingles are not holed for nailing : the nails are driven directly into the shingles at about 1 in. from the edge, and about 1 in. above the gauge line (that is to say, about 6 in. from the butt). The heads should not be driven into the wood. The nails may be ordinary galvanised slate nails, $1\frac{1}{2}$ in. long and of No. 12 or 13 gauge.

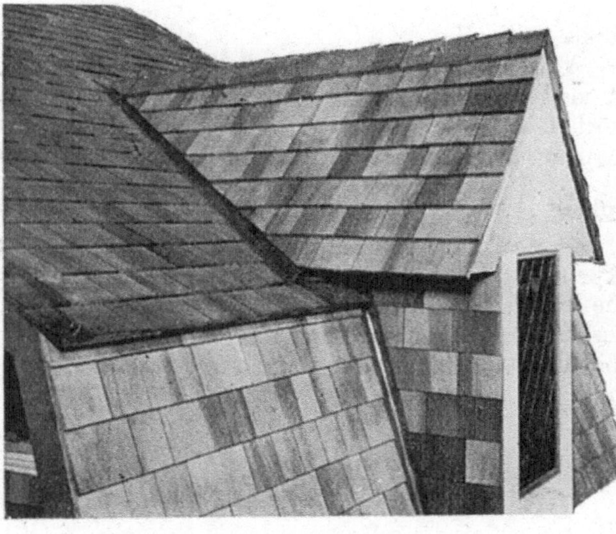

Fig. 2.—VERGES, RIDGES, ABUTMENTS, VALLEYS, AND VERTICAL WORK IN RED CEDAR SHINGLING. (*W H. Colt Ltd.*)

Laying

Fig. 1 illustrates the method of laying. A double course is laid at the eaves, as in plain tiling, projecting about 2 in. beyond the fascia. In continuing with the courses up the roof, care should be taken that a minimum side lap of $1\frac{1}{2}$ in. is given, but no attempt should be made to sort the shingles into widths. If they are used directly from the bundles, the correct random effect will be obtained. A gap of $\frac{1}{8}$ in. to $\frac{1}{4}$ in. should be allowed between adjacent shingles.

Hips and Ridges

Hips and ridges are best formed from the shingles themselves, using shingles of an even width of, say, 4 in. Wider ones may have to be cut down for this purpose. The method of butting the ridges at edges and overlapping at ends is clearly shown in Fig. 1. Lead or felt is not needed at ridges and hips. Alternatively, hips and ridges may be boarded, using timber not less than 4 in. wide.

Verges and Abutments

Wide shingles should be used in alternate courses at verges and abutments, as in Fig. 2.

Valleys

Valleys are formed with lead in the same way as for a tiled or slated roof. A good width of lead, say 15 in., should be used, with no tilting fillet.

Walls

Walls are frequently shingled in staggered courses: this variation in method may also be employed for roofs. The gauge on vertical work may be increased to $7\frac{1}{2}$ in., to which exposure the shingles on the mansard and vertical work of Fig. 2 have been fixed.

Colour

Both oak and red cedar-wood shingles improve greatly in appearance after a few months' exposure to the weather. The original red tinge of the latter changes to an attractive silver-grey. If any special colour is desired a good creosote stain should be used, but the user who dislikes the first appearance of a shingled roof is strongly recommended to wait until the roof has weathered before finally deciding whether or not to stain.

Chapter XI

EMERGENCY REPAIRS TO ROOFS

MUCH of the activity of the building trade is now taken up with the repair of houses which have sustained minor damage by air bombardment. These repairs are of an emergency and often of a temporary nature owing to shortage of materials and labour available.

Among the most vulnerable parts of a house to blast from bombs is the roof, and here it is essential that such damage be repaired promptly ; the longer such attention is delayed, the longer is the interior of the house exposed to the elements and the greater is the depreciation.

The actual roof repairs that require to be effected comprise mainly broken or stripped roofing slates or tiles. Minor holes in the roof covering are best replaced with the same material as the rest of the covering.

A roof completely stripped of its slate or tile covering but with the timbers intact can be re-covered with the same material if this is available. If not, it may be covered up with roofing felt, battened up at the edges, and given a coat of tar ; methods of covering with roofing felt, and other emergency materials, such as corrugated iron, are given later.

Inspect the Roof

Before commencing to retile or reslate, inspect the roof framing to see whether any rafters have lifted from the ridge by the force of the blast and that purlins and struts are in place and well secured. Where a rafter has been snapped by a piece of flying debris, a repair can be effected in most cases by fixing a new piece of timber to the broken one.

In cases where several roof members have collapsed, it may be necessary to remove all the covering and battens before respiking the members together again and replacing any damaged timbers.

In more drastic cases, it may be found necessary to dismantle what remains of the roof and re-erect. Consideration can be given to the possibility of replacing a pitched roof by a flat one, consisting of joists spaced fairly wide apart and covered with insulating board and roofing felt, the whole being given a coat of tar.

Repair of Slate Covering

Care has to be taken when replacing damaged slates to disturb the undamaged parts of the roof as little as possible. Old roofs which have proved satisfactory often become troublesome when disturbed. In such cases "slurrying" will prove helpful.

Another source of trouble is the difficulty in obtaining the necessary slates of the right size to effect a proper repair even if salvage can be obtained nearby. One method of overcoming this is to use whatever sizes are available on the damaged area. This will possibly necessitate rebattening and the forming of the junction between the two sections with a felt course, thus effectively breaking the bond without reducing the lap.

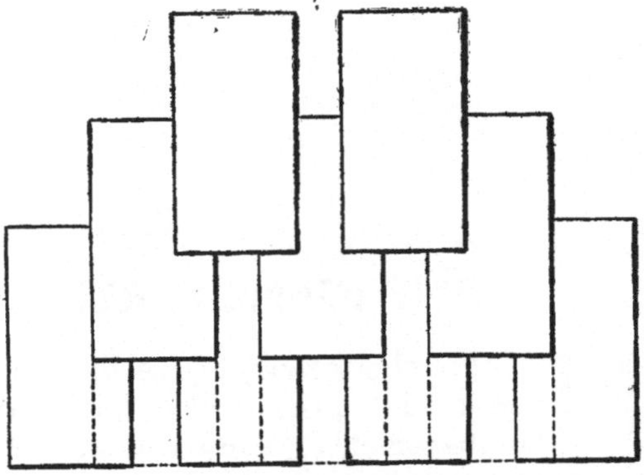

Fig. 1.—COVERING ROOF WITH SLATES IN EXTENDED ORDER

Slates shown dotted form double course at eaves.

Another method that can be adopted to overcome the shortage of the right size of slates is to cover the roof with slates in extended order, as a temporary measure. This method will allow a saving of one-third of the normal number of slates (see Fig. 1).

Where the damage is only slight, the slates may be replaced by asbestos-cement sheeting which has been cut to the right size.

Repair of Tile Covering

Repairs of a tiled roof may have to be made with tiles of a different curvature. In order to avoid leakage, torching with mortar from inside the roof at the junction between the new and old work may have to be resorted to.

COVERING ROOFS WITH BITUMEN ROOFING FELT

There are many kinds of bitumen roof coverings on the market that are a great improvement, both in the matter of handling and laying and in weathering qualities, over the old tarred and sanded " felting."

How to Cut the Felt

Unroll the material on a level, smooth surface, where no stones, etc., will cut through. Avoid walking on the roofing when unrolling. To cut, use a straight wood batten 3 ft. long, and a sharp, pointed knife —a lino knife is excellent. Draw the knife towards you when cutting.

As a rule roofings are supplied in rolls 3 ft. wide by 12 yds. long.

Fixing Felting Up and Down

The best arrangement of fixing felting on a boarded roof is to use it with the lap joints running in a vertical direction, and when employed in this way quite flat roof pitches, not exceeding say $\frac{1}{4}$ pitch, can be dealt with successfully (Fig. 2).

The provision of rolls or ribs underneath the felting introduces the principle of weather-tightness which is a feature of the long joints in corrugated-iron roofing. Water won't run uphill. Therefore if the 3-ft. wide covering is laid on ribs 1 ft. 5 in. apart, every alternate strip forming a joint-rail, the danger of water driving through vertical joints will be avoided.

Further, the wide corrugations formed in the roof will tend to prevent or lessen the rucking of the roofing material after a spell of really hot weather.

Double Covering

For a building requiring a better construction, viz. a double thickness of bitumen felting, the arrangement sketched in Fig. 3 may be adopted, quite the cheapest material being used for the undercoat and a " 2-ply " or even a superior stuff for the outer one. A detail of the finish at the gable end of a building is illustrated in Fig. 4.

Where the two thicknesses of roofing are employed the gable end would have the inner coating placed under the lifting batten, as shown in the sketch (Fig. 3).

The Battens

In all cases these battens must be chamfered or rounded on the top edges to prevent cutting the felting at the bends.

If there is any choice it is always as well to fix felting material in warm weather. There is less danger of it being cracked in the process of fitting up although of course it is softer and requires careful handling in other respects.

Undercoating

Where an undercoating is used this may be laid on with either horizontal or vertical joints, preferably the former on larger surfaces.

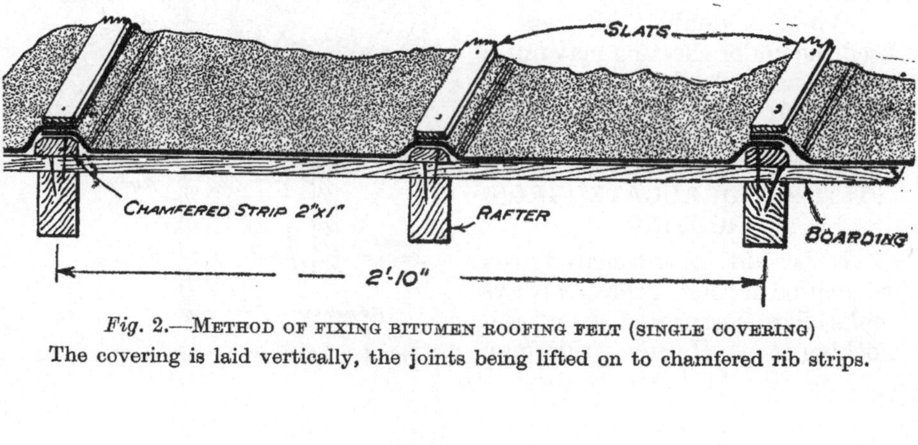

Fig. 2.—Method of fixing bitumen roofing felt (single covering)
The covering is laid vertically, the joints being lifted on to chamfered rib strips.

Covering Ridges

With ridges, two methods are possible. If the ridge board stands up well above the surface of the roof as shown in Fig. 5 (A), a common constructional detail, then each roof pitch may be dealt with by a separate length of felting, the joint at the top being as shown and the whole being covered by a zinc or other ridge capping.

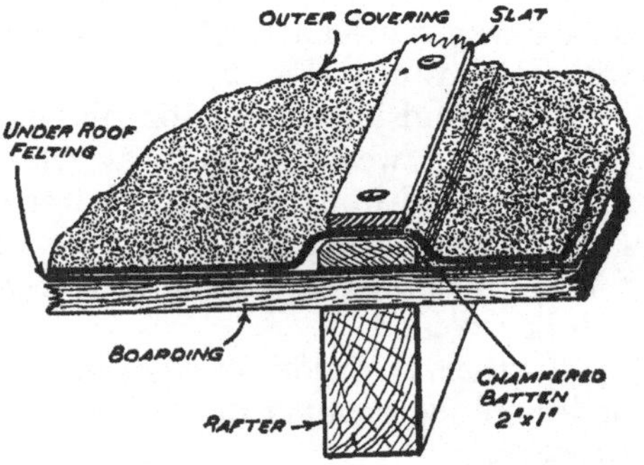

Fig. 3.—METHOD OF DOUBLE COVERING WITH ROOFING FELT

In some cases the writer has used a flush apex either by depressing the ridge board or using a half-lapped ridge joint for the top ends of the roof rafters. These two arrangements are indicated in the sketches B and C, Fig. 5. The roof felting may then pass over the ridge to the other pitch in one strip.

If the roofing is one of two coverings, the under layer should be tacked on with smaller clouts. Further, if the ridge does not lift the roofing to an amount equal to the thickness of the ribs, the latter must be chamfered off at the top.

Fixing Felting at Eaves

At the eaves of a shed the fixing of felting requires special care. If there is any " ripping off " in a gale of wind, it is here that the trouble usually starts. The roofing felt may be lapped over the metal guttering and secured by the usual slat, as indicated in Fig. 6. The slight tilt given to the covering is accomplished by planing off the top of the fascia board at an angle as shown. This raising of the bending line should be shown at A, which should be equivalent to the height of the " roll."

Where a double thickness is used the under sheeting may finish at the gutter back and the outer felting lap over, as depicted in Fig. 7.

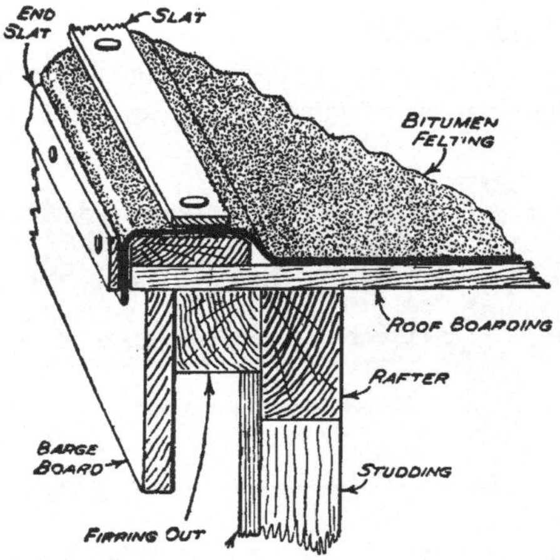

Fig. 4.—TREATMENT FOR GABLE ENDS

FITTING CORRUGATED-IRON ROOFING

It is said of corrugated iron when used as roofing that it always looks like corrugated iron and nothing else. However this may

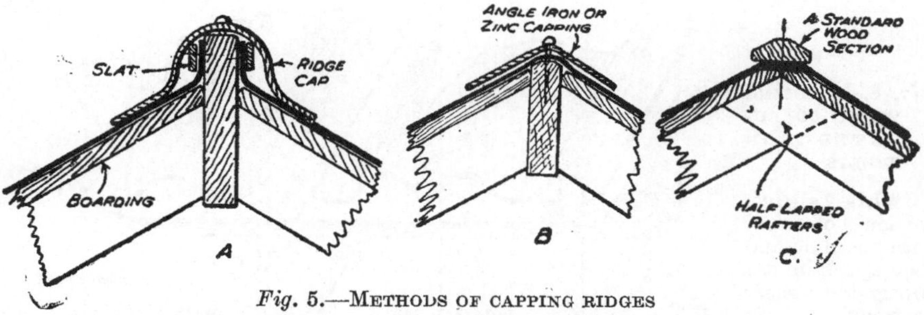

Fig. 5.—METHODS OF CAPPING RIDGES

A, with raised ridge board. B, with flush ridge board. C, without ridge board, using wood capping.

be where it is simply nailed on and left unembellished in any way at its edges, it can nevertheless be used in a manner which renders it both less distasteful and incongruous among other more traditional buildings.

Corrugated-iron roofs are very hot in summer and cold in winter. By combining corrugated iron with a layer of wood boarding (with or without a layer or roofing felt) or insulating board, a very much better roof and a more habitable interior can be obtained. If the ridge is capped with, say, a half-round tile set in cement, the iron painted a red or brown colour, and the sheeting used in one length as is possible in a small building, quite a respectable finish may be obtained, especially if the gables and eaves are provided with a barge board and a fascia board with guttering as illustrated in the accompanying Figs. 8, 9, and 10.

Further, the roof will be quite weather-tight, and the dead air space between the wood and the iron will form a fairly good heat insulation.

Laying Corrugated Sheets

Fig. 8 shows the line of roofing, illustrating on the left the treatment at the gable end, and on the right the joint between sheetings supported

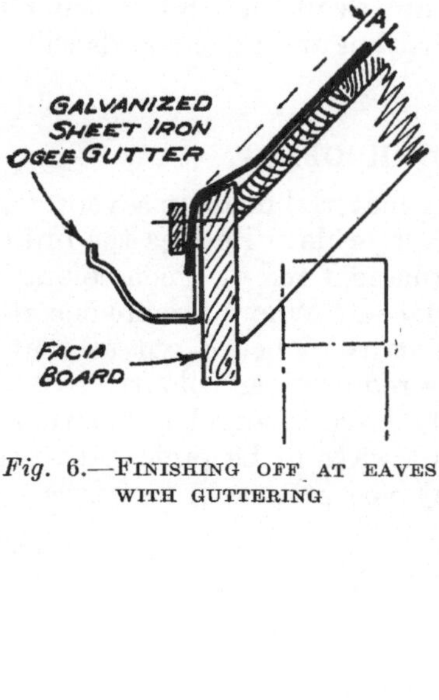

Fig. 6.—FINISHING OFF AT EAVES WITH GUTTERING

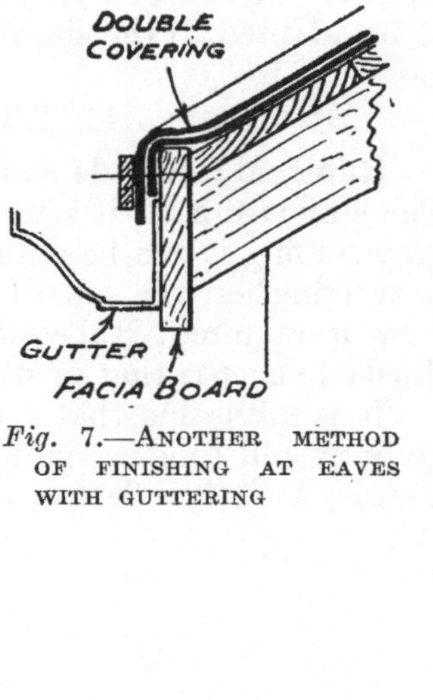

Fig. 7.—ANOTHER METHOD OF FINISHING AT EAVES WITH GUTTERING

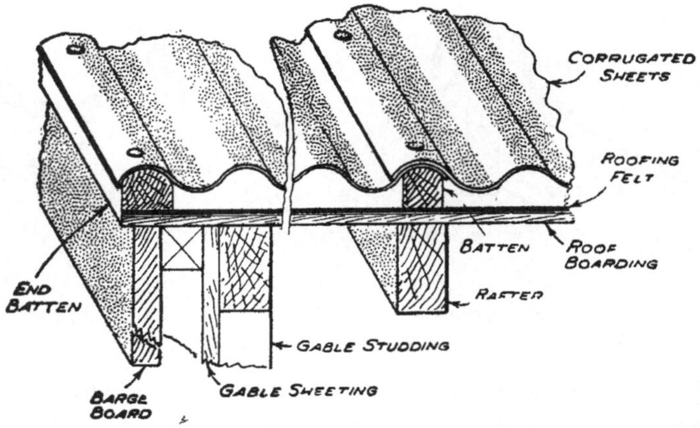

Fig. 8.—Roofing with corrugated-iron sheets

This shows section of roof with boarding and roofing felt under corrugated sheet covering.

by a continuous batten planed to fit in the hollow of the corrugations. Sheets up to 12 ft. long are obtainable, although 10 ft. is a more usual maximum length. This means that a span of about 18 or 19 ft. can be bridged by a single sheet on each side of the roof.

Treatment of Ridges and Eaves

At ridges and eaves the details can be arranged as shown in sketch (Fig. 9). At the ridges firring may be run along the ridge board as indicated to support the sheet, and the eaves fascia board may be raised up to support the other end of the sheeting. An alternative arrangement is indicated in Fig. 10, where the design demands an overhanging eaves and a more ornate guttering.

With single sheets only screw roofing nails will be required.

Corrugated iron is 2 ft. 3 in. wide and fits on battens placed at 2-ft. centres. Details of corrugated asbestos sheeting are given in Chapter VII. Various sizes of asbestos sheet are available, and if the above method of construction is adopted the battens and ridge boards will have to be adapted to the size of sheet.

FIXING RUBEROID ROOFING

Ruberoid is a trade name for a roofing material made in several forms. The standard stuff is sent out in rolls 3 ft. wide. Besides the ordinary grey roofing it can be obtained in a permanent red or green colour, and in two finishes, viz. smooth and slate surfaces. Where a more decorative form is required, Ruberoid is made in strips punched out so that the finished effect is that of slates of either a red or green colour.

It is advisable that Ruberoid should have a sound foundation. A grooved and tongued under-boarding is always to be preferred to sawn boards, as it lies flatter, in spite of any vee groove in its edges. For

Ruberoid, $\frac{3}{4}$-in. tongued and grooved floor-boarding is recommended, otherwise 1-in. close-butted sawn boarding should be used.

In either case, the board should be well nailed to the rafters or other supports, with the heads of all brads punched below the surface.

Where rough (sawn) boards are used, any upstanding edges should be planed off so that a relatively smooth, even surface is obtained. The supports for the board should be sufficiently stiff for the particular job in hand.

All arrises over which the covering has to be folded or bent should be chamfered off in a rounded form to prevent any tendency to cut through the material.

Preliminary Treatment

The material requires anything up to fourteen days' weathering before use. It should be laid in an open space, after being cut, so that it may expand, and, naturally, this treatment is more rapidly accomplished in the summer than in winter. The material is best laid in warm weather, and in any case periods of rain and snow should be avoided. In cold and frosty weather it may be necessary to heat the roof covering with a blow-lamp flame, used by rapidly passing it over the surface of the sheet at the required spot before attempting to bend or fold the material.

The outside of the roll of roofing should always be laid downwards, with that face next to the boarding.

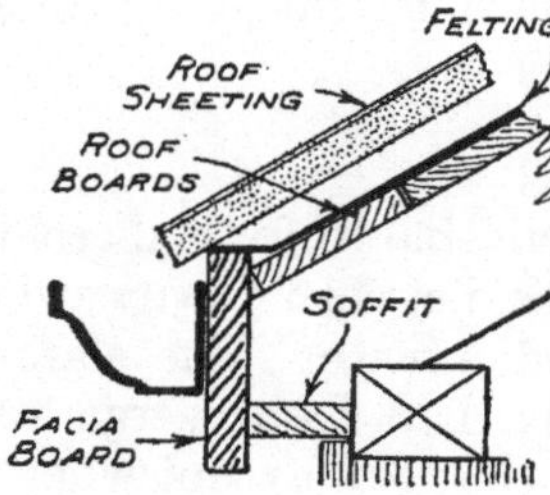

Fig. 10 (*above*).—ALTERNATIVE ARRANGEMENT OF CORRUGATED ROOF WITH OVERHANGING EAVES

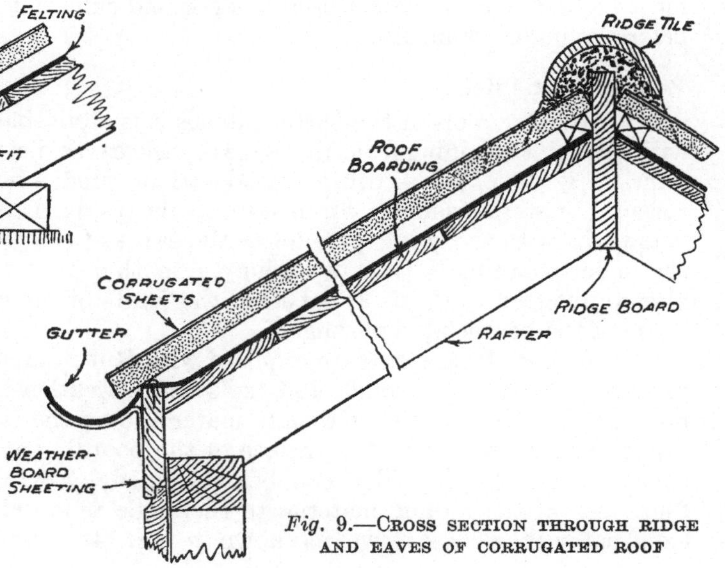

Fig. 9.—CROSS SECTION THROUGH RIDGE AND EAVES OF CORRUGATED ROOF

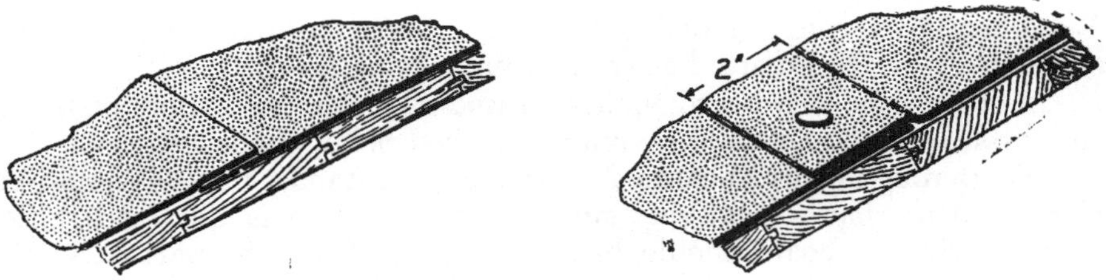

Incorrect *Correct*

Figs. 11 *and* 12.—How to lay Ruberoid roofing horizontally

Horizontal joints on a pitch roof or on a fall in a flat roof should be made as at Fig. 12, not as shown in Fig. 11. The lap should be 2 in. minimum.

Horizontal Joints

The proper way to arrange the horizontal lap joints is shown in Fig. 12.

After the lap joint is prepared and cemented, the nails—$\frac{3}{4}$-in. galvanised clouts are used in the ordinary course—may be driven through the joint. The extent of the lap should not be less than 2 in., and the pitch of the nails should be an equal amount. The seam of the two sheets is made water-tight with a solvent compound applied by a brush. This material must not be heated, although it is not quite so adhesive or free-flowing in very cold weather. It may be kept warm but must not be put over a fire like pitch. The compound does not adhere to a wet surface.

After rain or melting snow the roof must be allowed to dry off before proceeding with the work. In addition, work in completing the joints must be held over if the material has not had sufficient weathering time before laying is commenced.

Roof of Flat Pitch

On ordinary roofs of the flatter pitches it is advisable to fix Ruberoid with the joints running from the ridges to the eaves, i.e. with downwards joints (Fig. 13), unless other considerations predominate. The slate-surfaced material should, for instance, always be laid from verge to verge, viz. with the joints parallel to the eaves of the roof, except where the under-boarding is thin or springy. In this case, the arrangement already referred to (Fig. 13) is better, the joints of the covering crossing those of the boards at right angles.

No rolls or lifting strips are required with Ruberoid, as the cementing renders "down-roof" joints and nails quite weather-tight. There is no need therefore to run the roofing material over the ridge. The latter can be almost flush with the surface of the boarding and have any raw edges planed off, the ridge cap being formed by bending an 8-in. or 9-in. strip of the roofing material to the angle required, cementing and clout-nailing the edges down, as shown in Fig. 14.

Cementing the Joints

Each length of roofing material should lap 2 in. and, in applying the cement, first remove any powder from the edge or surface to be coated and put on the compound liberally, working it in with the brush, as shown in Fig. 13. Nails should be at least 1 in. from the edge of the sheet and, when laid, coat the nail heads with the cement. A good finish is obtained by painting a band 2 in. or $2\frac{1}{2}$ in. wide down the joint, using chalk lines to guide the brush in a neat straight course. For the slate-surfaced material, painting the nail heads is not recommended.

Gutters and Valleys

In covering a roof having gutters or valleys these parts should be fitted and finished before the run of the roof is commenced. For gutters, two thicknesses of Ruberoid, bedded together with the mastic compound, are recommended. The strips should be laid in as long a length as possible to reduce the number of joints to the minimum. It is important not to use any clout nails in the bottom of the gutter ; not in the upper layer at any rate. The only nailing that is necessary is at the joints. With this particular material, the carpenter need not provide any drip steps in the fall of the gutter such as are essential in providing the supporting woodwork for zinc or lead. Therefore, in calculating and marking off the fall of the gutter, there is no need to allow extra height for these drips. A straight fall from end to end of 2 in. in 10 ft. is all that is necessary.

Flashing to Brick Walls

For flashing a more or less horizontal joint where a brick wall abuts on to a flat roof or to a gutter, the brick joint not more than two courses up must be raked out to a depth of not less than 1 in. A strip of roofing

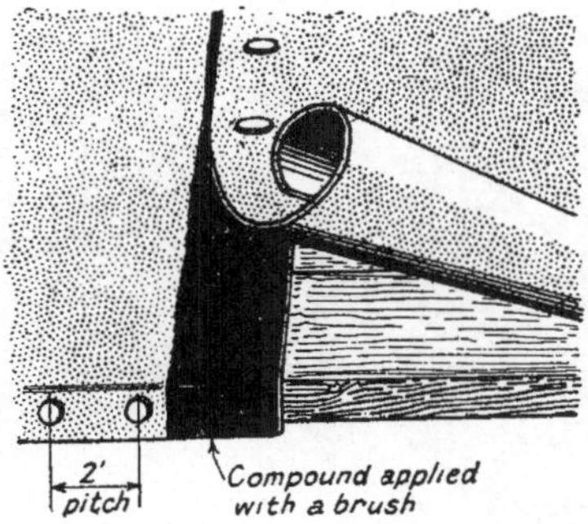

Fig. 13.—How Ruberoid down-roof seams are nailed and cemented

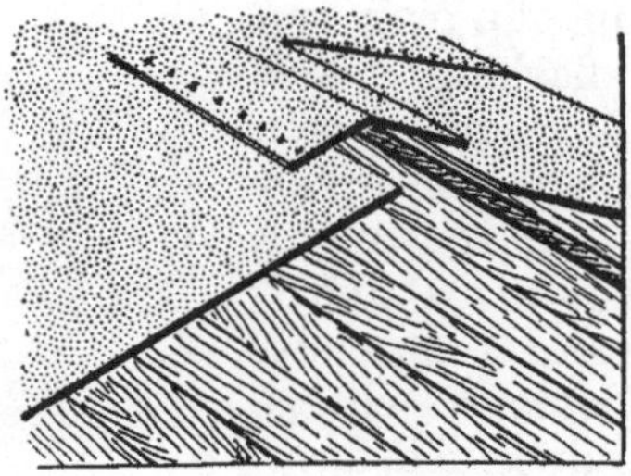

Fig. 14.—Ridge capping

This may be formed out of an 8- or 9-in. strip of the roofing material. Joint nailed and cemented.

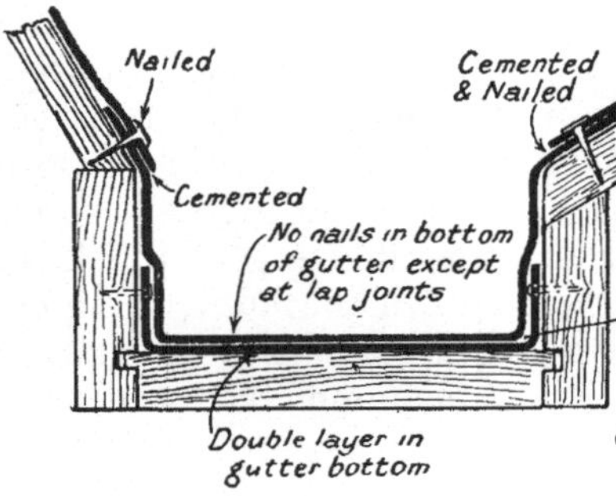

Fig. 15.—GUTTER BETWEEN SAW TOOTH ROOFS WITH DOUBLE BOTTOM OF RUBEROID

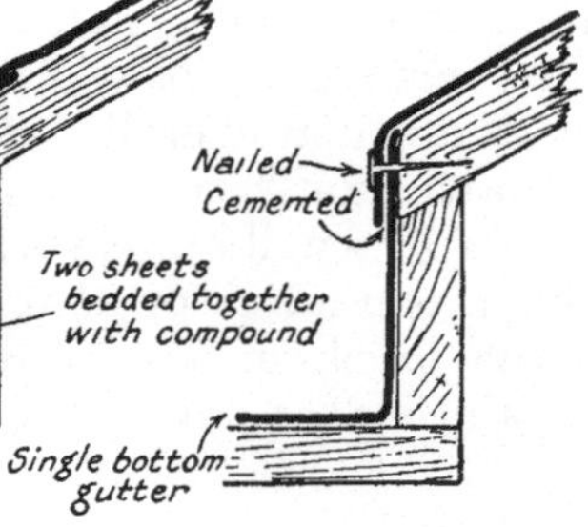

Fig. 16.—ALTERNATIVE ARRANGEMENT WITH SINGLE LAYER OF RUBEROID

material must then be cut off, in as long a length as possible and of such a width as will allow a ¾-in. bend into the wall and a 4-in. turn out on to the flat. If the weather is cold and frosty, the strip of Ruberoid may be warmed by a flash of a blow-lamp, as previously referred to.

The main roofing, or gutter bottom, as the case may be, should turn up the wall 2 in. or 3 in. at least, and be spiked into the nearest joint above the surface of the gutter or roof. The flashing strip, being fitted, can then be secured by wood or lead wedges, as shown in Fig. 19, at the "turn in" and with mastic compound and galvanised clouts along the lower flanged outer edge, as indicated. The job may then be passed back to the bricklayer to make good the top joint by Portland cement pointing. The flat joint and nail-heads should be painted over with the compound in the usual way to ensure water-tightness.

An internal angle is dealt with in the same manner, the flashings at the corner being cut out and laid as shown in Fig. 22. The left-hand piece of flashing, that cut at an angle as at A, overlaps the other. Wood or lead wedge plugs are used in the raked-out joint in the wall, as in the fixing of a plain run of flashing, clout nails being driven through the overlaps, as shown. A plumber's lead-dressing tool, or its equivalent, will be found useful in forming internal angles in the Ruberoid covering. An external angle is dealt with in a similar

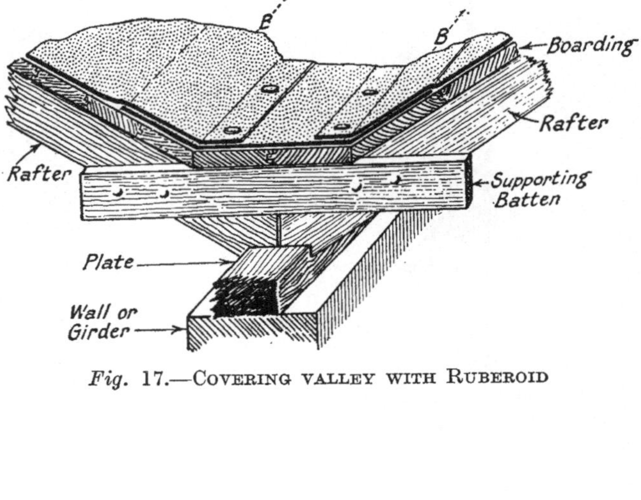

Fig. 17.—COVERING VALLEY WITH RUBEROID

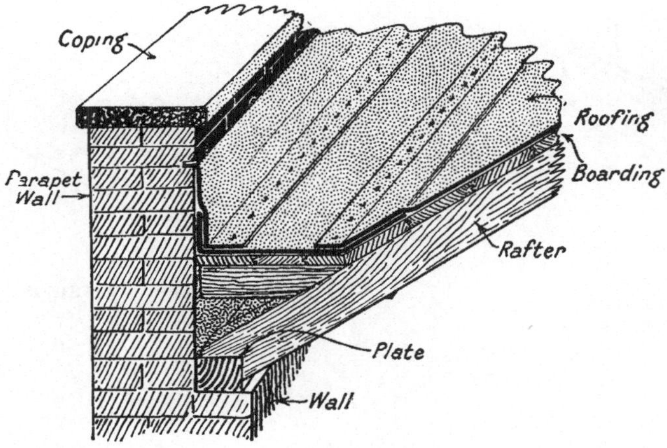

Fig. 18.—FLASHING OF RUBEROID TO BRICK WALL

manner, the details, Fig. 23, showing the cutting and the fixing.

Stepped Flashing

Stepped flashing can be arranged in Ruberoid just as easily as in lead or zinc. The flashing strips are cut out in triangular form, as illustrated in Figs. 20 and 21, and are fixed in the same way. At a ridge the piece is of a duplex form. The dimensions will depend on the pitch of the roof. If the upright wall is of wood, then the flashing may be clout-nailed instead of being turned into a brick joint.

Ridges, Eaves, and Verges

At ridges, the detail illustrated in Fig. 14 may be followed, the strip forming the capping being the last part to be fixed. Clout nails may be relied on to fix this roofing material on the vertical edges of eaves and verges (gable ends). The mechanical strength of Ruberoid is much superior to ordinary bitumen roofing felt, and as the heads of the nails may be painted over with the mastic compound after they are driven, there is no danger of wet-weather conditions rotting the fixings. At the same time it is important that the nails should be driven into wood of a thickness that will satisfactorily support them. Therefore the use of a thicker board, and an essentially sound one, at any edge formed in the roof around which the roofing has to be bent and nailed, are points which should be borne in mind. It is also obvious that nailing in or too near to a joint in the under-boarding should be avoided, and in any case, end grain is none too good, even where the nails are supporting roofing material.

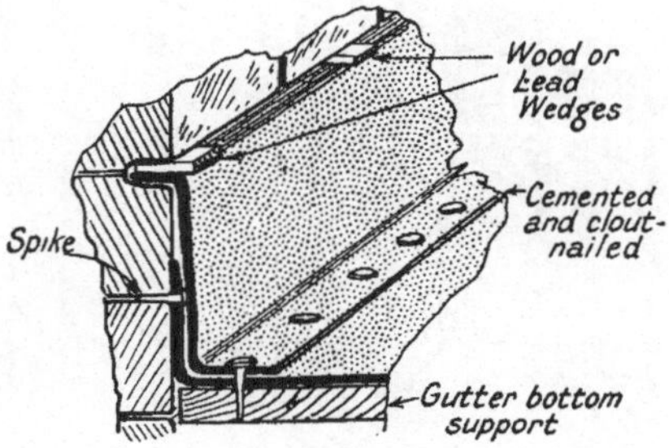

Fig. 19.—MAKING JOINT WITH WALL

The flashing strip is turned into the open joint, wedged, and the apron nailed and cemented down to the roof surface.

Double-layer Roofs

Where a double layer of material on a pitched roof is required, the

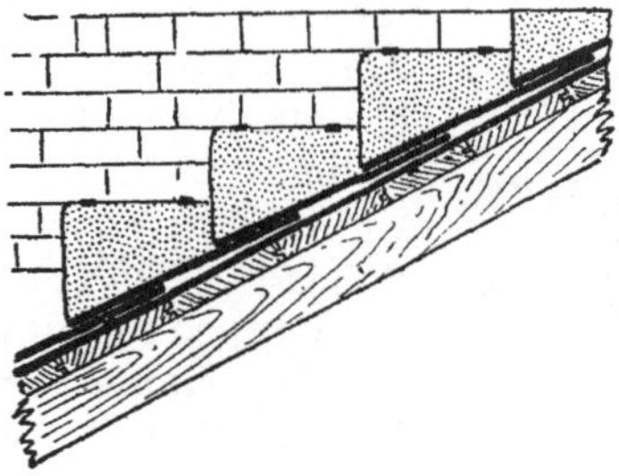

Fig. 20.—STEPPED FLASHINGS FOR AN INCLINED ROOF FIXED IN POSITION

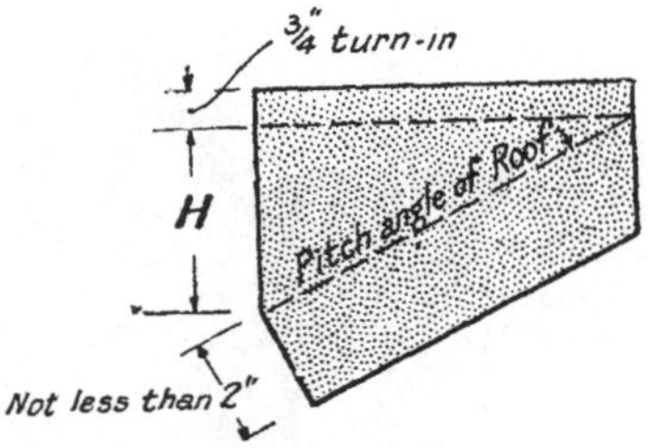

Fig. 21.—STEPPED FLASHINGS AS CUT

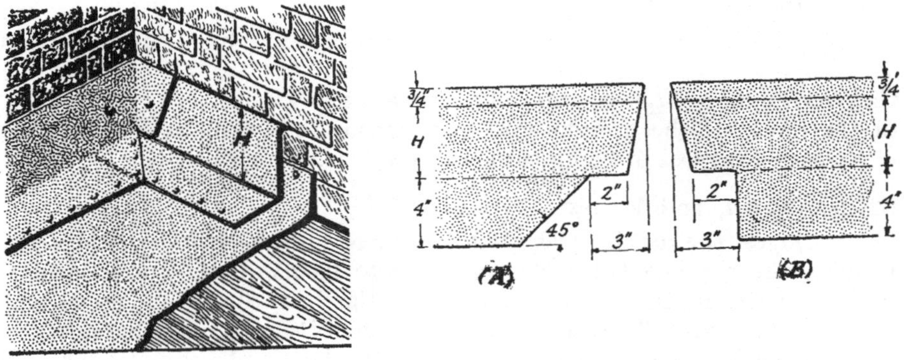

Fig. 22.—RUBEROID FLASHINGS TO AN INTERNAL ANGLE OF WALL

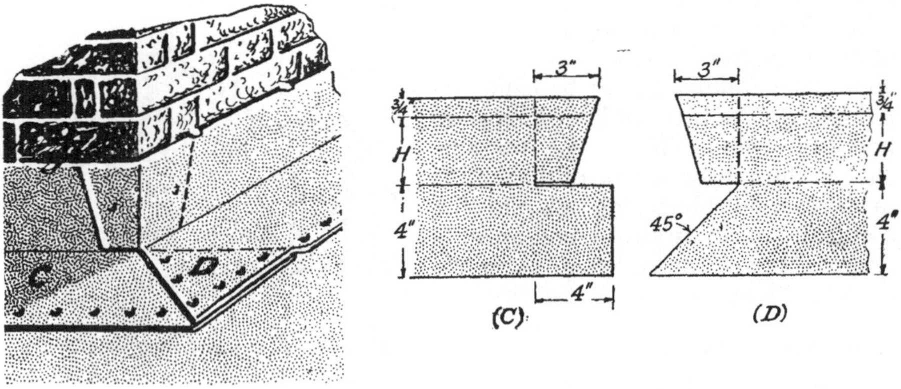

Fig. 23.—RUBEROID FLASHINGS FOR EXTERNAL ANGLE OF WALL

system often employed is illustrated in Fig. 24. The under layer is fixed with "down-roof" joints with nails only, and similarly secured at eaves and ridges. The second stage is to coat the whole surface with mastic compound and, as these processes extend, to put on the outer layer of covering. The usual 2-in. lap joint should be provided in fixing adjacent outer sheets, but all nailing may be omitted, weather-tightness being ensured by painting all edge joints with compound. Care must be taken to press out all bubbles of air in laying this outer covering. Ruberoid is absolutely air-tight if properly secured, but if the air is not squeezed out, it will remain trapped, causing expansion or contraction according to temperature.

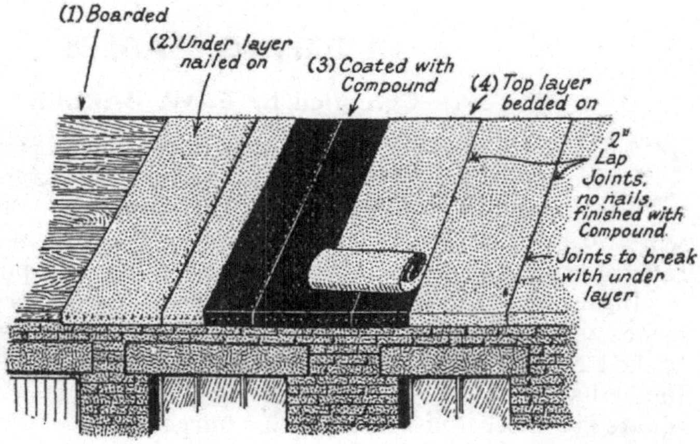

Fig. 24.—Laying roof with double thickness of Ruberoid

Covering Open Roofs

Where the material is required to cover roofs which are open underneath and in which the under-boards are not of the grooved and tongued form, it may be necessary to support the sheets by a strip of Ruberoid, 1½ in. wide, nailed and cemented down the centre of each sheet. This, of course, only applies to a roof covered with "down-roof" joints.

The Finish at Eaves

A feather-edge board, or its equivalent, can be used to ensure a sufficient thickness of wood in clout-nailing the turned-over edge of the Ruberoid at the eaves. The edge of the Ruberoid should overlap the back flange of metal gutters.

ROOFING TABLES

Compiled by E. W. BARBER

CERTAIN rules for finding sizes of roof members have already been given on p. 22. Calculations regarding strength and safe loads will be found in Chapter IV, which begins on p. 43. In the same chapter will also be found a method of obtaining the correct bevels for common rafters, hip rafters, jack rafters, roof boarding, and purlins.

In actual practice it is necessary for a carpenter to have a reliable means of ascertaining the lengths of common rafters, jack rafters, and backed hips to suit the particular roof truss upon which he is working. In the hands of anyone who is thoroughly familiar with its use, the steel square is a most useful tool for this purpose.

Readers who wish to make themselves acquainted with the method of using the steel square are advised to obtain a specialised book on the subject, e.g. *The Steel Square*, by Noel D. Green (George Newnes, Ltd.).

As an alternative, we give in the following pages a series of tables which may be used to obtain the same results.

HOW TO USE THE ROOFING TABLES

By the use of the roofing tables, roof members for a pitched roof (of any one of the eight pitches given) may be measured to the correct lengths and bevels found so that the members may be cut without the aid of the steel square or any other patent device, regardless of span. In compiling these tables, the span of the building has been taken as the overall dimension including the external walls.

The first table, which occupies pp. 128 and 129, gives the lengths of common rafter for spans ranging from 10 ft. to 30 ft. 11 in.

Table II, which occupies pp. 130 and 131, shows the correct lengths of backed hips for roofs of different pitches having any span between 10 ft. and 30 ft. 11 in.

Bevels for roof members can be obtained from the table on p. 132, whilst general data will be found on p. 133.

The following examples are worked out for a hip roof with a span of 22 ft. 4 in., the pitch to be $\frac{3}{8}$.

Length of Common Rafter

Refer to Table I, headed "Length of Common Rafter." On p. 129 find the column headed 22 (feet) and read downwards to the horizontal line corresponding to the required pitch (in this case $\frac{3}{8}$). This gives a length of common rafter 13 ft. 9 in. for a roof having a span of 22 ft. and a pitch of $\frac{3}{8}$. Read along the top of left-hand table to 22 ft., but as the span is 22 ft. 4 in. it is necessary to refer to the right hand of table, which deals with the inches. Read along the top of table to 4 in. and read down to required $\frac{3}{8}$ pitch. This reads $2\frac{1}{2}$ in. These two results are added together, thus 13 ft. 9 in. + $2\frac{1}{2}$ in. = 13 ft. $11\frac{1}{2}$ in., this being the length of common rafter for a roof with a span of 22 ft. with $\frac{3}{8}$ pitch.

Length of Backed Hips

Refer to Table II, headed "Length of Backed Hips," and repeat as for common rafter, the results reading 17 ft. $7\frac{5}{16}$ in. + $3\frac{3}{16}$ in. = 17 ft. $10\frac{1}{2}$ in. Valleys the same.

Length of Jack Rafters

Refer to Table III, last column, which is headed "Diminishing Length of Jack Rafters." Read downwards to the line corresponding to $\frac{3}{8}$ pitch at left of table, which is 1 ft. $3\frac{5}{16}$ in. This is marked on common rafter, starting from the long point of plumb cut and repeated along length of rafter. This gives the different lengths and number of jack rafters down the hip at 14-in. centres.

Length of Jack Rafters

The following example is worked out for a roof with a span of 16 ft., the pitch to be 45° Reference to Table I, headed "Length of Common Rafter," will show that the common rafter in this case will be 11 ft. $3\frac{3}{4}$ in.

Now refer to Table III, headed "Roof Members. Cuts in 8 Pitches." Read down column 1, which gives the slope of roof in degrees, and 45° ($\frac{1}{2}$ pitch of roof) will be found. Reading across the table to the final column, the diminishing length of jack rafter is given as 1 ft. $5\frac{1}{4}$ in. The jack rafters are centred down the hip at 14 in., so that it is now possible to determine both the length and number of jack rafters required.

The common rafter is 11 ft. $3\frac{3}{4}$ in., and the diminishing length of the jack rafter is 1 ft. $5\frac{1}{4}$ in. By simple subtraction we find that the length of the jack rafter (A) is 9 ft. $10\frac{1}{2}$ in. By repeating the process—9 ft. $10\frac{1}{2}$ in. less 1 ft. $5\frac{1}{4}$ in.—we get the length of rafter (B) as 8 ft. $5\frac{1}{4}$ in., and so on.

In actual practice the diminishing length of the jack rafter is marked on the common rafter, starting from the long point of plumb cut and repeated along the length of the rafter.

The Bevels of Roof Members

Refer to Table III, headed "Roof Members. Cuts in 8 Pitches." At the top of this section are the names of the members, and as each one is required read downwards to the required pitch on the left of this section. See below :

36° 52′	9	$\frac{3}{8}$	37°	53°	28°	62°	41°	65°	38°	58°	51°	1′ $3\frac{5}{16}$″

The jack rafter plumb cut and bevel cut is the same as the plumb cut and bevel cut of common rafter.

TABLE I.—LENGTH OF COMMON RAFTER

Feet ← *Span of the Building* → *Inches*

Slope of Roof in Degrees °	′	*Rise of Roof in 12 in. (½ Span)* in.	*Pitch of Roof*	10 ft.	10 in.	11 ft.	11 in.	12 ft.	12 in.	13 ft.	13 in.	14 ft.	14 in.
14	2	3	1/8	5	1 7/8	5	8	6	2 1/4	6	8 7/16	7	2 9/16
18	26	4	1/6	5	3 1/4	5	9 9/16	6	3 7/8	6	10 3/16	7	4 9/16
26	34	6	1/4	5	7 1/16	6	1 13/16	6	8 1/2	7	3 3/16	7	9 15/16
33	41	8	1/3	6	0 1/8	6	7 5/16	7	2 9/16	7	9 3/4	8	4 15/16
36	52	9	3/8	6	3	6	10 1/2	7	6	8	1 1/2	8	9
45	0	12	1/2	7	0 7/8	7	9 5/16	8	5 13/16	9	2 5/16	9	10 7/8
53	8	16	2/3	8	4	9	2	10	0	10	10	11	8
56	19	18	3/4	9	0 1/8	9	11	10	9 13/16	11	8 5/8	12	7 7/16

Slope of Roof in Degrees °	′	1 in.	2 in.	3 in.	4 in.	5 in.	6 in.	7 in.	8 in.	9 in.	10 in.	11 in.
14	2	1/2	1	1 9/16	2 1/16	2 9/16	3 1/16	3 9/16	4 1/8	4 5/8	5 1/8	5 11/16
18	26	1/2	1 1/16	1 9/16	2 1/8	2 5/8	3 3/16	3 11/16	4 3/16	4 3/4	5 1/4	5 13/16
26	34	9/16	1 1/8	1 11/16	2 1/4	2 13/16	3 3/8	3 15/16	4 1/2	5	5 9/16	6 1/8
33	41	5/8	1 3/16	1 13/16	2 3/8	3	3 5/8	4 3/16	4 13/16	5 3/8	6	6 5/8
36	52	5/8	1 1/4	1 7/8	2 1/2	3 1/8	3 3/4	4 3/8	5	5 5/8	6 1/4	6 7/8
45	0	11/16	1 7/16	2 1/8	2 13/16	3 9/16	4 1/4	4 15/16	5 11/16	6 3/8	7 1/16	7 3/4
53	8	13/16	1 11/16	2 1/2	3 5/16	4 3/16	5	5 13/16	6 11/16	7 1/2	8 5/16	9 3/16
56	19	7/8	1 13/16	2 11/16	3 5/8	4 1/2	5 7/16	6 5/16	7 3/16	8 1/8	9	9 15/16

Slope of Roof in Degrees °	′	*Rise of Roof in 12 in. (½ Span)* in.	*Pitch of Roof*	15 ft.	15 in.	16 ft.	16 in.	17 ft.	17 in.	18 ft.	18 in.	19 ft.	19 in.
14	2	3	1/8	7	8 3/4	8	2 15/16	8	9 1/8	9	3 5/16	9	9 1/2
18	26	4	1/6	7	10 7/8	8	5 3/16	8	11 1/2	9	5 13/16	10	0 3/16
26	34	6	1/4	8	4 5/8	8	11 5/16	9	6 1/4	10	0 3/4	10	7 7/16
33	41	8	1/3	9	0 3/16	9	7 3/8	10	2 9/16	10	9 13/16	11	5
36	52	9	3/8	9	4 1/2	10	0	10	7 1/2	11	3	11	10 1/2
45	0	12	1/2	10	7 5/16	11	3 3/4	12	0 1/4	12	8 3/4	13	5 3/16
53	8	16	2/3	12	6	13	4	14	2	15	0	15	10
56	19	18	3/4	13	6 1/4	14	5 1/16	15	3 7/8	16	2 11/16	17	1 1/2

Slope of Roof in Degrees °	′	1 in.	2 in.	3 in.	4 in.	5 in.	6 in.	7 in.	8 in.	9 in.	10 in.	11 in.
14	2	1/2	1	1 9/16	2 1/16	2 9/16	3 1/16	3 9/16	4 1/8	4 5/8	5 1/8	5 11/16
18	26	1/2	1 1/16	1 9/16	2 1/8	2 5/8	3 3/16	3 11/16	4 3/16	4 3/4	5 1/4	5 13/16
26	34	9/16	1 1/8	1 11/16	2 1/4	2 13/16	3 3/8	3 15/16	4 1/2	5	5 9/16	6 1/8
33	41	5/8	1 3/16	1 13/16	2 3/8	3	3 5/8	4 3/16	4 13/16	5 3/8	6	6 5/8
36	52	5/8	1 1/4	1 7/8	2 1/2	3 1/8	3 3/4	4 3/8	5	5 5/8	6 1/4	6 7/8
45	0	11/16	1 7/16	2 1/8	2 13/16	3 9/16	4 1/4	4 15/16	5 11/16	6 3/8	7 1/16	7 3/4
53	8	13/16	1 11/16	2 1/2	3 5/16	4 3/16	5	5 13/16	6 11/16	7 1/2	8 5/16	9 3/16
56	19	7/8	1 13/16	2 11/16	3 5/8	4 1/2	5 7/16	6 5/16	7 3/16	8 1/8	9	9 15/16

If span is in feet and inches, find result of feet span in left-hand table. Then find result of the inches of span in right-hand table and add two results together.

TABLE I (*contd.*)—LENGTH OF COMMON RAFTER

Feet ←—— *Span of the Building* ——→ *Inches*

Slope of Roof in Degrees		*Rise of Roof in 12 in. (½ Span)*	*Pitch of Roof*	20		21		22		23		24		1	2	3	4	5	6	7	8	9	10	11
°	′	*in.*		*ft.*	*in.*	*ft.*	*in.*	*ft.*	*in.*	*ft.*	*in.*	*ft.*	*in.*	*in.*	*in.*	*in.*	*in.*	*in.*	*in.*	*in.*	*in.*	*in.*	*in.*	*in.*
14	2	3	1/8	10	3 11/16	10	9 7/8	11	4 1/16	11	10 1/4	12	4 7/16	1/2	1	1 9/16	2 1/16	2 9/16	3 1/16	3 9/16	4 1/8	4 5/8	5 1/8	5 11/16
18	26	4	1/6	10	6 1/2	11	0 13/16	11	7 1/8	12	1 7/16	12	7 13/16	1/2	1 1/16	1 9/16	2 1/8	2 5/8	3 3/16	3 11/16	4 3/16	4 3/4	5 1/4	5 13/16
26	34	6	1/4	11	2 3/16	11	8 7/8	12	3 9/16	12	10 5/16	13	5	9/16	1 1/8	1 11/16	2 1/4	2 13/16	3 3/8	3 15/16	4 1/2	5	5 9/16	6 1/8
33	41	8	1/3	12	0 3/16	12	7 7/16	13	2 1/2	13	9 7/8	14	5 1/16	5/8	1 3/16	1 13/16	2 3/8	3	3 5/8	4 3/16	4 13/16	5 3/8	6	6 5/8
36	52	9	3/8	12	6	13	1 1/2	13	9	14	4 1/2	15	0 1/2	5/8	1 1/4	1 7/8	2 1/2	3 1/8	3 3/4	4 3/8	5	5 5/8	6 1/4	6 7/8
45	0	12	1/2	14	1 3/4	14	10 3/16	15	6 11/16	16	3 3/16	16	11 5/8	11/16	1 7/16	2 1/8	2 13/16	3 9/16	4 1/4	4 15/16	5 11/16	6 3/8	7 1/16	7 3/4
53	8	16	2/3	16	8	17	6	18	4	19	2	20	0	13/16	1 11/16	2 1/2	3 5/16	4 3/16	5	5 13/16	6 11/16	7 1/2	8 5/16	9 3/16
56	19	18	3/4	18	0 5/16	18	11 1/8	19	9 15/16	20	8 13/16	21	7 9/16	7/8	1 13/16	2 11/16	3 5/8	4 1/2	5 7/16	6 5/16	7 3/16	8 1/8	9	9 15/16

Slope of Roof in Degrees		*Rise of Roof in 12 in. (½ Span)*	*Pitch of Roof*	25		26		27		28		29		30		1	2	3	4	5	6	7	8	9	10	11
°	′	*in.*		*ft.*	*in.*	*ft.*	*in.*	*ft.*	*in.*	*ft.*	*in.*	*ft.*	*in.*	*ft.*	*in.*	*in.*	*in.*	*in.*	*in.*	*in.*	*in.*	*in.*	*in.*	*in.*	*in.*	*in.*
14	2	3	1/8	12	10 5/8	13	4 13/16	13	11	14	5 3/16	14	11 3/8	15	5 9/16	1/2	1	1 9/16	2 1/16	2 9/16	3 1/16	3 9/16	4 1/8	4 5/8	5 1/8	5 11/16
18	26	4	1/6	13	2 1/8	13	8 7/16	14	2 3/4	14	9 1/16	15	3 3/8	15	9 3/4	1/2	1 1/16	1 9/16	2 1/8	2 5/8	3 3/16	3 11/16	4 3/16	4 3/4	5 1/4	5 13/16
26	34	6	1/4	13	11 11/16	14	6 7/16	15	1 1/8	15	7 11/16	16	2 7/16	16	9 1/8	9/16	1 1/8	1 11/16	2 1/4	2 13/16	3 3/8	3 15/16	4 1/2	5	5 9/16	6 1/8
33	41	8	1/3	15	0 1/4	15	7 1/2	16	2 11/16	16	9 15/16	17	5 1/8	18	0 15/16	5/8	1 3/16	1 13/16	2 3/8	3	3 5/8	4 3/16	4 13/16	5 3/8	6	6 5/8
36	52	9	3/8	15	7 1/2	16	3	16	10 1/2	17	6	18	1 1/2	18	9	5/8	1 1/4	1 7/8	2 1/2	3 1/8	3 3/4	4 3/8	5	5 5/8	6 1/4	6 7/8
45	0	12	1/2	17	8 1/8	18	4 5/8	19	1 1/8	19	9 9/16	20	6 1/16	21	2 9/16	11/16	1 7/16	2 1/8	2 13/16	3 9/16	4 1/4	4 15/16	5 11/16	6 3/8	7 1/16	7 3/4
53	8	16	2/3	20	10	21	8	22	6	23	4	24	2	25	0	13/16	1 11/16	2 1/2	3 5/16	4 3/16	5	5 13/16	6 11/16	7 1/2	8 5/16	9 3/16
56	19	18	3/4	22	6 7/16	23	5 1/4	24	4 1/16	25	2 7/8	26	1 11/16	27	0 1/2	7/8	1 13/16	2 11/16	3 5/8	4 1/2	5 7/16	6 5/16	7 3/16	8 1/8	9	9 15/16

If span is in feet and inches, find result of feet span in left-hand table. Then find result of the inches of span in right-hand table and add two results together.

TABLE II.—LENGTH OF BACKED HIPS

Feet ←—— *Span of the Building* ——→ *Inches*

Slope of Roof in Degrees		*Rise of Roof in 12 in. (½ Span)*	*Pitch of Roof*	10		11		12		13		14	
°	′	*in.*		*ft.*	*in.*	*ft.*	*in.*	*ft.*	*in.*	*ft.*	*in.*	*ft.*	*in.*
14	2	3	1/8	7	2 3/16	7	10 13/16	8	7 3/8	9	4	10	0 5/8
18	26	4	1/6	7	3 3/16	7	11 7/8	8	8 5/8	9	5 5/16	10	2 1/16
26	34	6	1/4	7	6	8	3	9	0	9	9	10	6
33	41	8	1/3	7	9 13/16	8	7 3/16	9	4 9/16	10	1 15/16	10	11 5/16
36	52	9	3/8	8	0 1/16	8	9 5/8	9	7 1/4	10	4 7/8	11	2 7/16
45	0	12	1/2	8	7 15/16	9	6 5/16	10	4 11/16	11	3 1/8	12	1 1/2
53	8	16	2/3	9	8 5/8	10	8 1/4	11	7 15/16	12	7 5/8	13	7 1/4
56	19	18	3/4	10	3 11/16	11	2 7/8	12	4 7/16	13	4 13/16	14	5 3/16

Slope of Roof in Degrees		1	2	3	4	5	6	7	8	9	10	11
°	′	*in.*	*in.*	*in.*	*in.*	*in.*	*in.*	*in.*	*in.*	*in.*	*in.*	*in.*
14	2	11/16	1 7/16	2 1/8	2 7/8	3 9/16	4 5/16	5	5 3/4	6 7/16	7 3/16	7 7/8
18	26	3/4	1 7/16	2 3/16	2 7/8	3 5/8	4 3/8	5 1/16	5 13/16	6 9/16	7 1/4	8
26	34	3/4	1 1/2	2 1/4	3	3 3/4	4 1/2	5 1/4	6	6 3/4	7 1/2	8 1/4
33	41	13/16	1 9/16	2 3/8	3 1/8	3 15/16	4 11/16	5 1/2	6 1/4	7 1/16	7 13/16	8 5/8
36	52	13/16	1 9/16	2 3/8	3 3/16	4	4 13/16	5 5/8	6 7/16	7 3/16	8	8 13/16
45	0	7/8	1 3/4	2 5/8	3 1/2	4 5/16	5 3/16	6 1/16	6 15/16	7 13/16	8 11/16	9 9/16
53	8	15/16	1 15/16	2 15/16	3 7/8	4 15/16	5 13/16	6 13/16	7 3/4	8 3/4	9 11/16	10 11/16
56	19	1	2 1/16	3 1/16	4 1/8	5 1/8	6 3/16	7 3/16	8 1/4	9 1/4	10 5/16	11 5/16

Slope of Roof in Degrees		*Rise of Roof in 12 in. (½ Span)*	*Pitch of Roof*	15		16		17		18		19	
°	′	*in.*		*ft.*	*in.*	*ft.*	*in.*	*ft.*	*in.*	*ft.*	*in.*	*ft.*	*in.*
14	2	3	1/8	10	9 1/4	11	5 7/8	12	2 1/2	12	11 1/8	13	7 3/4
18	26	4	1/6	10	10 11/16	11	7 1/2	12	4 3/16	13	0 15/16	13	9 5/8
26	34	6	1/4	11	3	12	0	12	9	13	6	14	3
33	41	8	1/3	11	8 11/16	12	6 1/16	13	3 1/2	14	0 7/8	14	10 1/4
36	52	9	3/8	12	0 1/16	12	9 11/16	13	7 1/4	14	4 7/8	15	2 1/2
45	0	12	1/2	12	11 7/8	13	10 1/4	14	8 11/16	15	7 1/16	16	5 7/16
53	8	16	2/3	14	6 15/16	15	6 5/8	16	6 1/4	17	5 15/16	18	5 9/16
56	19	18	3/4	15	5 9/16	16	5 15/16	17	6 5/16	18	6 5/8	19	7

Slope of Roof in Degrees		1	2	3	4	5	6	7	8	9	10	11
°	′	*in.*	*in.*	*in.*	*in.*	*in.*	*in.*	*in.*	*in.*	*in.*	*in.*	*in.*
14	2	11/16	1 7/16	2 1/8	2 7/8	3 9/16	4 5/16	5	5 3/4	6 7/16	7 3/16	7 7/8
18	26	3/4	1 7/16	2 3/16	2 7/8	3 5/8	4 3/8	5 1/16	5 13/16	6 9/16	7 1/4	8
26	34	3/4	1 1/2	2 1/4	3	3 3/4	4 1/2	5 1/4	6	6 3/4	7 1/2	8 1/4
33	41	13/16	1 9/16	2 3/8	3 1/8	3 15/16	4 11/16	5 1/2	6 1/4	7 1/16	7 13/16	8 5/8
36	52	13/16	1 9/16	2 3/8	3 3/16	4	4 13/16	5 5/8	6 7/16	7 3/16	8	8 13/16
45	0	7/8	1 3/4	2 5/8	3 1/2	4 5/16	5 3/16	6 1/16	6 15/16	7 13/16	8 11/16	9 9/16
53	8	15/16	1 15/16	2 15/16	3 7/8	4 15/16	5 13/16	6 13/16	7 3/4	8 3/4	9 11/16	10 11/16
56	19	1	2 1/16	3 1/16	4 1/8	5 1/8	6 3/16	7 3/16	8 1/4	9 1/4	10 5/16	11 5/16

If span is in feet and inches, find result of feet span in left-hand table. Then find result of the inches of span in right-hand table and add two results together.

TABLE II (*contd.*)—LENGTH OF BACKED HIPS

Feet ←—— *Span of the Building* ——→ *Inches*

Slope of Roof in Degrees		Rise of Roof in 12 in. (½ Span)	Pitch of Roof	20		21		22		23		24		1	2	3	4	5	6	7	8	9	10	11
°	′	in.		ft.	in.	ft.	in.	ft.	in.	ft.	in.	ft.	in.	in.	in.	in.	in.	in.	in.	in.	in.	in.	in.	in.
14	2	3	1/8	14	4 5/16	15	0 15/16	15	9 9/16	16	6 3/16	17	2 13/16	11/16	1 7/16	2 1/8	2 7/8	3 9/16	4 5/16	5	5 3/4	6 7/16	7 3/16	7 7/8
18	26	4	1/6	14	6 3/8	15	3 1/16	15	11 13/16	16	8 1/2	17	5 1/4	3/4	1 7/16	2 3/16	2 7/8	3 5/8	4 3/8	5 1/16	5 13/16	6 9/16	7 1/4	8
26	34	6	1/4	15	0	15	9	16	6	17	3	18	0	3/4	1 1/2	2 1/4	3	3 3/4	4 1/2	5 1/4	6	6 3/4	7 1/2	8 1/4
33	41	8	1/3	15	7 5/8	16	5	17	2 3/8	17	11 3/4	18	9 1/8	13/16	1 9/16	2 3/8	3 1/8	3 15/16	4 11/16	5 1/2	6 1/4	7 1/16	7 13/16	8 5/8
36	52	9	3/8	16	0 1/16	16	9 11/16	17	7 5/16	18	4 15/16	19	2 1/2	13/16	1 9/16	2 3/8	3 3/16	4	4 13/16	5 5/8	6 7/16	7 3/16	8	8 13/16
45	0	12	1/2	17	3 7/8	18	2 1/4	19	0 5/8	19	11	20	9 7/16	7/8	1 3/4	2 5/8	3 1/2	4 5/16	5 3/16	6 1/16	6 15/16	7 13/16	8 11/16	9 9/16
53	8	16	2/3	19	5 1/4	20	4 15/16	21	4 1/2	22	4 3/16	23	3 7/8	15/16	1 15/16	2 15/16	3 7/8	4 15/16	5 13/16	6 13/16	7 3/4	8 3/4	9 11/16	10 11/16
56	19	18	3/4	20	7 3/8	21	7 3/4	22	8 1/8	23	8 1/2	24	8 7/8	1	2 1/16	3 1/16	4 1/8	5 1/8	6 3/16	7 3/16	8 1/4	9 1/4	10 5/16	11 5/16

Slope of Roof in Degrees		Rise of Roof in 12 in. (½ Span)	Pitch of Roof	25		26		27		28		29		30		1	2	3	4	5	6	7	8	9	10	11
°	′	in.		ft.	in.	ft.	in.	ft.	in.	ft.	in.	ft.	in.	ft.	in.	in.	in.	in.	in.	in.	in.	in.	in.	in.	in.	in.
14	2	3	1/8	17	11 7/16	18	8 1/16	19	4 11/16	20	1 1/4	20	9 7/8	21	6 1/2	11/16	1 7/16	2 1/8	2 7/8	3 9/16	4 5/16	5	5 3/4	6 7/16	7 3/16	7 7/8
18	26	4	1/6	18	1 15/16	18	10 11/16	19	7 3/8	20	4 1/8	21	0 13/16	21	9 9/16	3/4	1 7/16	2 3/16	2 7/8	3 5/8	4 3/8	5 1/16	5 13/16	6 9/16	7 1/4	8
26	34	6	1/4	18	9	19	6	20	3	21	0	21	9	22	6	3/4	1 1/2	2 1/4	3	3 3/4	4 1/2	5 1/4	6	6 3/4	7 1/2	8 1/4
33	41	8	1/3	19	6 1/2	20	3 15/16	21	1 1/4	21	10 11/16	22	8 1/16	23	5 7/16	13/16	1 9/16	2 3/8	3 1/8	3 15/16	4 11/16	5 1/2	6 1/4	7 1/16	7 13/16	8 5/8
36	52	9	3/8	20	0 1/8	20	9 3/4	21	7 5/16	22	4 15/16	23	2 9/16	24	0 1/8	13/16	1 9/16	2 3/8	3 3/16	4	4 13/16	5 5/8	6 7/16	7 3/16	8	8 13/16
45	0	12	1/2	21	7 13/16	22	6 3/16	23	4 9/16	24	3	25	1 3/8	25	11 3/4	7/8	1 3/4	2 5/8	3 1/2	4 5/16	5 3/16	6 1/16	6 15/16	7 13/16	8 11/16	9 9/16
53	8	16	2/3	24	3 9/16	25	3 3/16	26	2 7/8	27	2 9/16	28	2 3/16	29	1 7/8	15/16	1 15/16	2 15/16	3 7/8	4 15/16	5 13/16	6 13/16	7 3/4	8 3/4	9 11/16	10 11/16
56	19	18	3/4	25	9 1/4	26	9 5/8	27	10	28	10 9/16	29	10 11/16	30	11 1/16	1	2 1/16	3 1/16	4 1/8	5 1/8	6 3/16	7 3/16	8 1/4	9 1/4	10 5/16	11 5/16

If span is in feet and inches, find result of feet span in left-hand table. Then find result of the inches of span in right-hand table and add two results together.

TABLE III—ROOF MEMBERS. CUTS IN 8 PITCHES

Slope of Roof in Degrees	*Rise of Roof in 12 in.*	*Pitch of Roof*	*Common Rafter Level Cut*	*Common Rafter Plumb Cut*	*Backed Hips Level Cut*	*Backed Hips Plumb Cut*	*Backed Hips Edge Cut*	*Backed Hips Backing*	*Jack Rafters Edge Cut*	*Purlins Side Cut*	*Purlins Edge Cut*	*Diminishing Length of Jack Rafter*
												ft. in.
14° 2′	3	$\frac{1}{8}$	14°	76°	10°	80°	45°	81°	44°	77°	46°	1 0$\frac{9}{16}$
18° 26′	4	$\frac{1}{6}$	18°	72°	13°	77°	45°	78°	43°	72°	47°	1 0$\frac{7}{8}$
26° 34′	6	$\frac{1}{4}$	27°	63°	19°	71°	44°	74°	42°	65°	48°	1 1$\frac{11}{16}$
33° 41′	8	$\frac{1}{3}$	34°	56°	25°	65°	42°	66°	39°	60°	49°	1 2$\frac{11}{16}$
36° 52′	9	$\frac{3}{8}$	37°	53°	28°	62°	41°	65°	38°	58°	51°	1 3$\frac{5}{16}$
45° 0′	12	$\frac{1}{2}$	45°	45°	35°	55°	39°	60°	35°	55°	55°	1 5$\frac{1}{4}$
53° 8′	16	$\frac{2}{3}$	53°	37°	43°	47°	36°	55°	31°	50°	58°	1 8$\frac{3}{8}$
56° 19′	18	$\frac{3}{4}$	36°	34°	47°	43°	34°	54°	29°	48°	61°	1 9$\frac{7}{8}$

Read downwards for different cuts of roof members and across for required pitch. All cuts to nearest degree.

Start at long point of plumb cut of common rafter. Mark the diminishing jack rafter length and repeat along rafter for pattern, giving lengths and number of jack rafters required at 14-in. centres.

TABLE FOR CONVERSION OF INCHES TO DECIMALS OF A FOOT

Inch	*Inches*											
	0	1	2	3	4	5	6	7	8	9	10	11
—	—	0·0833	0·1667	0·2500	0·3333	0·4167	0·5000	0·5833	0·6667	0·7500	0·8333	0·9167
$\frac{1}{8}$	0·0104	0·0938	0·1771	0·2604	0·3438	0·4271	0·5104	0·5938	0·6771	0·7604	0·8438	0·9271
$\frac{1}{4}$	0·0208	0·1042	0·1875	0·2708	0·3542	0·4375	0·5208	0·6042	0·6875	0·7708	0·8542	0·9375
$\frac{3}{8}$	0·0313	0·1146	0·1979	0·2813	0·3646	0·4479	0·5313	0·6146	0·6979	0·7813	0·8646	0·9479
$\frac{1}{2}$	0·0417	0·1250	0·2083	0·2917	0·3750	0·4583	0·5417	0·6250	0·7083	0·7917	0·8750	0·9583
$\frac{5}{8}$	0·0521	0·1354	0·2188	0·3021	0·3854	0·4688	0·5521	0·6354	0·7188	0·8021	0·8854	0·9688
$\frac{3}{4}$	0·0625	0·1458	0·2292	0·3125	0·3958	0·4792	0·5625	0·6458	0·7292	0·8125	0·8958	0·9792
$\frac{7}{8}$	0·0729	0·1563	0·2396	0·3229	0·4063	0·4896	0·5729	0·6563	0·7396	0·8229	0·9063	0·9896

SLOPE OF ROOF	COMMON RAFTER FEET	HIP RAFTER FEET
14° 2′	0·5153	0·7180
18° 26′	0·5270	0·7264
26° 34′	0·5590	0·7500
33° 41′	0·6009	0·7817
36° 52′	0·6250	0·8003
45°	0·7071	0·8660
53° 8′	0·8333	0·9718
56° 19′	0·9014	1·0307

THIS TABLE GIVES A CONSTANT WHIGH WHEN MULTIPLIED BY SPAN IN FEET GIVES LENGTHS OF RAFTERS IN FEET AND DECIMAL PARTS OF A FOOT. SHOULD ODD INCHES BE IN THE SPAN THESE CAN BE TAKEN FROM APPROPRIATE LINE IN MAIN TABLE AND ADDED TO THIS RESULT.

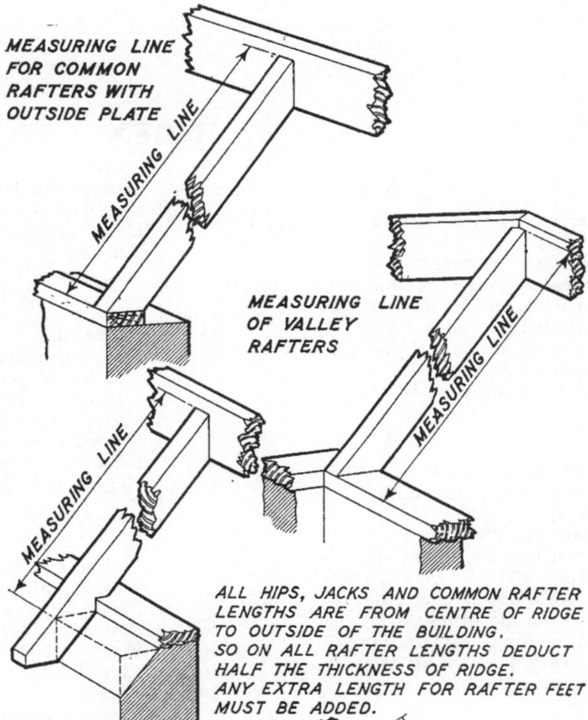

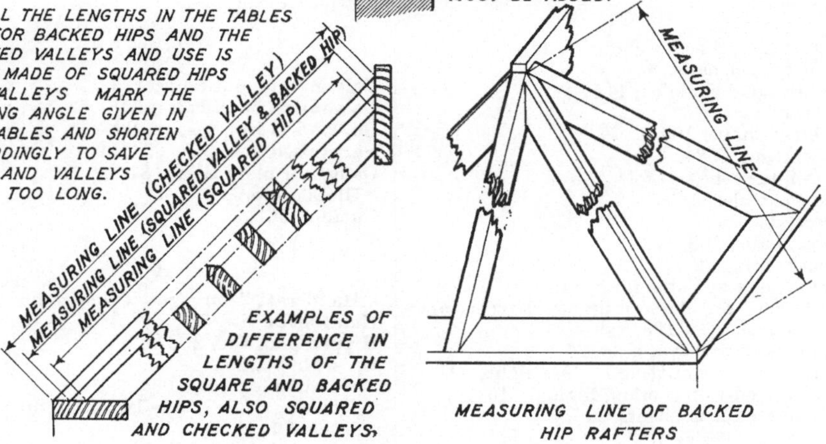

MEASURING LINES FOR ROOF MEMBERS

INDEX